VOLUME NINETY

ADVANCES IN PHARMACOLOGY

A Tribute to Paul Greengard (1925–2019)

VOLUME NINETY

ADVANCES IN PHARMACOLOGY

A Tribute to Paul Greengard (1925–2019)

Edited by

STEVIN H. ZORN
President and CEO,
MindImmune Therapeutics, Inc.,
Kingston, RI, United States

Serial Editor

S.J. ENNA
University of Kansas Medical Center,
Kansas City, KS, United States

Managing Editor

LYNN LeCOUNT
University of Kansas Medical Center,
School of Medicine, Kansas City, KS, United States

ELSEVIER

ACADEMIC PRESS
An imprint of Elsevier

Academic Press is an imprint of Elsevier
50 Hampshire Street, 5th Floor, Cambridge, MA 02139, United States
525 B Street, Suite 1650, San Diego, CA 92101, United States
The Boulevard, Langford Lane, Kidlington, Oxford OX5 1GB, United Kingdom
125 London Wall, London, EC2Y 5AS, United Kingdom

First edition 2021

ISBN: 978-0-12-822516-5
ISSN: 1054-3589

For information on all Academic Press publications
visit our website at https://www.elsevier.com/books-and-journals

Publisher: Zoe Kruze
Editorial Project Manager: Shellie Bryant
Production Project Manager: Denny Mansingh
Cover Designer: Greg Harris

Typeset by SPi Global, India

Contents

Contributors

Martin Bähler
Institute of Molecular Cell Biology, Cells in Motion Interfaculty Centre, University of Münster, Münster, Germany

Fabio Benfenati
Center for Synaptic Neuroscience and Technology, Istituto Italiano di Tecnologia; IRCCS Ospedale Policlinico San Martino; Department of Experimental Medicine, University of Genova, Genova, Italy

Victor Bustos
Laboratory of Cellular and Molecular Neuroscience, Rockefeller University, New York, NY, United States

Kyle R. Christensen
Department of Psychiatry, Yale University, School of Medicine, New Haven, CT, United States

Robert E. Davis
Intra-Cellular Therapies, Inc., The Alexandria Center for Life Science, New York, NY, United States

Allen Fienberg
Intra-Cellular Therapies, Inc., The Alexandria Center for Life Science, New York, NY, United States

Marc Flajolet
Laboratory of Cellular and Molecular Neuroscience; Acting Director of the Laboratory of Molecular and Cellular Neuroscience, a.k.a. the Greengard Lab, The Rockefeller University, New York, NY, United States

Jean-Antoine Girault
Inserm UMR-S 1270; Sorbonne Université, Faculty of Science and Engineering; Institut du Fer à Moulin, Paris, France

Arthur Godino
Nash Family Department of Neuroscience and Friedman Brain Institute, Icahn School of Medicine at Mount Sinai, New York, NY, United States

Hugh C. Hemmings Jr
Department of Anesthesiology; Department of Pharmacology, Weill Cornell Medicine, New York, NY, United States

Jose Ledo
Laboratory of Cellular and Molecular Neuroscience, Rockefeller University, New York, NY, United States

Angela M. Lee
Department of Psychiatry, Yale University; Yale Interdepartmental Neuroscience Program, New Haven, CT, United States

Peng Li
Intra-Cellular Therapies, Inc., The Alexandria Center for Life Science, New York, NY, United States

Sharon Mates
Intra-Cellular Therapies, Inc., The Alexandria Center for Life Science, New York, NY, United States

Angus C. Nairn
Department of Psychiatry, Yale University, School of Medicine; Department of Psychiatry, Yale School of Medicine, Connecticut Mental Health Center, New Haven, CT, United States

Eric J. Nestler
Nash Family Department of Neuroscience and Friedman Brain Institute, Icahn School of Medicine at Mount Sinai, New York, NY, United States

Thu Lan Nguyen
Laboratory of Cellular and Molecular Neuroscience, The Rockefeller University, New York, NY, United States

Francesca Palese
Department of Drug Discovery and Development, Istituto Italiano di Tecnologia, Genoa, Italy; Departments of Anatomy and Neurobiology, Pharmacology and Biological Chemistry, University of California, Irvine, CA, United States

Marina R. Picciotto
Department of Psychiatry, Yale University; Yale Interdepartmental Neuroscience Program, New Haven, CT, United States

Daniele Piomelli
Departments of Anatomy and Neurobiology, Pharmacology and Biological Chemistry, University of California, Irvine, CA, United States

Jimcy Platholi
Department of Anesthesiology; Feil Family Brain and Mind Research Institute, Weill Cornell Medicine, New York, NY, United States

Silvia Pontis
Department of Drug Discovery and Development, Istituto Italiano di Tecnologia, Genoa, Italy

Maria V. Pulina
Laboratory of Cellular and Molecular Neuroscience, Rockefeller University, New York, NY, United States

Natalia Realini
Department of Drug Discovery and Development, Istituto Italiano di Tecnologia, Genoa, Italy

Patricia Rodriguez-Rodriguez
Laboratory of Molecular and Cellular Neuroscience, The Rockefeller University, New York, NY, United States; Department of Neurobiology, Care Sciences and Society, Division of Neurogeriatrics, Karolinska Institutet, Solna, Sweden

Jean-Pierre Roussarie
Laboratory of Molecular and Cellular Neuroscience, The Rockefeller University, New York, NY, United States

Marine Salery
Nash Family Department of Neuroscience and Friedman Brain Institute, Icahn School of Medicine at Mount Sinai, New York, NY, United States

Vijay Kumar Siripuram
Laboratory of Cellular and Molecular Neuroscience, The Rockefeller University, New York, NY, United States

Gretchen L. Snyder
Intra-Cellular Therapies, Inc., The Alexandria Center for Life Science, New York, NY, United States

Yashoda Krishna Sunkari
Laboratory of Cellular and Molecular Neuroscience, The Rockefeller University, New York, NY, United States

Flavia Valtorta
IRCCS San Raffaele Scientific Institute; Vita-Salute San Raffaele University, Milan, Italy

Kimberly E. Vanover
Intra-Cellular Therapies, Inc., The Alexandria Center for Life Science, New York, NY, United States

James K.T. Wang
Dermalytica Inc., Wilmington, DE, United States

Preface: A Tribute to Paul Greengard (1925–2019)

Stevin H. Zorn

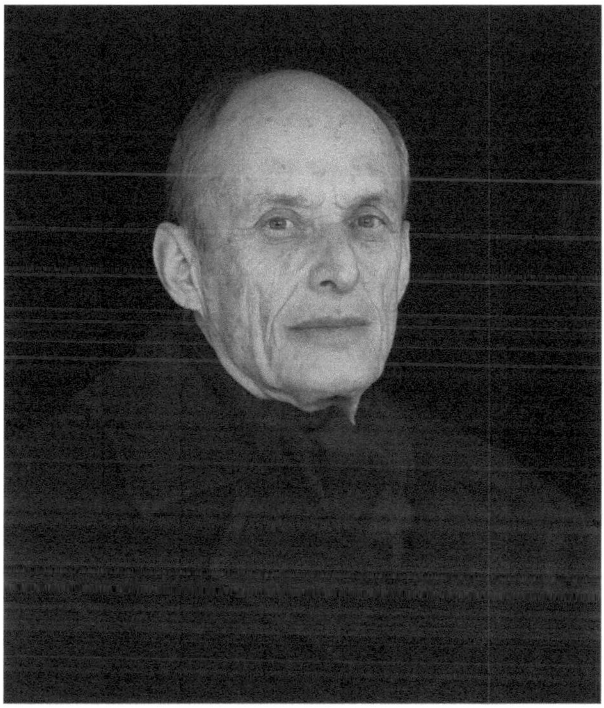

Fig. 1 Paul Greengard. *Photo credit: Personal communication from Ursula von Rydingsvard.*

On April 13, 2019, the world lost one of the most influential sculptors of neuroscience: Paul Greengard (Fig. 1). Paul was a friend and mentor who had a profound influence on my life; and I miss him dearly. On that day, a whole generation of former students, postdocs, and colleagues also lost their friend and mentor. Paul was described by Nestler (2019) as a "mentor extraordinaire," adding that "it is difficult to overstate the impact that Paul had on our understanding of cell signaling in general, and in the nervous system in particular."

This monograph is a tribute to the life and game-changing scientific contributions of Paul Greengard. Paul lived a long and consequential life to the golden age of 93. He influenced the understanding of how the nervous system works, how brain cells communicate on a molecular and cellular level, and left a legacy of students, postdocs, and scientists to expand innovative science as they continue to pave a path to a better understanding of the brain. Paul's influence was vast, integrating knowledge across many sciences such as biophysics, neurobiology, mathematics, and computational neuroscience—all coalescing to contributions that led to Paul's most significant work of understanding chemical transmission in the brain. In 2000, Paul received the Nobel Prize in Physiology or Medicine, which he shared with Arvid Carlsson and Eric Kandel, for his revolutionary advances in understanding signal transduction in the nervous system. His discoveries provided insights into how problems with brain cell communication could directly lead to brain disorders including schizophrenia, Parkinson's disease, bipolar disorder, drug addiction, and Alzheimer's disease. Paul's hundreds of mentees and associates have advanced to become top scientists and leaders themselves, forming a broad network of key future innovators and influencers in academia, medicine, government, pharmaceuticals, and biotechnology. His impact will live on for generations to come.

I first met Paul on a wintery day in the late 1980s when I interviewed with him for a postdoctoral position in his lab at the Rockefeller University in New York. The lab was on a holiday break, so I was fortunate to have uninterrupted time with Paul. It was the most intense interview that I have ever experienced. For 8 h, Paul sat with me and discussed my doctoral research to the minutest detail. Like others in this volume have described, Paul had a unique probing style beginning with the simplest and then drilling down to the most complex details. He then emerged with an awe-inspiring synthesis and expansion of thought. He did this with me and with countless graduate students and postdocs in his weekly lab meetings while we were all together in the lab (Fig. 2). Paul's thinking was like no other that I have ever met, and it influenced me greatly in life. He challenged me to think in the most deeply comprehensive ways imaginable. And it was fun! Discussing science with Paul, while extremely challenging, was always mixed with his unusual humor and his boundless curiosity, which eventually resulted in transformative thinking in ways that I simply could not have imagined alone. We talked science, a lot of science, went to movies, where he talked all the way through, had sushi on Second Avenue, walked our dogs

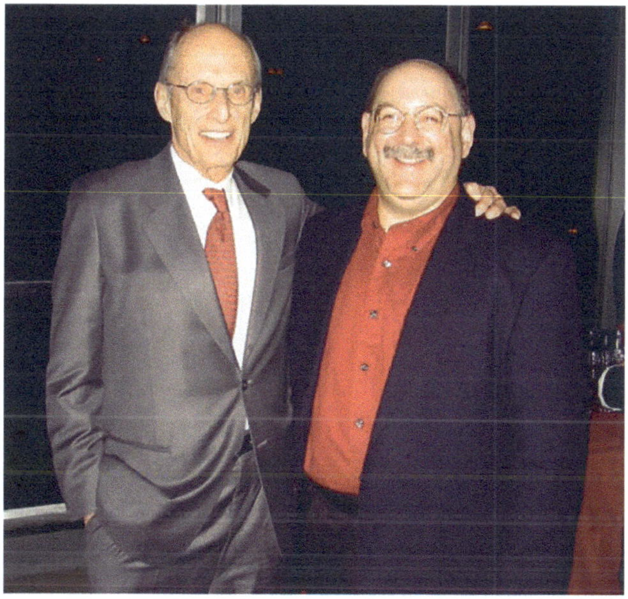

Fig. 2 Stevin H. Zorn and Paul Greengard. *Photo credit: Personal communication from Stevin Zorn.*

together—my poodle and his giant German Shepherd named Kara—and cooked together. I also had the pleasure of house sitting for Paul and his wife, Ursula von Rydingsvard (Fig. 3). The years I spent with Paul were among the most consequential and life changing of my career. I will always be the most grateful to Paul for his mentoring and dedication to helping me grow into my career. But as much time as Paul spent being my mentor, discussing science, life and love (he was at my wedding), he devoted himself to science and to those around him, leaving important pieces of himself in each and every colleague to carry forward. See also Gandy and Suzuki (2019), Nestler (2019), and Nestler and Huganir (2019).

This tribute work reviews science that emerged from Paul's lab and science that followed based on his influence. The chapters are authored/coauthored by members of the Greengard lab. This book summarizes the cellular signaling molecules that were mostly discovered in Paul's lab as well as how they work together to integrate electrical and chemical neurotransmission. In the first chapter, Flajolet and colleagues review Paul's persistent desire to comprehend and fix the brain. Benfenati, Bähler, and Valtorta review the molecular players in both synaptic transmission and plasticity.

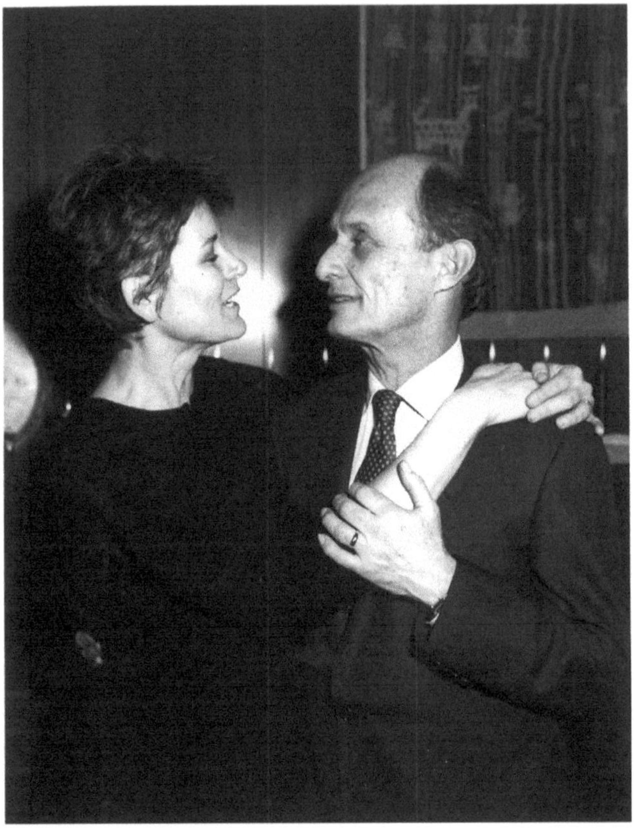

Fig. 3 Paul Greengard and Ursula von Rydingsvard, wedding. *Photo credit: Mariana Cook photography, supplied by Ursula von Rydingsvard.*

Christensen and Nairn, and Girault focus on the history, characterization, and function of cAMP-mediated regulation of serine/threonine protein phosphatases, including DARPP-32, and their role in dopamine-mediated signaling in striatal neurons. Lee and Picciotto follow with a review of the roles of DARPP-32 and CaMKII proteins with respect to systems and behaviors relevant to nicotine addiction. Platholi and Hemmings describe the modulation of dendritic spines by protein phosphatase-1 in health and disease. Roussarie and Rodriguez-Rodriguez describe the deciphering of cell type-specific signal transduction in the brain and highlight their linkage to brain disease. Salery, Godino, and Nestler review drug-activated cells—from immediate early genes to neuronal ensembles—and postulates how they will offer a more comprehensive understanding of drug addiction. Palese, Pontis, Realini, and Piomelli contribute new science in their

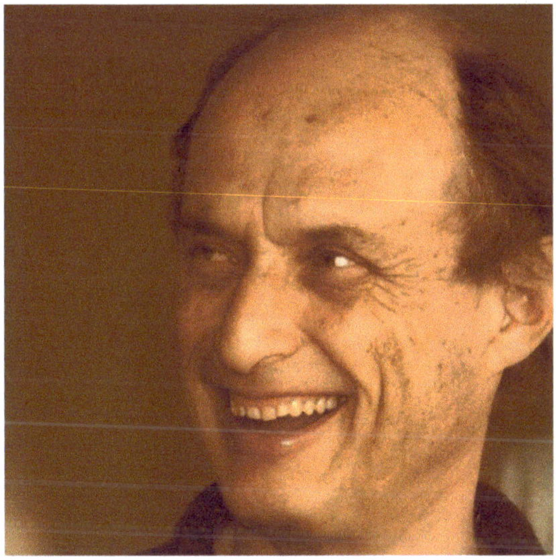

Fig. 4 Paul Greengard. *Photo credit: Personal communication from Stevin Zorn.*

chapter describing a signaling molecule, N-acylphosphatidylethanolamines (NAPE)-specific phospholipase D, and how it regulates LRRK2 association with neuronal membranes. This work has implications for Parkinson's disease.

In the later years in Paul's lab, a focus on Alzheimer's disease and increasingly on the translation of Paul's life work toward the development of therapeutics became a key focus. Thus, Bustos, Pulina, and Ledo summarize their work relating to Alzheimer's disease describing how presenilin-1 is both responsible for the creation as well as the destruction of beta-amyloid, a key pathologic element in Alzheimer's disease. Additional information on this period can be found in Gandy and Suzuki (2019). Snyder and colleagues review the pharmacological and clinical profile of a new drug that was recently approved for schizophrenia (Lumateperone), which was derived from an experimental approach envisioned by Paul Greengard. The last chapter by Wang is a forward-looking proposal for a new conceptual framework for drug discovery in neurodegenerative diseases (Fig. 4).

References

Gandy, S., & Suzuki, T. (2019). In memoriam. Paul Greengard, PhD. (1925–2019). *Alzheimer's & Dementia*, *15*, 1229–1235.

Nestler, E. (2019). In memoriam. Personal reflections on a mentor extraordinaire: Paul Greengard, Ph.D. (1925–2019). *Neuropsychopharmacology*, *44*, 1837–1838.

Nestler, E., & Huganir, R. (2019). Obituary. Paul Greengard (1925–2019). *Cell*, *177*, 1365–1366.

CHAPTER ONE

Paul Greengard: A persistent desire to comprehend the brain, and also to fix it

Marc Flajolet[a,b,*], Thu Lan Nguyen[a], Vijay Kumar Siripuram[a], and Yashoda Krishna Sunkari[a]

[a]Laboratory of Cellular and Molecular Neuroscience, The Rockefeller University, New York, NY, United States
[b]Acting Director of the Laboratory of Molecular and Cellular Neuroscience, a.k.a. the Greengard Lab, The Rockefeller University, New York, NY, United States
[*]Corresponding author: e-mail address: flajolm@rockefeller.edu

Contents

Abstract

Paul Greengard's name is and will remain profoundly associated with Neuroscience, with brain signaling and chemical transmission, with Parkinson's and Alzheimer's diseases, with fundamental discoveries and solving paradoxes, but much less perhaps with drug discovery. This should not be mistaken as disdain. Paul in fact did contemplate developing therapeutic avenues to actually treat brain diseases much more than it is known, perhaps during his entire career, and certainly over the last two decades. As a matter of fact, he did more than contemplate it, he directly and indirectly contributed in the development of treatments for neurological diseases and disorders. Paul's impact on fundamental aspects of the brain has been so gargantuan that any other aspect of Paul's life will have difficulty to shine. It is precisely this less known aspect of Paul's career

Advances in Pharmacology, Volume 90
ISSN 1054-3589
https://doi.org/10.1016/bs.apha.2020.09.008

that will be covered in this review. We will discover how Paul very early on moved away from biophysics to avoid working on nuclear weapons and instead started his career in the pharmacological spheres of a large pharmaceutical company.

Abbreviations

AD	Alzheimer's disease
ADHD	attention deficit hyperactivity disorder
APP	amyloid precursor protein
APP-C99	amyloid precursor protein—99 amino acid long C-terminal fragment
BacTRAP	bacterial artificial chromosome—translating ribosome affinity purification
CK1	casein kinase 1
DEL	DNA-encoded library
DARPP32	dopamine and cAMP regulated phosphoprotein MW 32 kDa
FAD	familial Alzheimer's disease
FDA	U.S. Food and Drug Administration
FGFR	fibroblast growth factor receptor
iDISCO	immunolabeling-enabled three-dimensional imaging of solvent-cleared organs
iPSC	induced pluripotent stem cell
MDD	major depression disorder
NADP$^+$	nicotinamide adenine dinucleotide phosphate
NGS	next generation sequencing
PD	Parkinson's disease
PP1	protein phosphatase 1
PP2C	protein phosphatase 2C
PS1	presenilin 1
WWII	world war II

1. Introduction

Paul Greengard was a giant in the field of neuroscience and internationally recognized for his fundamental work on how neurons communicate, and the importance of chemical transmission. Inspired by the work of Earl W. Sutherland (for a review see: Leongway & Sutherland, 1963) and of Edwin G. Krebs (Posner, Stern, & Krebs, 1965) on the signaling machinery (e.g., adenosine metabolites) involved in regulating the endocrine system and muscle activity, Paul thought early on that neurons cannot only be summarized as a complex cluster of wires performing merely electrical tasks. A number of apparent paradoxes were preventing him from proving this, but Paul and his colleagues methodically went through each of these paradoxes and demonstrated the importance of chemistry in neuronal signaling. For example, one important paradox addressed was to explain how chemistry, or slow signaling events, could mediate fast synaptic transmission? How biochemical strides that takes from minutes to hours to occur can mediate electrical signaling that takes less than 1/1000th of a second to happen? The answer was subtle and decidedly convincing. Paul wrote: "these slow signaling pathways don't *mediate* fast synaptic transmission. Rather they *modulate* fast synaptic transmission ..."

Paul was certainly one of the pioneers in asserting that chemical transmission was everywhere, and he went further, when he reminded the world in his Nobel lecture that 99% of all synapses in the brain use chemical transmission.

Paul trained as a mathematician and nothing discernable predisposed him at a young age to become someday a significant protagonist in the field of drug discovery. It is much less known than his fundamental adventures, but Paul had a strong desire not only to understand, to tame the brain but also to fix it. Drug discovery had been an integral part of Paul's intellect all along, and it came back to the surface regularly throughout his life and career.

2. No to atomic research and weapons development

Paul began his studies of math and physics at Hamilton College, from where he graduated in 1948. He then slowly moved away from physics to escape the resulting atomic research and weapons development which was heavily promoted at the exit of WWII, just 3 years after the horrific nuclear bombing of Hiroshima and Nagasaki.

It was in biophysics at Johns Hopkins that Paul had his first laboratory experience, in the laboratory of Keffer Hartline, the Chairman of the Department of Biophysics at the time and renowned for his work on vision; Hartline would later receive the Nobel Prize in Physiology or Medicine in 1967 (https://www.nobelprize.org/uploads/2018/06/hartline-lecture.pdf). After receiving his Ph.D. from Johns Hopkins in 1953, Paul moved to Europe for his post-doctoral studies, slipping more and more toward biochemistry and sliding away from hardcore biophysics. In Europe, he would work on electrical stimulation, nerve metabolites, and on the uptake/release of adenosine and adenine derivatives. During these years, in Dr. R.W. Straub's lab, Paul would also approach phosphorylation, a chemical modification of proteins and other metabolites (Greengard & Straub, 1958) that will become later on Paul's signature and favorite chemical alteration. However, his great work about phosphorylation and neuronal signaling had to wait for now.

3. Paul's first immersion into the world of drug development

Instead of plunging into the inner worlds of neuronal biochemistry, a different trajectory was awaiting Paul, at least at this point. While in Europe, he was solicitated by the American pharmaceutical company *Geigy Research Laboratories* (later *Ciba-Geigy* and then *Novartis* after the fusion with *Sandoz*). Paul came back to the States and accepted a job in Geigy's Department of Biochemistry. Already fascinated by the possibility of fixing biological problems, he was convinced, he recalled, that this was his chance to contribute something into the complex adventure of discovering useful drugs. At Geigy he researched primarily on steroid and nicotinamide metabolism in animal models ranging from bull frog adrenal glands to bovine adrenal cortex. This translated at the bench by working on the biosynthesis of hormones and their co-factors (e.g., Aldosterone, NAD/$NADP^+$) (Greengard, Kalinsky, Manning, & Zak, 1968; Greengard, Quinn, & Reid, 1964). Aldosterone, an important adrenocortical steroid regulating electrolyte metabolism, was isolated only 10 years prior to that. Medically, this work had direct relevance for blood pressure control (Psychoyos, Tallan, & Greengard, 1966). During his years at Geigy he grew frustrated about how little was known about the brain; most of the work performed at the time was performed on peripheral organs and on the peripheral nervous system, very rarely on brain tissue. Inspired by the work of Drs. Sutherland and Krebs, Paul started to formulate his own working hypothesis and developed the conviction that hormone-dependent signaling in the brain might work just as it works in the body. However, in a neuroscientific arena that was rather bare and nascent, challenges were numerous. In the 1960s many of the classical neurotransmitters were totally unidentified or have been only very recently discovered. For example, glutamate as a neurotransmitter has been introduced in 1952 by Dr. Hayashi but it took until the mid-1970s to be accepted. Of course, many of the crucial concepts were not known (e.g., transmitter storage and release, chemical synapses), but the knowledge of the brain itself was still quite approximative and many cell types and neuronal networks were totally unknown. Finally, from a technical point of view, the technical possibilities were also exceedingly limited. In the absence of most molecular tools, of individual gene cloning (will have to wait 1973), of countless biochemical reagents (e.g., antibodies, agonists, antagonists and inhibitors) and of important technological developments (e.g., real time measurement methods, imaging methodologies and equipment, genome wide studies, etc.), the challenges were colossal. Paul realized that what he initially saw as a temporary hindrance to study the brain, was in fact, an apparently insurmountable and unreachable highland.

During all these years, while working together with Paul on manuscripts, in the lab or at his home, sometimes even on the rejuvenating lawn at his treasured home in the woods of upstate New York, he would agreeably bring colleagues back in time with him, revisiting episodes of his life. He often started by asking questions, but his readiness to answer them, after a mere pause, was a vibrant indication that the questions were also addressed to himself. Routinely a back and forth between monologs and two-way conversations, those fascinating episodes would not last very long as he would not allow himself to stay away too long from his current work at hand.

Paul mentioned several times that he learned quickly that large pharmaceutical companies, just like many other large companies, were built on too many layers of bureaucratic weightiness and that projects were pushed forward based on political choices rather than effectiveness, quality or merit. He described scientific meetings at international conferences from the 1960s as political games to advance an agonist or an antagonist based on data points that he thought were missing so much substance, so much veracity. After 8 years, he was irrevocably convinced that too many key ingredients were missing in the great recipe of drug making. On top of the list, the main component clearly missing was knowledge, plain and basic knowledge about the brain. "How can we treat something that we don't understand?" he asked during one of our retrospective discussions. More research was needed to understand the brain, and much more was required to start designing winning drug strategies.

Fully convinced that the knowledge about neuroscience at that time was too rudimentary and not compatible with fully rational drug development, Paul left the drug discovery business and made yet another 180 degrees turn. Paul left *Geigy* in 1967, assured that he could bring more to the field of neuroscience by researching in academia, far away from the unnecessary pressure and personal interests of large pharmaceutical companies.

4. A brain region highly involved with diseases and disorders

Paul headed back to academia, this time to begin working officially on his own projects, following his own ideas. After sabbaticals at Albert Einstein College and Vanderbilt University, Paul started his own laboratory first at the Yale University, in 1968, as a full professor of pharmacology, and then, in 1983, at The Rockefeller University where he would pursue his research until April 2019 as the Vincent Astor Professor.

Paul really went far deep inside the brain, spending five impressively productive decades painstakingly dissecting every molecular step involved in the functioning of the brain system called the basal ganglia. The basal ganglia comprise the brain regions and neuronal circuits governing aspects of voluntary movement, learning and action selection. This system involves one important brain region called the striatum. The striatum is best known for its importance in motor control and reward. Those are dopamine territories. Disruption in various neurotransmitter systems (Brichta, Greengard, & Flajolet, 2013) and deficit in motor control (Kaplitt, 2019) are cardinal features of Parkinson's disease for example. Reward dysfunction due to dopamine imbalance represents the underlying engine of drug addiction (Nairn et al., 2004; Svenningsson, Nairn, & Greengard, 2005), and virtually all drugs of abuse interfere with dopaminergic signaling. Other diseases and disorders such as Attention Deficit Hyperactivity Disorder (ADHD) (Zhou et al., 2010, 2018), schizophrenia (Chuhma, Mingote, Kalmbach, Yetnikoff, & Rayport, 2017), major depression disorder (MDD) (Alexander et al., 2010; Cheng, Umschweif, Leung, Sagi, & Greengard, 2019; Warner-Schmidt et al., 2012) to some extent, are also largely involve dopamine (Walaas, Hemmings, Greengard, & Nairn, 2011). Paul liked to discuss how important dopamine was for the entire brain directly and indirectly, not just for the basal ganglia. Beside its general interest Paul fixated on the basal ganglia circuitry because it was not as intricate as other circuits, and, more importantly, because it was relevant for a number of disorders and diseases. I cannot tell if, at the beginning of his career, he worked consciously on this specific brain region to someday therapeutically tackle these diseases himself. However, he was certainly motivated later on by the idea that his research could make a difference for designing drug-like small molecular weight compounds, and therefore for patients. And slowly Paul's Lab was growing even bigger. Over the last 20 years, driven by internal discoveries, newly identified pathways and also new technical possibilities, a significant part of the lab worked on neuropsychiatric disorders and diseases such as drug addiction, MDD, schizophrenia and ADHD. In that context, a number of studies aimed at searching for other relevant signaling pathways, for novel proteins regulating G-protein coupled receptors (e.g., for metabotropic glutamate, serotonin and acetylcholine receptors) and their regulatory proteins were conducted because of their great therapeutic potential. This work led us to the identification of a number of proteins and pathways such as: protein phosphatase 2C or PP2C (Flajolet et al., 2003), fibroblast growth factor receptor of FGFR (Flajolet et al., 2008), p11 (Cheng et al., 2019; Chottekalapanda et al., 2020; Jin et al., 2019; Lee et al., 2015; Medrihan et al., 2020; Milosevic et al., 2017; Oh et al., 2013; Svenningsson et al., 2006; Warner-Schmidt et al., 2012), Norbin (Wang et al., 2009, 2015), AGAP1/AP3 (Bendor et al., 2010). The p11 program especially has been developed quite substantially over the last decade and was showing some strong relevance not only to MDD but also to PD and dyskinesia especially (Schintu et al., 2016). For example, an important study demonstrated that gene therapy blockade of p11 was beneficial in laboratory animals for motor function and dyskinesia (Marongiu et al., 2016). Similarly, a large body of work centered on cocaine addiction has been built over the last 20 years (Bateup et al., 2008; Bibb et al., 2001; Ceglia et al., 2017; Chergui, Svenningsson, & Greengard, 2004; Fienberg et al., 1998; Lee et al., 2006; Schaefer et al., 2010; Snyder et al., 2000). Cocaine was chosen to decipher the molecular mechanisms underlying addiction because of its importance in the field, because of the pathways involved and because self-cocaine administration is possible in laboratory animals.

5. A Rosetta Stone, a knockout mouse and a Nobel medal

The discovery, in Paul's lab, of how various neurotransmitters such as dopamine and other important ones, such as glutamate, serotonin, acetylcholine, etc., were integrated and lead to concerted actions inside the synapse lead to several hundred of publications (for reviews see: Greengard, Allen, & Nairn, 1999; Greengard, 2001). The centerpiece of this work, which Paul called the "Rosetta Stone," was DARPP-32 (dopamine and cyclic AMP regulated phosphoprotein MW=32 kDa), a protein highly expressed in the striatum and that can be phosphorylated on four different major sites creating a complex set of possible phosphorylation combinations (Greengard, 2001). Based on the combination, DARPP-32 can act as a positive or negative modulator for downstream events. The protein phosphatase 1 (PP1), a crucial component of the DARPP-32 signaling pathway and acting immediately downstream of DARPP-32, dictates the direction of the response (Greengard et al., 1999). Along the years, Paul and his colleagues, Dr. Angus Nairn leading the pack, demonstrated that DARPP-32 acted as an integrator for various neurotransmitters, and also that substances as well as FDA approved drugs targeting the striatum were modifying the DARPP-32 phosphorylation state. These findings became crystal clear when the gene coding for DARPP-32 was removed genetically from laboratory mice (Fienberg & Greengard, 2000). An array of scientists in Paul's lab and collaborators worked actively on this mouse model to characterize the importance of DARPP-32 in vivo. Indeed, all physiological and biochemical responses to dopamine were dramatically altered or abolished in mice missing DARPP-32. Furthermore, all pharmacological responses induced, for example, by psychostimulants or by drugs used in the case of schizophrenia were also altered or abolished in the genetically modified mice (Svenningsson et al., 2004).

This work culminated with the recognition in 2000 by the Nobel Prize Committee with the awarding of the Nobel Prize in Physiology or Medicine (https://www.nobelprize.org/uploads/2018/06/greengard-lecture.pdf). Remarkably, in the concluding remarks of his Nobel lecture Paul said the following: "it should be possible through the new-found knowledge of the intracellular signaling pathways by which dopamine produces its physiological effects, to develop various therapeutic substances that activate or inhibit these various intracellular components."

6. A fascination for Alzheimer's disease

During these years, while focusing on the basal ganglia system, Paul and his colleagues started developing a strong interest for another colossal problem: Alzheimer's disease (AD). In 1995, he helped the Fisher family, and Zachary Fisher especially, develop the Fisher Center for Alzheimer's research Foundation, a not-for-profit Foundation that, to this day, is exclusively devoted to Alzheimer's disease research. The holy grail search was, and still is, of course to find a cure for this terrible disease that started to become prominent in the 1990s, and that now has a staggering 50 million patients worldwide with millions of new patients each year. The disease is characterized by a slow and progressive cognitive deterioration that typically starts with short term memory deficits due to the deterioration of a brain region (hippocampal formation) largely involved in learning and memory. The disease exists in two versions (sporadic AD and the rare Familial AD or FAD) and remains an incurable mostly random threat that only increases with age. The two major AD culprits are amyloid plaques that are the consequence of Abeta peptide oligomerization and *tau* neurofibrillary tangles that are the results of hyper-phosphorylated *tau* aggregation. For a long time, Paul and his colleagues focused a large part of their research on the Amyloid hypothesis. Paul always had a strong preference for this hypothesis for a number of reasons, the main one being that mutations causing FAD were found in genes involved in the Amyloid pathway. Briefly, the Protein Precursor (APP) can be processed by two proteases namely gamma-secretase and beta-secretase. The successive cleavage of APP by each of these two proteases leads to the release of the toxic Abeta peptide. Over time, this highly hydrophobic peptide will aggregate into oligomers of increasing size and complexity, to ultimately form amyloid plaques. Paul was convinced that several of these crucial events were representing ideal therapeutic targets and could be blocked pharmacologically using drug-like molecules. That was another important reason to study this pathway; he was convinced all along that this was the path to a cure for AD. Reminiscent of his experience at Geigy, Paul needed to understand first what he was dealing with. It was compulsory to comprehend the fine tuning of all the steps involved, their spatiotemporal relevance, their role and importance in the pathophysiology of AD. Paul and colleagues did not leave a single stone uncovered. Using a complex set of state-of-the art techniques, they studied: APP metabolism, APP trafficking, APP phosphorylation, the gamma-secretase complex and its regulation/inhibition, Abeta peptide biology and its contribution to amyloid plaque formation (Bettayeb, Chang, et al., 2016; Bettayeb, Hooli, et al., 2016; Bustos, Pulina, Bispo, et al., 2017a, Bustos, Pulina, Bispo, et al., 2017b, Bustos, Pulina, Kelahmetoglu, et al., 2017; Ceglia et al., 2015; Flajolet et al., 2007; Liebmann et al., 2016; Pulina, Hopkins, Haroutunian, Greengard, & Bustos, 2019; Roussarie et al., 2020; Tian, Chang, Greengard, & Flajolet, 2014). The therapeutic strategy was to target APP cleavage directly, and also indirectly, by searching novel mechanisms that could regulate APP processing and/or Abeta accumulation/degradation (e.g., through phosphorylation, through novel accessory/regulatory proteins, through trafficking, etc.). Numerous relevant paths emerged from those studies including paths that aimed at therapeutic interventions identifying, for example, CK1, as an enzyme that had a direct influence on Abeta production (Flajolet et al., 2007). Another recent project was entirely devoted to

Presenilin-1 (PS1), the active component of the gamma-secretase complex (for a recent review see: Victor Bustos' chapter in this issue; see also: Bustos, Pulina, Bispo, et al., 2017a, Bustos, Pulina, Bispo, et al., 2017b, Bustos, Pulina, Kelahmetoglu, et al., 2017). This recent work led to implicating, in the disease, an APP metabolite called C99, in a way never seen before, and, more importantly, C99 became a putative novel diagnostic tool that correlates with neurodegeneration better than Abeta itself (Pulina et al., 2019). While Paul never intended to work in depth on diagnostic aspects of diseases, in his late 80s, he became very excited about the C99 story and did, indeed, seriously develop the C99 project. Later, Paul's lab greatly intensified work on Alzheimer's disease, also broadening significantly the topics, combining state-of-the-art technologies such as BacTRAP (see later), iDISCO (immunolabeling-enabled three-dimensional imaging of solvent-cleared organs) (Liebmann et al., 2016) and next generation sequencing (NGS) including single cell sequencing. The lab's current AD research focuses on Abeta and Tau of course, but also on accessory glia cells (e.g., microglia and astrocytes) demonstrating recently, for example, that PS1 phosphorylation regulates Abeta degradation by microglia (Ledo et al., 2020) and that it plays a role on microglia development (Ledo et al., 2020), on iPSCs derived from human patients, on various animal models of AD, on APP-C99 (Pulina et al., 2019), and more directly on drug discovery as well (see later).

Paul was never concerned by the disease himself, but he has been indirectly, and he thought that it was every neuroscientists' responsibility to work and research this terrifying memory-melting disease. Over the last few years, in our retrospective discussions, Paul wondered where the consciousness was, where was the memory, what does it mean when someone is forgetful or depressed... He still had so much he wanted to discover.

7. Forty years of knowledge stamped by an FDA approval

The early years of the 2000s mark perhaps the next 180 degrees turn in Paul's scientific career. His initial desire to not only understand the brain but also to fix it, coupled with his almost five decades of "new-found knowledge," brought his interest in drug discovery back to the surface. In 2002 he co-founded a biotechnology company (Intracellular Therapies, Inc.) with Dr. Sharon Mates and with Paul's former student Dr. Allen Fienberg who initiated some of this immediately after coming back from his post-doctoral experience at the Novartis institute in 2001. They proposed to leverage the discoveries made in Paul's laboratory over the years to create a novel type of drug discovery platform that addresses globally how small molecular weight compounds are altering intracellular cell signaling. The original concept was to take advantage of a large set of phospho-specific antibodies, many of which were unique, created and developed in Paul's lab, to probe intracellularly many signaling pathways at once in response to drug-like compounds. Molecules to be tested were categorized based on similarities, tested and compared to FDA approved drugs. This approach was first designed to identify the best possible hit molecules modifying a specific pathway. It was also designed to tackle the problem of side effects, by comparing newly discovered molecules to FDA approved drugs, grouping them in function of their known or suspected mode of action and also on the basis of their side effects. This effort lead to the Company's first FDA approval at the end of 2019 for a molecule to treat schizophrenia (Blair, 2020). The company's pipeline also includes molecules targeting a number of other indications that were very dear to Paul such as Parkinson's disease, MDD, treatment of opioid abuse, and other substance-use disorders, pain, mood disorder in general, and especially in the context of Alzheimer's disease. Unfortunately, Paul passed away just a few months prior to their first FDA approval... He would have been thrilled that finally his work was being successfully translated into a treatment to help patients. I believe this would have represented for Paul the final missing stone in his colossal edifice made of phospho-discoveries and chemical modifications, founded on many decades of breakthroughs, and crisscrossing a multi-dimensional labyrinth between neuronal cellular bodies and synaptic clefts, along dendrites and mushroom spines.

8. Ramping up novel therapeutic targets and pathways identification

Meanwhile, with a colleague at Rockefeller, Dr. Nathaniel Heintz, their two labs co-developed yet another revolutionary technique called BacTRAP (bacterial artificial chromosome—translating ribosome affinity purification) that allows the molecular dissection of intertwined neurons otherwise impossible to separate and study at the biochemical and molecular levels (Doyle et al., 2008; Heiman et al., 2008; Heiman, Kulicke, Fenster, Greengard, & Heintz, 2014). This technique has now been used very efficiently in Paul's lab, in the Heintz's lab, often in collaboration, as well as other collaborators such as Dr. Myriam Heiman who lead the BacTRAP team in the Greengard lab (Lee et al., 2020). In Paul's lab, BacTRAP has been used for various disease-related projects ranging from AD to PD, MDD and others (Brichta et al., 2015; Cheng et al., 2019; Medrihan et al., 2017). Very recently, our latest development using the BacTRAP technology was published in Neuron and illustrates how powerful this approach is to study for example resistant and vulnerable neurons in the case of Alzheimer's disease (Roussarie et al., 2020; see also review in this issue from Dr. Jean-Pierre Roussarie). Paul co-founded, with Dr. Heintz, a second biotechnology company (Envoy) based on the BacTRAP platform with the goal of identifying novel therapeutic pathways and molecular targets; this company and the patented technology associated with it was soon after acquired by Takeda Pharmaceuticals.

9. 85 Years old and starting an organic chemistry extension to his lab

Paul was well versed in math, physics, biophysics, biochemistry, biology but not yet in chemistry. Impatient and perhaps a little unsatisfied by not driving the chemistry side of things, well in his 85th years, he decided this had to change. Paul invested into chemistry and a new lab space dedicated for chemistry was allocated for Paul at The Rockefeller University. Because that was not enough, and because we recently initiated yet another ambitious project, a second lab space was dedicated 3 years ago also to chemistry, to actually build this time a wholly novel drug discovery platform based on a DNA-encoded library (DEL), once again, a totally entirely new project. This technology had been conceptualized Brenner and Lerner (1992), way before DNA synthesis was mainstream and almost 15 years before the invention of next generation sequencing (NGS), two technologies that were necessary for the DEL concept to work. Paul and Richard were very long-time friends and remained in close contact, in daily contact, until Paul passed away. After a discussion that Paul and Richard had together in person while vacationing three and a half years ago during the new-year break, Paul came back convinced that we should start using the DEL technology to search for drugs for the various targets that we had identified in the lab (for a recent reviews see: Cochrane et al., 2019; Neri & Lerner, 2018; Scheuermann & Neri, 2015; Yuen & Franzini, 2017; Zimmermann & Neri, 2016). He immediately grasped the power of this technology and the practical advantages compared to mainstream approaches. The DEL technology allows for very large libraries of compounds (millions to billions of compounds) to be screened easily in a single tube using very limited amount of target. Each compound is tagged with a specific and unique DNA sequence. Parallel screens can be performed all at once and the decoding of the target-bound compounds is performed by NGS. Paul immediately understood what this all meant, that large scale drug discovery was now possible in a regular laboratory setup. The same week that Paul came back to the lab from his winter break, we started exploring several commercial options, but nothing turned out to be satisfactory and not overly complicated. Dr. Marc Flajolet had to mention only once that "I am pretty sure that we can build it in-house Paul, this is heavily based on molecular biology, the DNA-encoding seems like a lot of fun to me," Paul's eyes sparkled, and he immediately agreed to embark on this new adventure. In a way the loop was closing, the pharmaceutical world that Paul left behind at Geigy exactly 50 years ago, was now coming back to him, but in a setup that looked much more favorable to Paul, in his own lab. He was not short of ideas regarding possible therapeutic targets to screen using our DEL platform. In a couple of brainstorming sessions, we put together a list of over 15 targets based on current work being performed in the lab. A majority of those targets were being studied in relation to AD, including MDD, inflammation and also PD. Soon after, we were acquiring serious chemistry equipment, enquiring for lab space at The Rockefeller University and planning to initiate our own DEL drug discovery platform. This platform is now well in place and up and running. Dr. Lerner remains a strong supporter of the Greengard Lab and also serves as an advisor for our DEL related projects. Just in Paul's final weeks, Paul and Marc were discussing projects to spin-off some of our recent drug developments about our DEL program into a novel company; because of recent chemistry developments the field needs more power to grow faster. Discussing these new long-term projects illuminated Paul's eyes every single time, it was one of his major driving forces.

10. Conclusion

Paul had no intention to stop, not even to slow down. His laboratory, 37 years after he joined The Rockefeller University, was still functioning at full capacity with about 55 persons. He relentlessly worked in his lab, 5 or 6 days a week; his lab remained his top professional priority until the very last day. The rest of the time, most of his free time, he would spend with his wife, the internationally celebrated artist and sculptor,

Ursula von Rydingsvard. In parallel, they each built their own incredible world, one molecular and abstract, made of chemical additions, pathways and arrows, the other one colossal and tri-dimensional, made of 4 in. × 4 in. cedar timbers and bronze, circular saw cuts and stacks, both extremely powerful and assembled to last an eternity. It is not obvious to the non-initiated, but the two worlds do overlap...

Paul loved science, he loved starting new projects, discovering new things and embracing novel technologies ... Starting new chapters always gave Paul an enormous burst of energy. While he will not participate physically in the next chapters, they will all remain a part of his legacy. He will not see the approval of drugs burgeoning from his work, he will not witness the many patients benefiting from those molecules, but he will be remembered as a giant explorer of the brain and his legacy will remain a great quarry of knowledge for drug development for a long time.

Acknowledgments

We thank the Fisher Center for Alzheimer's Research Foundation and the JPB Foundation for supporting this work. We thank Debra Poulter for proofreading and editing the present manuscript. We thank Adam Ogilvie for his administrative support. This review article is dedicated to the memory of Paul Greengard.

Conflict of interest

M.F. owns shares of Intracellular Therapies, Inc. No other conflicts of interest are noted.

References

Alexander, B., Warner-Schmidt, J., Eriksson, T., Tamminga, C., Arango-Lievano, M., Ghose, S., et al. (2010). Reversal of depressed behaviors in mice by p11 gene therapy in the nucleus accumbens. *Science Translational Medicine*, *2*(54), 54ra76.

Bateup, H. S., Svenningsson, P., Kuroiwa, M., Gong, S., Nishi, A., Heintz, N., et al. (2008). Cell type-specific regulation of DARPP-32 phosphorylation by psychostimulant and antipsychotic drugs. *Nature Neuroscience*, *11*(8), 932–939.

Bendor, J., Lizardi-Ortiz, J. E., Westphalen, R. I., Brandstetter, M., Hemmings, H. C., Jr., Sulzer, D., et al. (2010). AGAP1/AP-3-dependent endocytic recycling of M5 muscarinic receptors promotes dopamine release. *The EMBO Journal*, *29*(16), 2813–2826.

Bettayeb, K., Chang, J. C., Luo, W., Aryal, S., Varotsis, D., Randolph, L., et al. (2016). δ-COP modulates Aβ peptide formation via retrograde trafficking of APP. *Proceedings of the National Academy of Sciences of the United States of America*, *113*(19), 5412–5417.

Bettayeb, K., Hooli, B. V., Parrado, A. R., Randolph, L., Varotsis, D., Aryal, S., et al. (2016). Relevance of the COPI complex for Alzheimer's disease progression in vivo. *Proceedings of the National Academy of Sciences of the United States of America*, *113*(19), 5418–5423.

Bibb, J. A., Chen, J., Taylor, J. R., Svenningsson, P., Nishi, A., Snyder, G. L., et al. (2001). Effects of chronic exposure to cocaine are regulated by the neuronal protein Cdk5. *Nature*, *410*(6826), 376–380.

Blair, H. A. (2020). Lumateperone: First approval. *Drugs*, *80*(4), 417–423.

Brenner, S., & Lerner, R. A. (1992). Encoded combinatorial chemistry. *Proceedings of the National Academy of Sciences of the United States of America, 89*(12), 5381–5383.

Brichta, L., Greengard, P., & Flajolet, M. (2013). Advances in the pharmacological treatment of Parkinson's disease: Targeting neurotransmitter systems. *Trends in Neurosciences, 36*(9), 543–554.

Brichta, L., Shin, W., Jackson-Lewis, V., Blesa, J., Yap, E. L., Walker, Z., et al. (2015). Identification of neurodegenerative factors using translatome-regulatory network analysis. *Nature Neuroscience, 18*(9), 1325–1333.

Bustos, V., Pulina, M. V., Bispo, A., Lam, A., Flajolet, M., Gorelick, F. S., et al. (2017a). Phosphorylated Presenilin 1 decreases beta-amyloid by facilitating autophagosome-lysosome fusion. *Proceedings of the National Academy of Sciences of the United States of America, 114*(27), 7148–7153. https://doi.org/10.1073/pnas.1705240114.

Bustos, V., Pulina, M. V., Bispo, A., Lam, A., Flajolet, M., Gorelick, F. S., et al. (2017b). Phosphorylated Presenilin 1 decreases β-amyloid by facilitating autophagosome–lysosome fusion. *Proceedings of the National Academy of Sciences of the United States of America, 114*, 201705240.

Bustos, V., Pulina, M. V., Kelahmetoglu, Y., Sinha, S. C., Gorelick, F. S., Flajolet, M., et al. (2017). Bidirectional regulation of Aβ levels by Presenilin 1. *Proceedings of the National Academy of Sciences of the United States of America, 114*(27), 7142–7147.

Ceglia, I., Lee, K. W., Cahill, M. E., Graves, S. M., Dietz, D., Surmeier, D. J., et al. (2017). WAVE1 in neurons expressing the D1 dopamine receptor regulates cellular and behavioral actions of cocaine. *Proceedings of the National Academy of Sciences of the United States of America, 114*(6), 1395–1400.

Ceglia, I., Reitz, C., Gresack, J., Ahn, J. H., Bustos, V., Bleck, M., et al. (2015). APP intracellular domain-WAVE1 pathway reduces amyloid-β production. *Nature Medicine, 21*(9), 1054–1059.

Cheng, J., Umschweif, G., Leung, J., Sagi, Y., & Greengard, P. (2019). HCN2 channels in cholinergic interneurons of nucleus accumbens shell regulate depressive behaviors. *Neuron, 101*(4), 662–672.e5.

Chergui, K., Svenningsson, P., & Greengard, P. (2004). Cyclin-dependent kinase 5 regulates dopaminergic and glutamatergic transmission in the striatum. *Proceedings of the National Academy of Sciences of the United States of America, 101*(7), 2191–2196.

Chottekalapanda, R. U., Kalik, S., Gresack, J., Ayala, A., Gao, M., Wang, W., et al. (2020). AP-1 controls the p11-dependent antidepressant response. *Molecular Psychiatry, 25*(7), 1364–1381.

Chuhma, N., Mingote, S., Kalmbach, A., Yetnikoff, L., & Rayport, S. (2017). Heterogeneity in dopamine neuron synaptic actions across the striatum and its relevance for schizophrenia. *Biological Psychiatry, 81*(1), 43–51.

Cochrane, W. G., Malone, M. L., Dang, V. Q., Cavett, V., Satz, A. L., & Paegel, B. M. (2019). Activity-based DNA-encoded library screening. *ACS Combinatorial Science, 21*(5), 425–435.

Doyle, J. P., Dougherty, J. D., Heiman, M., Schmidt, E. F., Stevens, T. R., Ma, G., et al. (2008). Application of a translational profiling approach for the comparative analysis of CNS cell types. *Cell, 135*(4), 749–762.

Fienberg, A. A., & Greengard, P. (2000). The DARPP-32 knockout mouse. *Brain Research. Brain Research Reviews, 31*(2–3), 313–319.

Fienberg, A. A., Hiroi, N., Mermelstein, P. G., Song, W., Snyder, G. L., Nishi, A., et al. (1998). DARPP-32: Regulator of the efficacy of dopaminergic neurotransmission. *Science, 281*(5378), 838–842.

Flajolet, M., He, G., Heiman, M., Lin, A., Nairn, A. C., & Greengard, P. (2007). Regulation of Alzheimer's disease amyloid-beta formation by casein kinase I. *Proceedings of the National Academy of Sciences of the United States of America, 104*(10), 4159–4164.

Flajolet, M., Rakhilin, S., Wang, H., Starkova, N., Nuangchamnong, N., Nairn, A. C., et al. (2003). Protein phosphatase 2C binds selectively to and dephosphorylates metabotropic glutamate receptor 3. *Proceedings of the National Academy of Sciences of the United States of America, 100*(26), 16006–16011.

Flajolet, M., Wang, Z., Futter, M., Shen, W., Nuangchamnong, N., Bendor, J., et al. (2008). FGF acts as a co-transmitter through adenosine A(2A) receptor to regulate synaptic plasticity. *Nature Neuroscience, 11*(12), 1402–1409.

Greengard, P. (2001). The neurobiology of slow synaptic transmission. *Science, 294*(5544), 1024–1030.

Greengard, P., Allen, P. B., & Nairn, A. C. (1999). Beyond the dopamine receptor: The DARPP-32/protein phosphatase-1 cascade. *Neuron, 23*(3), 435–447.

Greengard, P., Kalinsky, H., Manning, T. J., & Zak, S. B. (1968). Prevention and remission by adrenocortical steriods of nicotinamide deficiency disease. II. A study of the mechanism. *The Journal of Biological Chemistry, 243*(16), 4216–4221.

Greengard, P., Quinn, G. P., & Reid, M. B. (1964). Pituitary influence of pyridine nucleotide metabolism of rat liver. *The Journal of Biological Chemistry, 239*, 1887–1892.

Greengard, P., & Straub, R. W. (1958). Effect of electrical stimulation on the concentration of phosphorylated intermediary metabolites in mammalian non-myelinated fibres. *The Journal of Physiology, 140*(1), 18-9P.

Heiman, M., Kulicke, R., Fenster, R. J., Greengard, P., & Heintz, N. (2014). Cell type-specific mRNA purification by translating ribosome affinity purification (TRAP). *Nature Protocols, 9*(6), 1282–1291.

Heiman, M., Schaefer, A., Gong, S., Peterson, J. D., Day, M., Ramsey, K. E., et al. (2008). A translational profiling approach for the molecular characterization of CNS cell types. *Cell, 135*(4), 738–748.

Jin, J., Bhatti, D. L., Lee, K. W., Medrihan, L., Cheng, J., Wei, J., et al. (2019). Ahnak scaffolds p11/Anxa2 complex and L-type voltage-gated calcium channel and modulates depressive behavior. *Molecular Psychiatry, 25*(5), 1035–1049.

Kaplitt, M. G. (2019). Gene-targeting approaches for movement disorders: Recent advances. *Current Opinion in Neurology, 32*(4), 566–570.

Ledo, J. H., Liebmann, T., Zhang, R., Chang, J. C., Azevedo, E. P., Wong, E., et al. (2020). Presenilin 1 phosphorylation regulates amyloid-β degradation by microglia. *Molecular Psychiatry*, 1–16.

Ledo, J. H., Zhang, R., Mesin, L., Mourão-Sá, D., Azevedo, E. P., Troyanskaya, O. G., et al. (2020). Lack of a site-specific phosphorylation of Presenilin 1 disrupts microglial gene networks and progenitors during development. *PLoS One, 15*(8), e0237773.

Lee, H., Fenster, R. J., Pineda, S. S., Gibbs, W. S., Mohammadi, S., Davila-Velderrain, J., et al. (2020). Cell type-specific transcriptomics reveals that mutant Huntingtin leads to mitochondrial RNA release and neuronal innate immune activation. *Neuron, 107*, 891–908. S0896-6273(20)30475-X.

Lee, K. W., Kim, Y., Kim, A. M., Helmin, K., Nairn, A. C., & Greengard, P. (2006). Cocaine-induced dendritic spine formation in D1 and D2 dopamine receptor-containing medium spiny neurons in nucleus accumbens. *Proceedings of the National Academy of Sciences of the United States of America, 103*(9), 3399–3404.

Lee, K. W., Westin, L., Kim, J., Chang, J. C., Oh, Y. S., Amreen, B., et al. (2015). Alteration by p11 of mGluR5 localization regulates depression-like behaviors. *Molecular Psychiatry, 20*(12), 1546–1556.

Leongway, E., & Sutherland, V. C. (1963). Pharmacologically active brain substances and their relation to endocrine effects. *Anesthesiology, 24*, 543–562.

Liebmann, T., Renier, N., Bettayeb, K., Greengard, P., Tessier-Lavigne, M., & Flajolet, M. (2016). Three-dimensional study of Alzheimer's disease hallmarks using the iDISCO clearing method. *Cell Reports, 16*(4), 1138–1152.

Marongiu, R., Arango-Lievano, M., Francardo, V., Morgenstern, P., Zhang, X., Cenci, M. A., et al. (2016). Gene therapy blockade of dorsal striatal p11 improves motor function and dyskinesia in Parkinsonian mice. *Proceedings of the National Academy of Sciences of the United States of America, 113*(5), 1423–1428.

Medrihan, L., Sagi, Y., Inde, Z., Krupa, O., Daniels, C., Peyrache, A., et al. (2017). Initiation of behavioral response to antidepressants by cholecystokinin neurons of the dentate gyrus. *Neuron, 95*(3), 564–576.

Medrihan, L., Umschweif, G., Sinha, A., Reed, S., Lee, J., Gindinova, K., et al. (2020). Reduced Kv3.1 activity in dentate gyrus parvalbumin cells induces vulnerability to depression. *Biological Psychiatry, 88*(5), 405–414. S0006-3223(20)31291-9.

Milosevic, A., Liebmann, T., Knudsen, M., Schintu, N., Svenningsson, P., & Greengard, P. (2017). Cell- and region-specific expression of depression-related protein p11 (S100a10) in the brain. *The Journal of Comparative Neurology, 525*(4), 955–975.

Nairn, A. C., Svenningsson, P., Nishi, A., Fisone, G., Girault, J. A., & Greengard, P. (2004). The role of DARPP-32 in the actions of drugs of abuse. *Neuropharmacology, 47*(Suppl. 1), 14–23.

Neri, D., & Lerner, R. A. (2018). DNA-encoded chemical libraries: A selection system based on endowing organic compounds with amplifiable information. *Annual Review of Biochemistry, 87*, 479–502.

Oh, Y. S., Gao, P., Lee, K. W., Ceglia, I., Seo, J. S., Zhang, X., et al. (2013). SMARCA3, a chromatin-remodeling factor, is required for p11-dependent antidepressant action. *Cell, 152*(4), 831–843.

Posner, J. B., Stern, R., & Krebs, E. G. (1965). Effects of electrical stimulation and epinephrine on muscle phosphorylase, phosphorylase b kinase, and adenosine 3′,5′-phosphate. *The Journal of Biological Chemistry, 240*, 982–985.

Psychoyos, S., Tallan, H. H., & Greengard, P. (1966). Aldosterone synthesis by adrenal mitochondria. *The Journal of Biological Chemistry, 241*(12), 2949–2956.

Pulina, M. V., Hopkins, M., Haroutunian, V., Greengard, P., & Bustos, V. (2019). C99 selectively accumulates in vulnerable neurons in Alzheimer's disease. *Alzheimer's & Dementia, 16*(2), 273–282.

Roussarie, J. P., Yao, V., Rodriguez-Rodriguez, P., Oughtred, R., Rust, J., Plautz, Z., et al. (2020). Selective neuronal vulnerability in Alzheimer's disease: A network-based analysis. *Neuron, 107*(5), 821–835. S0896-6273(20) 30439-6.

Schaefer, A., Im, H. I., Venø, M. T., Fowler, C. D., Min, A., Intrator, A., et al. (2010). Argonaute 2 in dopamine 2 receptor-expressing neurons regulates cocaine addiction. *The Journal of Experimental Medicine, 207*(9), 1843–1851.

Scheuermann, J., & Neri, D. (2015). Dual-pharmacophore DNA-encoded chemical libraries. *Current Opinion in Chemical Biology, 26*, 99–103.

Schintu, N., Zhang, X., Alvarsson, A., Marongiu, R., Kaplitt, M. G., Greengard, P., et al. (2016). p11 modulates L-DOPA therapeutic effects and dyskinesia via distinct cell types in experimental Parkinsonism. *Proceedings of the National Academy of Sciences of the United States of America, 113*(5), 1429–1434.

Snyder, G. L., Allen, P. B., Fienberg, A. A., Valle, C. G., Huganir, R. L., Nairn, A. C., et al. (2000). Regulation of phosphorylation of the GluR1 AMPA receptor in the neostriatum by dopamine and psychostimulants in vivo. *The Journal of Neuroscience, 20*(12), 4480–4488.

Svenningsson, P., Chergui, K., Rachleff, I., Flajolet, M., Zhang, X., El Yacoubi, M., et al. (2006). Alterations in 5-HT1B receptor function by p11 in depression-like states. *Science, 311*(5757), 77–80.

Svenningsson, P., Nairn, A. C., & Greengard, P. (2005). DARPP-32 mediates the actions of multiple drugs of abuse. *The AAPS Journal, 7*(2), E353–E360.

Svenningsson, P., Nishi, A., Fisone, G., Girault, J. A., Nairn, A. C., & Greengard, P. (2004). DARPP-32: An integrator of neurotransmission. *Annual Review of Pharmacology and Toxicology*, *44*, 269–296.

Tian, Y., Chang, J. C., Greengard, P., & Flajolet, M. (2014). The convergence of endosomal and autophagosomal pathways: Implications for APP-CTF degradation. *Autophagy*, *10*(4), 694–696.

Walaas, S. I., Hemmings, H. C., Jr., Greengard, P., & Nairn, A. C. (2011). Beyond the dopamine receptor: Regulation and roles of serine/threonine protein phosphatases. *Frontiers in Neuroanatomy*, *5*, 50.

Wang, H., Warner-Schmidt, J., Varela, S., Enikolopov, G., Greengard, P., & Flajolet, M. (2015). Norbin ablation results in defective adult hippocampal neurogenesis and depressive-like behavior in mice. *Proceedings of the National Academy of Sciences of the United States of America*, *112*(31), 9745–9750.

Wang, H., Westin, L., Nong, Y., Birnbaum, S., Bendor, J., Brismar, H., et al. (2009). Norbin is an endogenous regulator of metabotropic glutamate receptor 5 signaling. *Science*, *326*(5959), 1554–1557.

Warner-Schmidt, J. L., Schmidt, E. F., Marshall, J. J., Rubin, A. J., Arango-Lievano, M., Kaplitt, M. G., et al. (2012). Cholinergic interneurons in the nucleus accumbens regulate depression-like behavior. *Proceedings of the National Academy of Sciences of the United States of America*, *109*(28), 11360–11365.

Yuen, L. H., & Franzini, R. M. (2017). Achievements, challenges, and opportunities in DNA-encoded library research: An academic point of view. *Chembiochem*, *218*(9), 829–836.

Zhou, M., Gresack, J., Cheng, J., Uryu, K., Brichta, L., Greengard, P., et al. (2018). CK1δ over-expressing mice display ADHD-like behaviors, frontostriatal neuronal abnormalities and altered expressions of ADHD-candidate genes. *Molecular Psychiatry*, 1–15. PMID: 31363163 https://doi.org/10.1038/s41380-018-0233-z.

Zhou, M., Rebholz, H., Brocia, C., Warner-Schmidt, J. L., Fienberg, A. A., Nairn, A. C., et al. (2010). Forebrain overexpression of CK1delta leads to down-regulation of dopamine receptors and altered locomotor activity reminiscent of ADHD. *Proceedings of the National Academy of Sciences of the United States of America*, *107*(9), 4401–4406.

Zimmermann, G., & Neri, D. (2016). DNA-encoded chemical libraries: Foundations and applications in lead discovery. *Drug Discovery Today*, *21*(11), 1828–1834.

CHAPTER TWO

Giving names to the actors of synaptic transmission: The long journey from synaptic vesicles to neural plasticity

Fabio Benfenati[a,b,c,*], Martin Bähler[d], and Flavia Valtorta[e,f]

[a]Center for Synaptic Neuroscience and Technology, Istituto Italiano di Tecnologia, Genova, Italy
[b]IRCCS Ospedale Policlinico San Martino, Genova, Italy
[c]Department of Experimental Medicine, University of Genova, Genova, Italy
[d]Institute of Molecular Cell Biology, Cells in Motion Interfaculty Centre, University of Münster, Münster, Germany
[e]IRCCS San Raffaele Scientific Institute, Milan, Italy
[f]Vita-Salute San Raffaele University, Milan, Italy
[*]Corresponding author: e-mail address: fabio.benfenati@iit.it

Contents

Abstract

More than a scientific paper or a review article, this is a remembrance of a unique time of science and life that the authors spent in Paul Greengard's laboratory at the Rockefeller University in New York in the 1980s and 1990s, forming the so-called *synaptic vesicle group*. It was a time in which the molecular mechanisms of synaptic transmission and the nature of the organelles in charge of storing and releasing neurotransmitter were just beginning to be understood. It was an exciting time in which the protein composition of synaptic vesicles started to be identified. It turned out that the interactions of synaptic vesicle proteins with the cytoskeleton and the presynaptic membrane and their modulation by protein phosphorylation represented an essential network regulating the efficiency of neurotransmitter release and thereby synaptic strength and plasticity. This is also a description of the distinct scientific journeys that the three authors

Advances in Pharmacology, Volume 90
ISSN 1054-3589
https://doi.org/10.1016/bs.apha.2020.09.007

took on going back to Europe and how they were strongly influenced by the generous and outstanding mentorship of Paul Greengard, his genuine interest in their lives and careers and the life-long friendship with him.

1. Introduction

1.1 The synaptic vesicle: The unknown nanomachine

1.1.1 The impact of signal transduction and protein phosphorylation in neurophysiology

In 2000 Arvid Carlsson, Paul Greengard and Eric R. Kandel were jointly awarded the Nobel Prize in Physiology or Medicine "*for their discoveries concerning signal transduction in the nervous system.*" Indeed, before them the study of signal transmission in the brain was largely considered to be the realm of electrophysiologists, since it was known, through the work of Hodgkin and Huxley and many others, that in the brain as well as in peripheral neurons rapid information transfer is achieved by means of electrical signals. In the 1950s it was already known that within neurons information is transported by means of action potentials, which can be considered digital signals of constant amplitude: information is coded solely by their frequency. However, across neurons, information transfer takes place through the release of chemical neurotransmitters, which stimulate receptors on the receiving neuron, thus giving rise to the generation of synaptic potentials: analog electrical signals of variable amplitude that, upon reaching a certain threshold, produce action potentials.

Tackling the problem from distinct points of view, Greengard, Carlsson and Kandel understood that the great complexity of information processing in the brain cannot be achieved simply through electric signals: by extrapolating to brain research the principles of what was being discovered for non-neuronal cells, they elucidated the intricate network of chemical messages that finely modulate neuronal activities, allowing the integration of the multitude of signals that impinge on a single neuron and the plasticity phenomena which underlie distinct brain features such as learning and memory.

Neurons are endowed with a variety of ion channels and transporters that move charges (ions) across the plasma membrane, generating an electrochemical imbalance which gives rise to the resting membrane potential. In the axons, transient depolarizations of the membrane potential produce self-regenerating signals (action potentials), which are conducted rapidly along nerve cells. At the nerve terminal, changes in membrane potential trigger the opening of Ca^{2+} channels which cause the release of chemical neurotransmitters. Such idea was predicted by Luigi Galvani from Bologna in 1794 in stating that "...*in the animal there is a particular machine capable of generating such disequilibrium, and it will be convenient to refer to this form of electricity as to animal electricity to denote, not a type of electricity whatsoever, but a particular one referred to a particular machine totally occult to the most acute sight.*"

A fundamental breakthrough in neurobiology occurred when the Nobel laureate Sir Bernard Katz proposed that the neurotransmitter acetylcholine released from motor neurons to activate muscle cells was released in uniform doses (quanta). Single quanta could be released spontaneously in the absence of stimuli, or synchronously in response to depolarization of the nerve terminal (Del Castillo & Katz, 1954). Katz had noticed that, at the neuromuscular junction, small spontaneous depolarizations (miniature endplate potential; mEPP) occur in relatively uniform sizes, and the larger depolarizations resulting from electrical stimulation of the nerve (endplate potential; EPP) occur in sizes which are multiples of the size of a mEPP. Thus, the mEPP may be considered the elementary unit, or "*quantum*," of neurotransmitter release.

In independent studies, De Robertis and Bennett (1955) and Palay (1956) had observed by transmission electron microscopy the presence in nerve terminals of densely packed vesicular structures of uniform size. In motor nerve terminals, such "*synaptic vesicles*" were clustered in areas of the presynaptic membrane (active zones) juxtaposed to infoldings of the postsynaptic membrane where acetylcholine receptors were thought to be concentrated. Katz proposed that the quantal nature of neurotransmitter release stemmed from the uniform capacity for neurotransmitter cargo of such "*synaptic vesicles*." In 1973, both Heuser and Reese, and Ceccarelli, Hurlbut and Mauro independently demonstrated that synaptic vesicles can be locally recycled at nerve terminals, undergoing an *exo*-endocytotic cycle. In subsequent years a considerable amount of evidence accumulated in support of the "*vesicle hypothesis*" of neurotransmitter release, i.e., the one-to-one correspondence between vesicles and transmitter quanta. The most convincing studies in support of this theory employed a combination of electrophysiological and morphological techniques (including immunocytochemistry to trace the movements of vesicle-specific proteins, and quick freezing to provide "snap-shots" of nerve endings with a millisecond time resolution). By the end of the 1980s the vesicular nature of quantal release was universally acknowledged.

1.1.2 *The key of protein phosphorylation: From glycogen to brain*

To respond to the stimuli coming from the external environment, each cell undergoes continuous changes in its physiological state. This high degree of plasticity is made possible by a fine modulation of the biological properties of cellular proteins through a set of processes known as post-translational modifications. Protein phosphorylation is recognized as the most common form of post-translational modification responsible for regulating the biological properties of proteins. Compared to other forms of post-translational modification of proteins, phosphorylation offers the advantage of greater versatility, linked to the property of being readily reversible. The introduction of one or more phosphate groups in the molecule of a protein, through modifications in charge or conformation, alters its properties, increasing or decreasing the activity if it is an enzyme, and/or modifying its ability to interact with other molecules in other cases.

Our understanding of protein phosphorylation in the transduction of signals coming from the environment stemmed from work on the regulation of metabolism. In this context, the Nobel laureate Earl Sutherland discovered cAMP and hence second messengers, and Edmond Fischer and Edwin Krebs identified reversible protein phosphorylation activated by second messengers. A discovery for which they were awarded the Nobel Prize in 1992.

The intuition that second messengers and protein phosphorylation could operate also in the brain as powerful mechanisms to reversibly modulate protein function was Paul Greengard's major achievement. Indeed, the identification of protein phosphorylation as a means to modulate neuronal activity and to integrate the numerous signals that impinge on a neuron at any time has constituted a conceptual framework for the many seminal achievements by Paul's group in the study of brain physiology and of human neurological and psychiatric disorders.

In the late 1970s and early 1980s Greengard's laboratory identified several brain proteins able to incorporate phosphate upon various stimulations. In the beginning, these proteins were no more than "bands on a gel," but some of them were soon given a name and discovered to be of paramount importance for neuronal function. One of these proteins, initially called Protein I and later renamed synapsin I, was a prominent brain phosphoprotein regulated by increases in both Ca^{2+} and cAMP concentrations (for review, see De Camilli, Benfenati, Valtorta, & Greengard, 1990).

1.1.3 *The "synaptic vesicle group" on the upper east side*

With a great intuition, Paul decided to assemble a group in the lab studying the biochemistry and physiology of synaptic vesicles. The key of this idea came from the observation that protein I, one of the most abundant phosphoproteins in brain tissue, was demonstrated by Huttner and De Camilli to be strictly localized to synapses, particularly to presynaptic terminals in association with synaptic vesicles.

Beautiful work by Huttner and De Camilli established that the phosphoprotein synapsin I is a synaptic vesicle associated protein (De Camilli, Harris, Huttner, & Greengard, 1983; Huttner, Schiebler, Greengard, & De Camilli, 1983). This finding raised the question as to why synapsin I specifically associates with synaptic vesicles. The naïve assumption was that a transmembrane synaptic vesicle protein would be responsible for the recruitment of synapsin I. Schiebler established a purification protocol for synapsin I under non-denaturing conditions and showed that it bound with high affinity to purified synaptic vesicles depleted of endogenous synapsin I (Schiebler, Jahn, Doucet, Rothlein, & Greengard, 1986). These experiments benefited from the generation of monoclonal antibodies against synaptophysin, one of the first synaptic vesicle components to be identified by Jahn, and the development of a dot-immunobinding assay that allowed for quantification of the concentrations of synapsin I and synaptic vesicles (Jahn, Schiebler, & Greengard, 1984; Jahn, Schiebler, Ouimet, & Greengard, 1985). Benfenati then went on showing that synapsin I bound with high affinity to small phospholipid vesicles (Benfenati, Greengard, Brunner, & Bähler, 1989). Essentially, the affinity of synapsin I for phospholipid vesicles was comparable to that for synaptic vesicles. This fact greatly complicated the search for a protein receptor, as reconstitution of proteins into lipid vesicles would not be expected to alter the binding affinity significantly. Nevertheless, because the membrane of synaptic vesicles did not appear to have a unique lipid composition, and therefore, did not readily explain the specific association of synapsin I with synaptic vesicles in vivo, the search for a protein receptor continued. One approach included the fragmentation of synapsin I to possibly separate domains involved in lipid binding from those involved in "receptor" binding (Benfenati, Bähler, Jahn, & Greengard, 1989; Benfenati, Greengard, et al., 1989). These original studies were later confirmed by the identification of three distinct regions in the evolutionary conserved synapsin domain C that insert into the hydrophobic core of the phospholipid bilayer and that are surface-exposed in the crystal structure of domain C of synapsin I (Cheetham et al., 2001; Esser et al., 1998). The idea of a strong and specific interaction of synapsin I with synaptic vesicle phospholipids was further strengthened, few years later, by the identification in the synapsin domain B of an amphipathic lipid packing sensor (ALPS) motif characterized by high affinity for highly curved membrane surfaces, as those of synaptic vesicles (Krabben et al., 2011).

The fact that synapsin I covered the surface of synaptic vesicles and was a phosphoprotein suggested that it might control retention, clustering and trafficking of synaptic vesicles within the presynaptic nerve terminal in a phosphorylation regulated manner. Since actin filaments were reported to form a scaffold within the presynaptic nerve terminal, it was hypothesized that synapsin I serves as an adaptor between synaptic vesicles and actin filaments. Indeed, a phosphorylation-dependent interaction of synapsin I with actin filaments could be shown (Bähler, Benfenati, Valtorta, Czernik, & Greengard, 1989; Bähler & Greengard, 1987). Subsequent studies revealed that synapsin I crosslinks synaptic vesicles to the actin-based cytoskeleton and nucleates actin at the vesicle surface (Benfenati, Valtorta, Chieregatti, & Greengard, 1992; Fesce, Benfenati, Greengard, & Valtorta, 1992; Valtorta, Greengard, Fesce, Chieregatti, & Benfenati, 1992). These activities of synapsin I are regulated by phosphorylation through CaM kinases. Phosphorylation of synapsin I leads to the dissociation of synaptic vesicles from the cytoskeleton preparing them for release (Benfenati et al., 1992; Ceccaldi et al., 1995). Further biophysical studies on purified synaptic vesicles demonstrated that synapsin I also triggers vesicle clustering and stabilizes the membrane bilayer, thus contributing to the remarkable uniform size of synaptic vesicles (Awizio, Onofri, Benfenati, & Bonaccurso, 2007; Benfenati et al., 1993; Monaldi et al., 2010; Pera, Stark, Kappl, Butt, & Benfenati, 2004). The role of synapsins in the assembly and maintenance of the functional synaptic vesicle pools was subsequently confirmed by an array of studies showing that ATP binding to a highly conserved site in the synapsin domain C favors cluster formation through synapsin oligomerization (Orlando et al., 2014) and that synapsins induce liquid phase separation within nerve terminals in a phosphorylation-dependent fashion that participates in the segregation of vesicle clusters (Milovanovic, Wu, Bian, & De Camilli, 2018).

A few decades passed by from those pioneering times. We now know that synaptic vesicles are fascinating biological nanomachines. These tiny organelles are perfect multisensor-actuators. Vesicles have a fusion protein, synaptobrevin, as an actuator that, upon binding to presynaptic membrane partners (syntaxin and SNAP-25), triggers fusion and neurotransmitter release. Vesicles have nano-switches that are turned on by phosphorylation and, based on the activation of the intracellular signaling pathways, regulate their life cycle and their competence for release. In addition, they bear a Ca^{2+}-sensor to trigger their fusion with the membrane and the associated release of neurotransmitter in the synaptic cleft.

Marcello Malpighi, professor at Alma Mater University of Bologna, while studying the kidney wrote in 1697: *"To carry out the marvelous operations in animals and plants, Nature has been pleased to construct their organized bodies with a very large number of machines, which are of necessity made up of extremely minute parts so shaped and situated as to form a marvelous organ, the structure and composition of which are usually invisible to the naked eye without the aid of a microscope."* In his text, Malpighi was referring to the kidney glomeruli. Nevertheless, his description of biological nanomachines perfectly fits to synaptic vesicles. Nowadays, synaptic vesicles are among the best-known intracellular organelles in cell biology. We now know that a complex molecular machinery regulates synaptic vesicle *exo*-endocytosis, and a multitude of studies have revealed the molecules involved in the processes by which synaptic vesicles are loaded with neurotransmitter, positioned at active zones, prepared and triggered to exocytose their neurotransmitter content upon nerve terminal depolarization, and finally retrieved from the plasma membrane to be used again. The synaptic vesicle proteome has been clarified, we know now protein by protein their composition, and for each protein the number of copies that sit on a single vesicle (Takamori et al., 2006). We know that mutations in several genes encoding synaptic vesicle proteins can cause severe neurological diseases such as epilepsy or autism and, in some cases, the pathogenesis of such diseases is triggered by an initial synaptic vesicle dysfunction. However, the pioneering studies on the functional role of synapsins, nerve terminal cytoskeleton and protein phosphorylation are still completely valid and demonstrate how structure (the organelle) and regulation of function (phosphorylation of its components) are strictly interconnected and determine the efficiency of information transfer within brain circuits. Our knowledge of such molecular mechanisms, of their relevance to synaptic physiology and pathology, and of the various modulatory possibilities has increased greatly thanks to the work initiated in Paul Greengard's laboratory, which was subsequently independently expanded by some of his former students and collaborators as well as by many other research teams worldwide.

2. The follow-up research directions

After the unforgettable and life-changing experience in Paul's lab, each of us took his/her scientific journey that was greatly inspired by the great experience and friendship that each of us acquired working a few years in the "synaptic vesicle group."

2.1 Fabio's journey: From synaptopathies to hybrid neuronal interfaces

The detachment from Paul's laboratory was very smooth. Indeed, Paul wanted the project on synapsin to be continued in collaboration by Flavia and me in Italy. This was a great opportunity for us in the difficult time of our return from NY. Although Flavia and I were in two different cities, the collaboration worked very well. Within this collaboration, we went back and forth many times between Italy and NYC—we were called "*the lab commuters*"—and this gave us the opportunity to be part of Paul's lab for a much longer time, knowing the new people of the lab and the new research projects going on. From that time, a nice series of papers came out that clarified the structure-function relationships between synapsin, synaptic vesicles and actin and the role of synapsins and their phosphorylation in the regulation of presynaptic plasticity and synaptic strength. A picture emerged in which synaptic vesicles were like entities navigating in an ocean of sticky cytoskeletal nets, with ATP-phosphorylation fueling them to find a site where to dock and fuse with the plasma membrane, releasing their message to the postsynaptic neuron (Baldelli, Fassio, Valtorta, & Benfenati, 2007; Farisello et al., 2013; Forte, Binda, Contestabile, Benfenati, & Baldelli, 2020; Medrihan et al., 2013; Medrihan, Ferrea, Greco, Baldelli, & Benfenati, 2015; Michetti, Caruso, et al., 2017; Perlini et al., 2015; Piccini et al., 2017; Valente et al., 2012; Verstegen et al., 2014). Meanwhile, the fusion of the great expertise of the group of Montecucco in Padua on clostridial neurotoxins with the deep knowledge of synaptic vesicles, identified for the first time a group of vesicle and presynaptic membrane proteins that were specific substrates of the Zn^{2+}-protease activity of these toxins known to irreversibly block quantal neurotransmitter release. This finding was a cornerstone in that the identified proteins VAMP/synaptobrevin on the vesicles and SNAP-25/syntaxin on the presynaptic membrane (SNARE proteins) were essential for the fusion of synaptic vesicles (Schiavo, Poulain, et al., 1992; Schiavo, Benfenati, et al., 1992; Schiavo et al., 1993). Similar results were obtained with an independent approach by the Rothman group (Söllner et al., 1993).

The availability of synapsin knockout mice brought me to study more thoroughly the physiological role of synapsins and their phosphorylation by multiple kinases with electrophysiological techniques, by concentrating on synaptic transmission and plasticity. A picture emerged in which the lack or dysfunction of synapsins causes a specific impairment of inhibitory transmission that causes hyperexcitability generating seizure propensity (Baldelli et al., 2007; Farisello et al., 2013; Valente et al., 2012; Medrihan et al., 2013; Verstegen et al., 2014; Medrihan et al., 2015; Perlini et al., 2015; Piccini et al., 2017; Michetti, Caruso, et al., 2017; Michetti, Castroflorio, et al., 2017; Forte et al., 2020). These studies on the synapsin model became very important when several cases of loss-of-function mutations in the SYN1 gene were identified in patients with reflex epilepsy that also presented autism-spectrum disorder symptoms (Corradi et al., 2014; Fassio et al., 2011; Lignani et al., 2013; Nguyen et al., 2015). More recently, the research on the cellular mechanisms of synaptic function and plasticity was further progressed by extending to other presynaptic proteins, such as PRRT2 or APache (Fruscione et al., 2018; Michetti, Castroflorio, et al., 2017; Piccini et al., 2017; Valente et al., 2016; Valente et al., 2019), or to fundamental transcription factors controlling the neuronal phenotype and homeostatic plasticity such as REST/NRSF (Paonessa et al., 2016; Pecoraro-Bisogni et al., 2018; Pozzi et al., 2013).

Subsequently, the great opportunity to start Neuroscience laboratories at the newly established Italian Institute of Technology in Genova brought me toward more technologically oriented topics, such as optogenetics and interfaces of smart materials with neurons. In the latter field, I focused my activity on the field of light-controlled organic nanoactuators (semiconductive polymers) to trigger light-driven neuronal activation. This allowed to interrogate specific brain circuits and compensate for nervous system pathologies in which neuronal degeneration has induced a loss of function. These results were particularly promising in the case of degenerative blindness, in which retina loses its photoreceptors, but preserves the inner retinal neurons. Indeed, in a series of papers, we demonstrated that neurons grown onto the polymeric interface could be stimulated to fire action potentials with high fidelity (Ghezzi et al., 2011). The same interface could rescue light sensitivity in blind retinas in contact with the polymer, with bursts of action potentials by retinal ganglion cells in response to daylight-intensity stimuli (Ghezzi et al., 2013). The same device layered onto an organic silk fibroin substrate, or later administered as sub-μm nanoparticles, was able to rescue light sensitivity, light-driven behaviors and visual acuity in a murine model of human *Retinitis pigmentosa* (Maya-Vetencourt et al., 2017).

While exploring additional non-genetic strategies for neuronal photo-stimulation, interesting results were produced by using novel membrane-targeted azobenzene photo-switches as light-driven nanomachines to perturb membrane dynamics, and thereby the passive and active properties of the neuronal membrane (DiFrancesco et al., 2020). In summary, a long journey initiated with Paul and with the deep friends who are co-authoring this paper. Going back to Italy, Flavia and I initially experienced some difficult times with paucity of funds but working together let us overcome the initial shock and build, brick by brick, our laboratories in Genoa and Milan that evolved under Paul's eyes watching us from the distance. We always kept in mind his life-long lesson to work hard and extend research and knowledge beyond the strict disciplinary borders, aware that we are members of a big world family who shared the unique experience to be in contact with him. A feeling like reaching the top of one of the highest 8000-m peaks.

2.2 Martin's journey: The unconventional myosins

Towards the end of my stay in the lab, Paul allowed me to work half-time independently on a topic of my own choice not related to the work in his lab. I decided to start working on actin-based molecular motors combining the area of my PhD thesis in muscle biology with that of the work in Paul's lab. At that time, only conventional myosin II and brush border myosin I were known in mammals. However, based on the assumption that there might be many different actin-based motors (myosins) in each cell and particularly in neurons that would exert directed mechanical force along actin filaments and thereby regulate the elaborate cellular membrane traffic, I set out to identify new myosins expressed in developing and adult brain tissue. By the time I left Paul's lab to start my own lab, I had identified two new class I myosins whose expression is developmentally regulated in brain tissue. Needless to say that, without these preliminary results in hand thanks to the generosity of Paul, I might not have been able to convince the search committee that there is a large superfamily of myosin molecules waiting to be discovered. Surprisingly, my lab discovered also two hybrid motor-signaling molecules that constituted the class IX of myosins (Chieregatti, Gärtner, Stöffler, & Bähler, 1998; Reinhard et al., 1995). These two class IX myosins are GTPase activating proteins (GAPs) for the small monomeric GTPase RhoA that switch RhoA from its active GTP-bound state to its inactive GDP-bound state. Thanks to these two class IX myosins, cell signaling remained of continued interest in my work (Hanley, Vollmer, & Bähler, 2020).

Many myosins have in common with synapsin I that they bind with high affinity to negatively charged phospholipids. Therefore, expert knowledge gained by work done on synapsin I together with Fabio and Flavia in Paul's lab was very helpful to avoid pitfalls in the later study of myosins. Actually, we recently determined that the myosin Myo19 which is localized on the outer mitochondrial membrane is interacting with lipids and an outer mitochondrial transmembrane protein called Miro (Oeding et al., 2018). Binding to Miro, a GTP- and Ca^{2+}-binding protein, stabilizes Myo19 and prevents it from getting degraded. Interestingly, Miro is not only the mitochondrial receptor for Myo19, but also for the microtubule-based motor proteins kinesin KIF5 and dynein, thereby coordinating actin- and microtubule-based force generation.

In essence, the time spent in Paul's lab was a very formative time for both my future scientific and personal life. I feel privileged that I was a member of Paul's lab for 6 years. During that time, I had the opportunity to get to know, work together and become friends with an amazing number of great scientists.

2.3 Flavia's journey: Membrane trafficking in developing and mature neurons

When I joined Greengard's laboratory, I was interested in the mechanisms that allow recycling of synaptic vesicles. I graduated in Milan with Ceccarelli, a pioneer in the study of neurotransmitter release and synaptic vesicle recycling. Although the results obtained by Ceccarelli, Hurlbut, and Mauro (1973) and by Heuser and Reese (1973) were essentially similar, the authors developed profoundly divergent models for their interpretation. Thus, Heuser and Reese, by analogy with endocytosis observed in non-neuronal cells, theorized a complete collapse of the vesicle membrane into the neuronal plasma membrane, with intermixing of molecular components followed by coated vesicle-mediated recycling. In contrast, Ceccarelli and co-workers suggested that synaptic vesicles might release neurotransmitter without fully fusing with the axolemma, and be directly retrieved, via a process that we later dubbed "kiss and run" (Fesce, Grohovaz, Valtorta, & Meldolesi, 1994; Valtorta, Meldolesi, & Fesce, 2001). According to Ceccarelli's view, membrane retrieval through coated vesicles would operate as a rescue pathway activated by a disproportion between the rates of exocytosis and direct recycling. To demonstrate this hypothesis, it was necessary to have markers for the synaptic vesicles and the presynaptic plasma membrane. During my thesis, I identified the first protein specific for the presynaptic plasma membrane (Valtorta, Madeddu, Meldolesi, & Ceccarelli, 1984).

The identification by the Greengard lab of proteins which are specific to synaptic vesicles, in particular p38/synaptophysin, provided the possibility to use antibodies to such proteins as markers, and therefore to follow the fate of the synaptic vesicle membrane during *exo*-endocytosis. Thanks to De Camilli, I was able to join Paul's lab and perform studies on synaptic vesicle recycling that I continued also when back in Milan. These studies showed that integral proteins of the synaptic vesicle membrane become exposed to the outer surface of the axolemma. However, under defined conditions of stimulation, synaptic vesicles can be quickly retrieved and their proteins never accumulate in the plasma membrane, thus supporting the possibility of a direct recycling after fusion (Torri Tarelli et al., 1990; Valtorta, Jahn, Fesce, Greengard, & Ceccarelli, 1988). Similar studies showed that, in contrast to integral proteins, synapsin I leaves the synaptic vesicle membrane during high frequency exo-endocytosis, as a result of its phosphorylation, thus adding support to the view of synapsin as a phosphorylation-dependent regulator of synaptic vesicle trafficking (Torri Tarelli, Bossi, Fesce, Greengard, & Valtorta, 1992).

In Paul's lab I met the other people of the "synaptic vesicle group." To each of them I owe a lot, since we all had distinct backgrounds and expertise that were willing to share. The interaction with Fabio and Martin was particularly intense. The interaction with Martin was close since the beginning, since the lab was crowded and, for several months, we had to share both the bench and the desk. This could have led to a continuous fighting, instead we became good friends and he introduced me and Fabio to the world of actin and the cytoskeleton, allowing the development of a first model for synapsin function, which was further refined in the following years (see above).

With Fabio I started an intense collaboration which has been going on for 35 years and which thus far has led to nearly 90 joint publications, mainly concerning the role of synapsins in health and disease (see Fabio's story). In addition to continue the work on synapsins, after going back to Italy I also worked on the mechanisms underlying protein sorting in nerve terminals, showing an essential role for synaptophysin in directing the correct sorting of the SNARE VAMP2 to synaptic vesicles (Pennuto, Bonanomi, Benfenati, & Valtorta, 2003; Pennuto, Dunlap, Contestabile, Benfenati, & Valtorta, 2002).

I also contributed to the elucidation of several aspects of membrane trafficking in developing neurons, from the identification of the membrane and cytoskeletal mechanisms underlying the first steps in neuronal development (in collaboration with Carlos Dotti; Gärtner et al., 2012; Gärtner, Fornasiero, Valtorta, & Dotti, 2014), to the regulation of membrane trafficking in growth cones (Bonanomi et al., 2005; Bonanomi et al., 2008).

Since it is now accepted that impairment of synaptic function is an early event also in diseases previously thought to be essentially neurodegenerative (e.g., Parkinson's disease) or neuroinflammatory (e.g., multiple sclerosis), I am currently building on my expertise in the study of synapse development and function to continue the study of the molecular mechanisms underlying various synaptopathies (Guarnieri et al., 2018; Sassone et al., 2017). Thirty-five years after starting my journey with Paul, I can say that he has shaped all my scientific career, and strongly influenced also my personal life, since from him I learned that even when working hard there is always space for human interactions, and in his lab I actually met some of my best friends.

3. Conclusion

3.1 The unforgettable Paul

It is difficult to concentrate long years of relationship with Paul in few lines. Getting in his lab for the first time was a shocking experience, we had never been in such a large lab, with hectic people working round the clock. Lab life was very hard in the very beginning, but after a while, the hard became exciting, things were moving on and we became intimately convinced to be part of a unique and exclusive community, with the consciousness of working on fundamental problems. Paul focused our projects on synaptic physiology at the cellular and molecular level, building-up a group devoted to the study of synaptic neurobiology and the role of phosphorylation in synaptic transmission. This was how we started to study the most abundant phosphoproteins, the synapsins. Paul was always present, curious, open to new ideas, able to watch results under diverse angles and making creative connections among them. This was evident in the correction of papers with him, an unbelievable school of thought that soon became a legend. Spending the whole afternoon on a single paragraph whose message was not clear;

spending hours to explain the smallest experimental detail. Paul kept asking a wealth of questions, pretending he did not understand the data or the rationale behind the experiment. And you had to explain to him many times, until he eventually got satisfied. Although this was sometimes making the unfortunate fellow nervous, it was an incredibly precious exercise to dissect bugs in the data, and a unique learning experience to follow logic paths in research and link apparently distant findings in a unifying picture, that's to say intuition and creativity in science. During these writing sessions one also learned to appreciate Paul's humor and philanthropy. From time to time Paul took a break and told hilarious stories, often making fun of himself. Here is an example of the timeline of this Socratic "*Odissey*" for the poor fellow:

1. *Postdoc has the feeling at the lab seminar that his/her data are worth publishing;*
2. *Very proud postdoc prepares a comprehensive draft of the paper;*
3. *Very happy postdoc finally gets a date for meeting with Paul;*
4. *The collective reading of the draft starts;*
5. *Paul pretends not to understand rationale, methods, results and conclusions, asking the postdoc to explain to him in the finest details;*
6. *Point 5 goes over and over again. Postdoc is getting nervous;*
7. *Paul starts dismantling the draft, brick after brick, and starts recomposing it;*
8. *All of a sudden, the results, seen under a different perspective, can easily be explained by a very simple model;*
9. *Postdoc is very happy and thinks the session is over;*
10. *An exhausting refinement of the text starts. Hours and hours to discuss about the tense of a verb, the appropriateness of a noun, whether use "a" or "the", deleting unnecessary words, ... until the text is considered crystal clear and easily understandable.*

Time has passed by, and many of us have been successful in our respective countries. We are now (authentic) senior scientists over 60, with large labs and academic duties, but we continue to feel proud of being part of the Greengard School, a life changing and unforgettable experience that, as a spider canvas, connects all of us through time and space. Cantimori (1904–66), an Italian historian at the Scuola Normale Superiore in Pisa, said "*... a real mentor is the one who takes your mind in his hands and escorts you for a while.*" Paul was a real mentor, we would say a "*Maestro,*" who helped us to become what we are. We believe this is true for many, if not all, his past and present associates.

Conflict of interest statement

The authors have no conflicts of interest to declare.

References

Awizio, A. K., Onofri, F., Benfenati, F., & Bonaccurso, E. (2007). Influence of synapsin I on synaptic vesicles: An analysis by force-volume mode of the atomic force microscope and dynamic light scattering. *Biophysical Journal, 93*, 1051–1060.

Bähler, M., Benfenati, F., Valtorta, F., Czernik, A. J., & Greengard, P. (1989). Characterization of synapsin I fragments produced by cysteine-specific cleavage: A study of their interactions with F-actin. *The Journal of Cell Biology, 108*, 1841–1849.

Bähler, M., & Greengard, P. (1987). Synapsin I bundles F-actin in a phosphorylation-dependent manner. *Nature, 326*, 704–707.

Baldelli, P., Fassio, A., Valtorta, F., & Benfenati, F. (2007). Lack of synapsin I reduces the readily releasable pool of synaptic vesicles at central inhibitory synapses. *The Journal of Neuroscience, 27*, 13520–13531.

Benfenati, F., Bähler, M., Jahn, R., & Greengard, P. (1989). Interactions of synapsin I with small synaptic vesicles: Distinct sites in synapsin I bind to vesicle phospholipids and vesicle proteins. *The Journal of Cell Biology, 108*, 1863–1872.

Benfenati, F., Greengard, P., Brunner, J., & Bähler, M. (1989). Electrostatic and hydrophobic interactions of synapsin I and synapsin I fragments with phospholipid bilayers. *The Journal of Cell Biology, 108*, 1851–1862.

Benfenati, F., Valtorta, F., Chieregatti, E., & Greengard, P. (1992). Interaction of free and synaptic vesicle-bound synapsin I with F-actin. *Neuron, 8*, 377–386.

Benfenati, F., Valtorta, F., Rossi, M. C., Onofri, F., Sihra, T., & Greengard, P. (1993). Interactions of synapsin I with phospholipids: Possible role in synaptic vesicle clustering and in the maintenance of bilayer structures. *The Journal of Cell Biology, 123*, 1845–1855.

Benfenati, F., Valtorta, F., Rubenstein, J. L., Gorelick, F. S., Greengard, P., & Czernik, A. J. (1992). Synaptic vesicle-associated Ca2+/calmodulin-dependent protein kinase II is a binding protein for synapsin I. *Nature, 359*, 417–420.

Bonanomi, D., Fornasiero, E. F., Valdez, G., Halegoua, S., Benfenati, F., Menegon, A., et al. (2008). Identification of a developmentally regulated pathway of membrane retrieval in neuronal growth cones. *Journal of Cell Science, 121*, 3757–3769.

Bonanomi, D., Menegon, A., Miccio, A., Ferrari, G., Corradi, A., Kao, H. T., et al. (2005). Phosphorylation of synapsin I by cAMP-dependent protein kinase controls synaptic vesicle dynamics in developing neurons. *The Journal of Neuroscience, 25*, 7299–7308.

Ceccaldi, P. E., Grohovaz, F., Benfenati, F., Chieregatti, E., Greengard, P., & Valtorta, F. (1995). Dephosphorylated synapsin I anchors synaptic vesicles to actin cytoskeleton: An analysis by videomicroscopy. *The Journal of Cell Biology, 128*, 905–912.

Ceccarelli, B., Hurlbut, W. P., & Mauro, A. (1973). Turnover of transmitter and synaptic vesicles at the frog neuromuscular junction. *The Journal of Cell Biology, 57*, 499–524.

Cheetham, J. J., Hilfiker, S., Benfenati, F., Weber, T., Greengard, P., & Czernik, A. J. (2001). Identification of synapsin I peptides that insert into lipid membranes. *The Biochemical Journal, 354*(Pt. 1), 57–66.

Chieregatti, E., Gärtner, A., Stöffler, H. E., & Bähler, M. (1998). Myr 7 is a novel myosin IX-RhoGAP expressed in rat brain. *Journal of Cell Science, 111*, 3597–3608.

Corradi, A., Fadda, M., Piton, A., Patry, L., Marte, A., Rossi, P., et al. (2014). SYN2 is an autism predisposing gene: Loss-of-function mutations alter synaptic vesicle cycling and axon outgrowth. *Human Molecular Genetics, 23*, 90–103.

De Camilli, P., Benfenati, F., Valtorta, F., & Greengard, P. (1990). The synapsins. *Annual Review of Cell Biology, 6*, 433–460.

De Camilli, P., Harris, S. M., Jr., Huttner, W. B., & Greengard, P. (1983). Synapsin I (Protein I), a nerve terminal-specific phosphoprotein. II. Its specific association with synaptic vesicles demonstrated by immunocytochemistry in agarose-embedded synaptosomes. *The Journal of Cell Biology, 96*, 1355–1373.

De Robertis, E. D. P., & Bennett, H. L. (1955). Some features of the submicroscopic morphology of synapses in frog and earthworm. *The Journal of Biophysical and Biochemical Cytology*, *1*, 47–58.

Del Castillo, J., & Katz, B. (1954). Quantal components of the end-plate potential. *The Journal of Physiology*, *124*, 560–573.

Reinhard, J., Scheel, A. A., Diekmann, D., Hall, A., Ruppert, C., & Bähler, M. (1995). A novel type of myosin implicated in signalling by Rho family GTPases. *The EMBO Journal*, *14*, 697–704.

DiFrancesco, M. L., Lodola, F., Colombo, E., Maragliano, L., Bramini, M., Paternò, G. M., et al. (2020). Neuronal firing modulation by a membrane-targeted photoswitch. *Nature Nanotechnology*, *15*, 296–306.

Esser, L., Wang, C. R., Hosaka, M., Smagula, C. S., Südhof, T. C., & Deisenhofer, J. (1998). Synapsin I is structurally similar to ATP-utilizing enzymes. *The EMBO Journal*, *17*, 977–984.

Farisello, P., Boido, D., Nieus, T., Medrihan, L., Cesca, F., Valtorta, F., et al. (2013). Synaptic and extrasynaptic origin of the excitation/inhibition imbalance in the hippocampus of synapsin I/II/III knockout mice. *Cerebral Cortex*, *23*, 581–593.

Fassio, A., Patry, L., Congia, S., Onofri, F., Piton, A., Gauthier, J., et al. (2011). SYN1 loss-of-function mutations in autism and partial epilepsy cause impaired synaptic function. *Human Molecular Genetics*, *20*, 2297–2307.

Fesce, R., Benfenati, F., Greengard, P., & Valtorta, F. (1992). Effects of the neuronal phosphoprotein synapsin I on actin polymerization. II. Analytical interpretation of kinetic curves. *The Journal of Biological Chemistry*, *267*, 11289–11299.

Fesce, R., Grohovaz, F., Valtorta, F., & Meldolesi, J. (1994). Neurotransmitter release: Fusion or 'kiss-and-run'? *Trends in Cell Biology*, *4*, 1–4.

Forte, N., Binda, F., Contestabile, A., Benfenati, F., & Baldelli, P. (2020). Synapsin I synchronizes GABA release in distinct interneuron subpopulations. *Cerebral Cortex*, *30*, 1393–1406.

Fruscione, F., Valente, P., Sterlini, B., Romei, A., Baldassari, S., Fadda, M., et al. (2018). PRRT2 controls neuronal excitability by negatively modulating Na+ channel 1.2/1.6 activity. *Brain: A Journal of Neurology*, *141*, 1000–1016.

Gärtner, A., Fornasiero, E. F., Munck, S., Vennekens, K., Seuntjen, E., Huttner, W. B., et al. (2012). N-cadherin specifies first asymmetry in developing neurons. *The EMBO Journal*, *31*, 1893–1903.

Gärtner, A., Fornasiero, E. F., Valtorta, F., & Dotti, C. G. (2014). Distinct temporal hierarchies in membrane and cytoskeleton dynamics precede the morphological polarization of developing neurons. *Journal of Cell Science*, *127*, 4409–4419.

Ghezzi, D., Antognazza, M. R., Dal Maschio, M., Lanzarini, E., Benfenati, F., & Lanzani, G. (2011). A hybrid bioorganic interface for neuronal photoactivation. *Nature Communications*, *2*, 166.

Ghezzi, D., Antognazza, M. R., Maccarone, R., Bellani, S., Lanzarini, E., Martino, N., et al. (2013). A polymer optoelectronic interface restores light sensitivity in blind rat retinas. *Nature Photonics*, *7*, 400–406.

Guarnieri, F. C., Bellani, S., Yekhlef, L., Bergamaschi, A., Finardi, A., Fesce, R., et al. (2018). Synapsin I deletion reduces neuronal damage and ameliorates clinical progression of experimental autoimmune encephalomyelitis. *Brain, Behavior, and Immunity*, *68*, 197–210.

Hanley, P. J., Vollmer, V., & Bähler, M. (2020). Class IX myosins: Motorized RhoGAP signaling molecules. *Advance in Experimental Medicine and Biology*, *1239*, 381–389. https://doi.org/10.1007/978-3-030-38062-5_16.

Heuser, J. E., & Reese, T. S. (1973). Evidence for recycling of synaptic vesicle membrane during transmitter release at the frog neuromuscular junction. *The Journal of Cell Biology*, *57*, 315–344.

Huttner, W. B., Schiebler, W., Greengard, P., & De Camilli, P. (1983). Synapsin I (protein I), a nerve terminal-specific phosphoprotein. III. Its association with synaptic vesicles studied in a highly purified synaptic vesicle preparation. *The Journal of Cell Biology*, *96*, 1374–1388.

Jahn, R., Schiebler, W., & Greengard, P. (1984). A quantitative dot-immunobinding assay for proteins using nitrocellulose membrane filters. *Proceedings of the National Academy of Sciences of the United States of America*, *81*, 1684–1687.

Jahn, R., Schiebler, W., Ouimet, C., & Greengard, P. (1985). A 38,000-dalton membrane protein (p38) present in synaptic vesicles. *Proceedings of the National Academy of Sciences of the United States of America*, *82*, 4137–4141.

Krabben, L., Fassio, A., Bhatia, V. K., Pechstein, A., Onofri, F., Fadda, M., et al. (2011). Synapsin I senses membrane curvature by an amphipathic lipid packing sensor motif. *The Journal of Neuroscience*, *31*, 18149–18154.

Lignani, G., Raimondi, A., Ferrea, E., Rocchi, A., Paonessa, F., Cesca, F., et al. (2013). Epileptogenic Q555X SYN1 mutant triggers imbalances in release dynamics and short-term plasticity. *Human Molecular Genetics*, *22*, 2186–2199.

Maya-Vetencourt, J. F., Ghezzi, D., Antognazza, M. R., Colombo, E., Mete, M., Feyen, P., et al. (2017). A fully organic retinal prosthesis restores vision in a rat model of degenerative blindness. *Nature Materials*, *16*, 681–689.

Medrihan, L., Cesca, F., Raimondi, A., Lignani, G., Baldelli, P., & Benfenati, F. (2013). Synapsin II desynchronizes neurotransmitter release at inhibitory synapses by interacting with presynaptic calcium channels. *Nature Communications*, *4*, 1512.

Medrihan, L., Ferrea, E., Greco, B., Baldelli, P., & Benfenati, F. (2015). Asynchronous GABA release is a key determinant of tonic inhibition and controls neuronal excitability: A study in the synapsin II-/- mouse. *Cerebral Cortex*, *25*, 3356–3368.

Michetti, C., Caruso, A., Pagani, M., Sabbioni, M., Medrihan, L., David, G., et al. (2017). The knockout of synapsin II in mice impairs social behavior and functional connectivity generating an ASD-like phenotype. *Cerebral Cortex*, *27*, 5014–5023.

Michetti, C., Castroflorio, E., Marchionni, I., Forte, N., Sterlini, B., Binda, F., et al. (2017). The PRRT2 knockout mouse recapitulates the neurological diseases associated with PRRT2 mutations. *Neurobiology of Disease*, *99*, 66–83.

Milovanovic, D., Wu, Y., Bian, X., & De Camilli, P. (2018). A liquid phase of synapsin and lipid vesicles. *Science*, *361*, 604–607.

Monaldi, I., Vassalli, M., Bachi, A., Giovedì, S., Millo, E., Valtorta, F., et al. (2010). The highly conserved synapsin domain E mediates synapsin dimerization and phospholipid vesicle clustering. *The Biochemical Journal*, *426*, 55–64.

Nguyen, D. K., Rouleau, I., Sénéchal, G., Ansaldo, A. I., Gravel, M., Benfenati, F., et al. (2015). X-linked focal epilepsy with reflex bathing seizures: Characterization of a distinct epileptic syndrome. *Epilepsia*, *56*, 1098–1108.

Oeding, S. J., Majstrowicz, K., Hu, X. P., Schwarz, V., Freitag, A., Honnert, U., et al. (2018). Identification of Miro1 and Miro2 as mitochondrial receptors for myosin XIX. *Journal of Cell Science*, *131*, 219469.

Orlando, M., Lignani, G., Maragliano, L., Fassio, A., Onofri, F., Baldelli, P., et al. (2014). Functional role of ATP binding to synapsin I in synaptic vesicle trafficking and release dynamics. *Journal of Neuroscience*, *34*, 14752–14768.

Palay, S. L. (1956). Synapses in the central nervous system. *The Journal of Biophysical and Biochemical Cytology*, *2*, 193–202.

Paonessa, F., Criscuolo, S., Sacchetti, S., Amoroso, D., Scarongella, H., Pecoraro-Bisogni, F., et al. (2016). Regulation of neural gene transcription by optogenetic inhibition of the RE1-silencing transcription factor. *Proceedings of the National Academy of Sciences of the United States of America*, *113*, E91–100.

Pecoraro-Bisogni, F., Lignani, G., Contestabile, A., Castroflorio, E., Pozzi, D., Rocchi, A., et al. (2018). REST-dependent presynaptic homeostasis induced by chronic neuronal hyperactivity. *Molecular Neurobiology*, *55*, 4959–4972.

Pennuto, M., Bonanomi, D., Benfenati, F., & Valtorta, F. (2003). Synaptophysin I controls the targeting of VAMP2/synaptobrevin II to synaptic vesicles. *Molecular Biology of the Cell*, *14*, 4909–4919.

Pennuto, M., Dunlap, D., Contestabile, A., Benfenati, F., & Valtorta, F. (2002). Fluorescence resonance energy transfer detection of synaptophysin I and vesicle-associated membrane protein 2 interactions during exocytosis from single live synapses. *Molecular Biology of the Cell*, *13*, 2706–2717.

Pera, I., Stark, R., Kappl, M., Butt, H. J., & Benfenati, F. (2004). Using the atomic force microscope to study the interaction between two solid supported lipid bilayers and the influence of synapsin I. *Biophysical Journal*, *87*, 2446–2455.

Perlini, L. E., Szczurkowska, J., Ballif, B. A., Piccini, A., Sacchetti, S., Giovedì, S., et al. (2015). Synapsin III acts downstream of semaphorin 3A/CDK5 signaling to regulate radial migration and orientation of pyramidal neurons in vivo. *Cell Reports*, *11*, 234–248.

Piccini, A., Castroflorio, E., Valente, P., Guarnieri, F. C., Aprile, D., Michetti, C., et al. (2017). APache is an AP2-interacting protein involved in synaptic vesicle trafficking and neuronal development. *Cell Reports*, *21*, 3596–3611.

Pozzi, D., Lignani, G., Ferrea, E., Contestabile, A., Paonessa, F., D'Alessandro, R., et al. (2013). REST/NRSF-mediated intrinsic homeostasis protects neuronal networks from hyperexcitability. *The EMBO Journal*, *32*, 2994–3007.

Sassone, J., Serratto, G., Valtorta, F., Silani, V., Passafaro, M., & Ciammola, A. (2017). The synaptic function of Parkin. *Brain: A Journal of Neurology*, *140*, 2265–2272.

Schiavo, G., Benfenati, F., Poulain, B., Rossetto, O., Polverino de Laureto, P., DasGupta, B. R., et al. (1992). Tetanus and botulinum-B neurotoxins block neurotransmitter release by proteolytic cleavage of synaptobrevin. *Nature*, *359*, 832–835.

Schiavo, G., Poulain, B., Rossetto, O., Benfenati, F., Tauc, L., & Montecucco, C. (1992). Tetanus toxin is a zinc protein and its inhibition of neurotransmitter release and protease activity depend on zinc. *The EMBO Journal*, *11*, 3577–3583.

Schiavo, G., Santucci, A., Dasgupta, B. R., Mehta, P. P., Jontes, J., Benfenati, F., et al. (1993). Botulinum neurotoxins serotypes A and E cleave SNAP-25 at distinct COOH-terminal peptide bonds. *FEBS Letters*, *335*, 99–103.

Schiebler, W., Jahn, R., Doucet, J. P., Rothlein, J., & Greengard, P. (1986). Characterization of synapsin I binding to small synaptic vesicles. *The Journal of Biological Chemistry*, *261*, 8383–8390.

Söllner, T., Whiteheart, S. W., Brunner, M., Erdjument-Bromage, H., Geromanos, S., Tempst, P., et al. (1993). SNAP receptors implicated in vesicle targeting and fusion. *Nature*, *362*, 318–324.

Takamori, S., Holt, M., Stenius, K., Lemke, E. A., Grønborg, M., Riedel, D., et al. (2006). Molecular anatomy of a trafficking organelle. *Cell*, *127*, 831–846.

Torri Tarelli, F., Bossi, M., Fesce, R., Greengard, P., & Valtorta, F. (1992). Synapsin I partially dissociates from synaptic vesicles during exocytosis induced by electrical stimulation. *Neuron*, *9*, 1143–1153.

Torri Tarelli, F., Villa, A., Valtorta, F., De Camilli, P., Greengard, P., & Ceccarelli, B. (1990). Redistribution of synaptophysin and synapsin I during alpha-latrotoxin-induced release of neurotransmitter at the neuromuscular junction. *The Journal of Cell Biology*, *110*, 449–459.

Valente, P., Casagrande, S., Nieus, T., Verstegen, A. M., Valtorta, F., Benfenati, F., et al. (2012). Site-specific synapsin I phosphorylation participates in the expression of post-tetanic potentiation and its enhancement by BDNF. *The Journal of Neuroscience*, *32*, 5868–5879.

Valente, P., Castroflorio, E., Rossi, P., Fadda, M., Sterlini, B., Cervigni, R. I., et al. (2016). PRRT2 is a key component of the Ca(2+)-dependent neurotransmitter release machinery. *Cell Reports*, *15*, 117–131.

Valente, P., Romei, A., Fadda, M., Sterlini, B., Lonardoni, D., Forte, N., et al. (2019). Constitutive inactivation of the PRRT2 gene alters short-term synaptic plasticity and promotes network hyperexcitability in hippocampal neurons. *Cerebral Cortex*, *29*, 2010–2033.

Valtorta, F., Greengard, P., Fesce, R., Chieregatti, E., & Benfenati, F. (1992). Effects of the neuronal phosphoprotein synapsin I on actin polymerization. I. Evidence for a phosphorylation-dependent nucleating effect. *The Journal of Biological Chemistry*, *267*, 11281–11288.

Valtorta, F., Jahn, R., Fesce, R., Greengard, P., & Ceccarelli, B. (1988). Synaptophysin (p38) at the frog neuromuscular junction: Its incorporation into the axolemma and recycling after intense quantal secretion. *The Journal of Cell Biology*, *107*, 2717–2727.

Valtorta, F., Madeddu, L., Meldolesi, J., & Ceccarelli, B. (1984). Specific localization of the alpha-latrotoxin receptor in the nerve terminal plasma membrane. *The Journal of Cell Biology*, *99*, 124–132.

Valtorta, F., Meldolesi, J., & Fesce, R. (2001). Synaptic vesicles: Is kissing a matter of competence? *Trends in Cell Biology*, *11*, 324–328.

Verstegen, A. M., Tagliatti, E., Lignani, G., Marte, A., Stolero, T., Atias, M., et al. (2014). Phosphorylation of synapsin I by cyclin-dependent kinase-5 sets the ratio between the resting and recycling pools of synaptic vesicles at hippocampal synapses. *The Journal of Neuroscience*, *34*, 7266–7280.

CHAPTER THREE

cAMP-regulated phosphoproteins DARPP-32, ARPP16/19, and RCS modulate striatal signal transduction through protein kinases and phosphatases

Kyle R. Christensen and Angus C. Nairn*
Department of Psychiatry, Yale University, School of Medicine, New Haven, CT, United States
*Corresponding author: e-mail address: angus.nairn@yale.edu

Contents

Abstract

Decades of research led by Paul Greengard identified protein phosphorylation as a ubiquitous and vital post-translational modification involved in many neuronal signaling pathways. In particular, his discovery that second messenger-regulated protein phosphorylation plays a central role in the propagation and transduction of signals in the nervous system has been essential in understanding the molecular mechanisms of neuronal communication. The establishment of dopamine (DA) as an essential neurotransmitter in the central nervous system, combined with observations that DA activates G-protein-coupled receptors to control the production of cyclic adenosine monophosphate (cAMP) in postsynaptic neurons, has provided fundamental insight into the regulation of neurotransmission. Notably, DA signaling in the striatum is involved in many neurological functions such as control of locomotion, reward, addiction, and learning, among others. This review focuses on the history, characterization, and function of cAMP-mediated regulation of serine/threonine protein phosphatases and their

Advances in Pharmacology, Volume 90
ISSN 1054-3589
https://doi.org/10.1016/bs.apha.2020.09.005

role in DA-mediated signaling in striatal neurons. Several small, heat- and acid-stable proteins, including DARPP-32, RCS, and ARPP-16/19, were discovered by the Greengard laboratory to be regulated by DA- and cAMP signaling, and found to undergo a complex but coordinated sequence of phosphorylation and dephosphorylation events. These studies have contributed significantly to the establishment of protein phosphorylation as a ubiquitous and vital process in signal propagation in neurons, paradigm shifting discoveries at the time. Understanding DA-mediated signaling in the context of signal propagation has led to numerous insights into human conditions and the development of treatments and therapies.

Abbreviations

AC	adenylyl cyclase
ARPP-16/19/21	cAMP-regulated phosphoprotein, 16/19/21 kiloDaltons
CaM	calmodulin
cAMP	cyclic adenosine monophosphate
Cdk1	cyclin-dependent kinase 1
CK	casein kinase
CNS	central nervous system
DA	dopamine
DARPP-32	dopamine- and cAMP-regulated phosphoprotein, 32 kiloDaltons
ENSA	α-endosulfine
GABA	γ-aminobutyric acid
Gwl	greatwall kinase
I-1	inhibitor-1
MAST	microtubule-associated serine/threonine kinase
MSN	medium spiny neuron
PKA	cAMP-dependent protein kinase
PP1	protein phosphatase 1
PP2A	protein phosphatase 2A
protein phosphatase 2ARCS	regulator of calmodulin signaling

1. Introduction

The human brain has popularly been called "the most complex object in the known universe" due to its estimated 86 billion neurons, each of which on average communicates with 1000 other neurons (Azevedo et al., 2009; Greengard, 2001). Communication between neurons is essential for our perception of the world and how we interact with it. Neurons communicate through synapses, which are classified into two types: the electrical gap junction where ions diffuse from one neuron to the next in a bidirectional manner, and in mammals the much more common chemical synapse where neurotransmitters are released into the synaptic cleft and interact with receptors on the postsynaptic neuron (Connors & Long, 2004; Farsad & De Camilli, 2002). Two categories of chemical transmission exist, fast and slow. In fast synaptic transmission, neurotransmitters bind to ion channel receptors present on the surface of the postsynaptic membrane, resulting in a conformational change where the channel opens and allows a flux of specific ions across the membrane. Both excitatory and inhibitory signals propagate through fast synaptic transmission, most commonly through the action of glutamate and γ-aminobutyric acid (GABA) respectively (Greengard, 2001; Hendry, Schwark, Jones, & Yan, 1987; Watkins, 2000). In contrast, as elucidated by Paul Greengard, slow synaptic transmission transduces signals relayed from presynaptic neurotransmitter release and subsequent binding to receptors via metabotropic second messenger systems. The discovery of these second messengers and their ability to modulate numerous aspects of neuronal physiology proved to be a paradigm shift in the history of neuroscience.

The work performed by Paul Greengard and his colleagues and trainees in the central nervous system (CNS) built on studies that investigated hormone signaling in liver and muscle cells (Graves & Krebs, 1999; Greengard, 2001; Sutherland, 1972). In the 1950s, Sutherland and colleagues discovered cyclic adenosine monophosphate (cAMP) synthesis increased in response to epinephrine and glucagon during the activation of glycogenolysis (Berthet, Rall, & Sutherland, 1957; Sutherland & Rall, 1958). This led to the discovery by Krebs and Fisher that cAMP activates a protein kinase in skeletal muscle tissue, and that activity of this kinase was essential for epinephrine to stimulate glycogenolysis (Walsh, Perkins, & Krebs, 1968). As a result, it was hypothesized by Paul Greengard that a similar signaling mechanism through the regulation of protein kinases and phosphorylation of substrates could influence and control diverse physiological effects in neurons. Early experiments investigating this phenomenon in the rabbit superior cervical sympathetic ganglion discovered that stimulation of the preganglionic fibers caused a several-fold increase in cAMP concentration in the ganglion (Kebabian & Calne, 1979; Kebabian & Greengard, 1971). Conversely, stimulation of the postganglionic fibers had no effect. It was therefore proposed that synaptic transmission within the ganglion resulted in the observed increase in cAMP, presumably in the postsynaptic neurons (McAfee, Schorderet, & Greengard, 1971).

Follow-up studies investigated the mechanism by which postsynaptic cAMP levels could be regulated. Through the 1970s, numerous studies found evidence that many actions of cAMP involved regulation of protein kinase activity (Greengard, 1978; Kuo & Greengard, 1969). Similar to the findings of Sutherland and colleagues, stimulation of ganglion neurons by dopamine (DA) resulted in an increase of cAMP concentration in the postsynaptic cell through the action of adenylyl cyclase (AC) (Kebabian & Greengard, 1971). This was the first description of a neurotransmitter-sensitive ACAC in the nervous system. The discovery of the same cAMP-dependent protein kinase (i.e. protein kinase A or PKA) in brain tissue (Miyamoto, Kuo, & Greengard, 1969), originally described in rabbit skeletal muscle (Walsh et al., 1968), although at much higher levels, led to the conclusion that cAMP, AC, and PKA constituted a signaling cascade essential for transducing information in slow synaptic transmission (Greengard, 1978, 2001). Additionally, PKA has the highest specific activity in cytosolic and synaptosomal fractions (Walter, Kanof, Schulman, & Greengard, 1978), and is enriched in synaptic structures (Kelly, Cotman, & Largen, 1979; Ueda et al., 1979; Weller & Morgan, 1976). Taken together, these results suggested an integral role for cAMP and PKA signaling in synaptic transmission (Maeno, Johnson, & Greengard, 1971).

Over the past several decades, the complexities of the control of protein phosphorylation became appreciated and understood to be a ubiquitous and vital process involved in numerous physiological functions and cell types (Leslie & Nairn, 2019; Nairn, Hemmings, & Greengard, 1985; Nestler, Walaas, & Greengard, 1984; Walaas, Hemmings, Greengard, & Nairn, 2011). However, despite many important studies, much work remains to be done to fully understand the molecular details of the roles of protein phosphorylation in intracellular mechanisms of communication. Due to the rapid and reversible nature of phosphorylation through the action of kinases and phosphatases, it is paramount that the proper balance of these modifications is maintained to ensure optimal function and health in living cells and organisms. In this review, we focus on the history and importance of three major kinase/phosphatase signaling pathways in the CNS in the context of DA signaling.

2. Dopamine signaling in the basal ganglia: A brief overview

The basal ganglia in primates is a collection of subcortical nuclei with important roles in regulating motor function and reward learning.

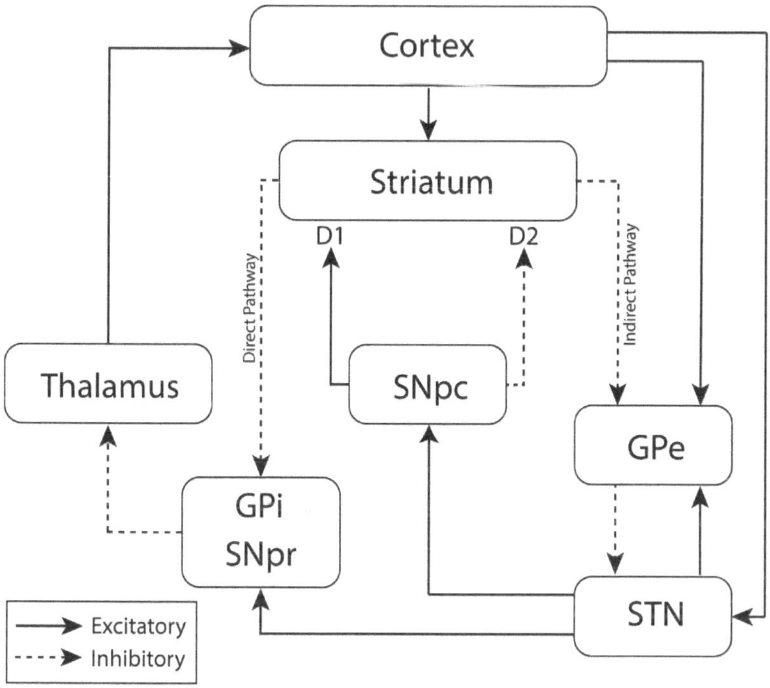

Fig. 1 Schematic of basal ganglia circuitry. The healthy adult brain shows a balance of excitatory and inhibitory innervation throughout the basal ganglia system. Solid lines represent excitatory efferents and dashed lines represent inhibitory efferents. Abbreviations: GPe, globus pallidus external segment; GPi, globus pallidus internal segment; SNpc, substantia nigra pars compacta; SNpr, substantia nigra pars reticulata; STN, subthalamic nucleus.

Composed of the striatum (consisting of the putamen, caudate, and nucleus accumbens), subthalamic nucleus, globus pallidus, ventral pallidum, and substantia nigra, the basal ganglia relay and integrate signals from around the brain (Fig. 1), the anatomy and circuitry of which has been well studied and reviewed elsewhere (Bostan, Dum, & Strick, 2018; Quartarone et al., 2020; Walaas et al., 2011). DA is the major modulatory neurotransmitter regulating basal ganglia circuits. DA fibers originating in the substantia nigra pars compacta (SNpc) innervate the striatum by terminating on medium spiny neurons (MSN), which compose an estimated 95% of total neurons there (Andén, Fuxe, Hamberger, & Hökfelt, 1966; Björklund & Dunnett, 2007). Seminal studies demonstrated the presence of DA receptors enriched in the striatum capable of producing high levels of cAMP when stimulated by DA, presumably from the presynaptic neuron (Clement-Cormier, Kebabian, Petzold, & Greengard, 1974; Kebabian & Greengard, 1971; (Kebabian & Calne, 1979; Kebabian, Petzold, & Greengard, 1972).

The specific effect of DA on the postsynaptic neuron depends on which DA receptor is expressed. Two main subtypes of DA receptors have been extensively characterized in the striatum, termed D1 and D2. In conjunction with excitatory cortical glutamatergic input, DA stimulates MSNs expressing D1 receptors (the "direct pathway") but inhibits MSNs expressing D2 receptors (the "indirect pathway") (Redgrave et al., 2010). Balance between these two DA signaling pathways allows for coordinated and smooth movements, and dysfunction and unbalanced DA basal ganglia signaling is linked to Parkinson's disease, schizophrenia, drug abuse, and other psychiatric conditions (Carlsson, 2001). Additionally, cortical efferents from motor-related areas innervate the STN directly (the "hyperdirect pathway") (Nambu et al., 2000). The discovery and functional characterization of this third pathway in non-human primates and humans led to a new proposed model of basal ganglia circuitry and information processing (Brunenberg et al., 2012; Nambu, 2004). This new model proposes three steps of motor signal processing where cortical inputs are processed through the STN via the hyperdirect pathway, followed by the direct pathway and finally the indirect pathway. The direct pathway facilitates movements by disinhibiting the thalamus whereas the hyperdirect and indirect pathways prevent movements by increasing thalamic inhibition. (Nambu, Tokuno, & Takada, 2002; Sano, Chiken, Hikida, Kobayashi, & Nambu, 2013).

Striatal interneurons also play a key role in DA signaling. Four types of these interneurons are well characterized: cholinergic, fast-spiking, calretinin-expressing, and persistent and low threshold spiking, with other types continuously being investigated (Zhai, Tanimura, Graves, Shen, & Surmeier, 2018). These interneurons modulate MSN activity through GABAergic innervation (Straub et al., 2016). Additionally, all striatal interneurons express various combinations of DA receptors, adding increased complexity in DA and striatal signaling (Clarke & Adermark, 2015). However, the relatively simple and well-understood role of MSN function within the anatomical circuity of the basal ganglia, combined with DA's implication in several areas of human health and disease, provided for an ideal focus of investigation of the biochemical signaling mechanisms involved in neural transmission and transduction (Greengard, 2001). Importantly, in MSNs both types of DA receptors regulate AC activity through G proteins. D1 stimulates AC activity through $G\alpha_s$ while D2 receptors decrease AC activity through $G\alpha_i$ (Beaulieu & Gainetdinov, 2011; Enjalbert & Bockaert, 1983; Kebabian & Calne, 1979).

3. Identification and characterization of brain region-specific phosphoproteins

Differential regulation of direct and indirect MSNs by DA and cAMP has major implications for the directional control of cAMP/PKA signaling mediated by a complex network of protein phosphorylation and dephosphorylation. However, biochemical appreciation of such bidirectional control was limited by the intermingled nature of different sub-types of MSNs. Indeed, in the late 1970s, studies of neuronal phosphoproteins were largely done at a whole brain level. For example, these types of experiments led to the discovery of the synapsins, a phosphoprotein family widely distributed in the CNS that plays an essential role of regulating the docking and release of synaptic vesicles and neurotransmitters into the synaptic cleft (De Camilli, Benfenati, Valtorta, & Greengard, 1990; Greengard, Valtorta, Czernik, & Benfenati, 1993). Building on this work, and extension of the technique for identifying phosphoproteins through studies of second messenger-mediated phosphorylation using γ-^{32}P-ATP and autoradiography to visualize phosphorylated proteins on SDS-PAGE gels, studies in the Greengard laboratory systematically identified many brain region- and neuron-specific phosphoproteins (Aswad & Greengard, 1981a, 1981b; Walaas, Aswad, & Greengard, 1983; Walaas & Greengard, 1984; Walaas, Nairn, & Greengard, 1983a, 1983b). These included three cAMP/PKA-regulated phosphoproteins that were enriched in striatum and named by their apparent molecular weight as ^{32}P-labeled proteins, namely 32 kDa (now termed DARPP-32), 21 kDa (ARPP-21; now termed Regulator of Calmodulin Signaling, or RCS), and 16 kDa (now termed ARPP-16). Subsequent purification from striatal homogenates that made use of the stability of the three proteins to acidic pH, followed by several sequential chromatography steps (Hemmings & Greengard, 1989; Hemmings, Nairn, Aswad, & Greengard, 1984; Horiuchi, Williams, Kurihara, Nairn, & Greengard, 1990), led to the discoveries that each regulated, either directly or indirectly, three of the four major types of serine/threonine protein phosphatases (Hemmings, Greengard, Tung, & Cohen, 1984; Hemmings, Nairn, Aswad, & Greengard, 1984; Horiuchi et al., 1990; Walaas, Aswad, & Greengard, 1983). The molecular roles of DARPP-32, RCS, and ARPP-16 will be briefly reviewed.

4. PKA phosphorylates DARPP-32 and inhibits PP1 in striatal neurons

The discovery of DARPP-32 in the early 1980s and its continued characterization over the last ~40 years has provided great insight into DA signaling in striatal MSNs. DARPP-32 was identified as an ~200 amino acid, heat-, and acid-stable protein that is phosphorylated by PKA at Thr34 (Hemmings, Nairn, Aswad, & Greengard, 1984; Hemmings, Nairn, & Greengard, 1984; Ouimet, Miller, Hemmings, Walaas, & Greengard, 1984; Walaas, Aswad, & Greengard, 1983; (Walaas & Greengard, 1984). DARPP-32 is highly expressed in all types of MSNs irrespective of DA receptor sub-type (Beaulieu & Gainetdinov, 2011; (Walaas & Greengard, 1984). Within MSNs, DARPP-32 is a cytosolic protein displaying prominent immunoreactivity throughout the somatodendritic compartment (Glausier et al., 2010; Ouimet & Greengard, 1990; Ouimet, Langley-Gullion, & Greengard, 1998; Ouimet et al., 1984), but also shuttles in and out of the cell nucleus (Stipanovich et al., 2008). In regions innervated by MSNs, DARPP-32 is strongly immunoreactive in nerve terminals (Walaas & Ouimet, 1989). Other brain regions such as layer VI of the cortex and the cerebellum show weaker immunoreactivity for DARPP-32 (Berger, Febvret, Greengard, & Goldman-Rakic, 1990; Ouimet, LaMantia, Goldman-Rakic, Rakic, & Greengard, 1992), as well as several non-neuronal tissues with varying effects on downstream targets (Walaas et al., 2011).

Studies into the biochemistry of DARPP-32 revealed strong similarities in structure and function to inhibitor-1 (I-1), a known potent inhibitor of protein phosphatase 1 (PP1). Both DARPP-32 and I-1 share a conserved domain in their respective N-terminus that is phosphorylated by PKA (Thr34 in DARPP-32 and Thr35 in I-1). This phosphorylation event allows DARPP-32 and I-1 to bind PP1 as a pseudosubstrate, thereby inhibiting PP1 by physically blocking the active site (Leslie & Nairn, 2019); Nairn et al., 2004; Svenningsson, Nairn, & Greengard, 2005; Svenningsson et al., 2004). PP1 is a highly conserved serine/threonine protein phosphatase abundant in all eukaryotic organisms (Cohen, 2002; Gibbons, Kozubowski, Tatchell, & Shenolikar, 2007). Four isoforms of PP1 (α, β, γ1, and γ2) exist in mammals encoded by three genes (*PPP1CA, PPP1CB,* and *PPP1CC)* with alternative splicing occurring to yield γ1 and γ2, with γ1 being most prevalent in the CNS (da Cruz e Silva et al., 1995; Kitagawa et al., 1990; Ouimet, da Cruz e Silva, & Greengard, 1995; Shima et al., 1993).

The primary structure across each isoform is more than ~85% conserved, with the most variable regions existing at the N- and C- termini (Fardilha, Esteves, Korrodi-Gregório, da Cruz e Silva, & da Cruz e Silva, 2010). Since these isoforms are localized to different subcellular compartments and exhibit different functions regarding interacting partners, it is reasonable to hypothesize that these variable termini dictate different functions of the isoforms. Related, PP1α and γ1 isoforms display strong immunoreactivity in striatal neurons, with high enrichment in dendritic spines, implying an important role in postsynaptic signal transduction (da Cruz e Silva et al., 1995; Ouimet et al., 1995).

PP1 possesses a vast interactome, estimated to contain over 200 protein interacting partners, with more continuing to be found (Korrodi-Gregório, Esteves, & Fardilha, 2014). Proteins bind to PP1 through several interaction motifs; DARPP-32 and I-1 utilize two such domains. First, most proteins that interact with PP1 contain a short sequence of ~6 amino acids called the RVxF motif that associates via charged and hydrophobic interactions with a docking site on the surface of PP1 located away from the catalytic site (Egloff et al., 1997; Goldberg et al., 1995; Kwon et al., 1997). The RVxF motif follows the general sequence of [K/R][K/R][V/I][x][F/W], where X is any residue except phenylalanine, isoleucine, methionine, tyrosine, proline, or aspartic acid, however, not all interacting partners conform exactly to this formula (Bollen, Peti, Ragusa, & Beullens, 2010; Hendrickx et al., 2009; Meiselbach, Sticht, & Enz, 2006; Wakula, Beullens, Ceulemans, Stalmans, & Bollen, 2003). For example, the RVxF motif located at amino acids 6-11 in DARPP-32 is RKKIQF (Kwon et al., 1997). The second interaction domain in DARPP-32 and I-1 includes the region around the PKA phosphorylation site (Thr34 or Thr35, respectively). Once docked via the RVxF motif, DARPP-32 wraps around the surface of PP1 and likely follows a groove of acid side chains to the active site (Goldberg et al., 1995). Phosphorylated Thr34 is likely to position itself in the catalytic site as if it were a substrate, thereby preventing PP1 from dephosphorylating other proteins (Hemmings, Nairn, Aswad, & Greengard, 1984; Huang et al., 1999). Interestingly, DARPP-32 that is dephosphorylated at Thr34 can still interact with PP1 at the RVxF site, but this interaction does not inhibit PP1. Therefore, the combination of RVxF docking and Thr34 phosphorylation is required for the regulatory function of DARPP-32 as a potent PP1 inhibitor (Desdouits et al., 1995; Huang et al., 1999).

While the PP1 inhibitory function of DARPP-32 is well known and characterized, and believed to be its primary role, the cellular environmental

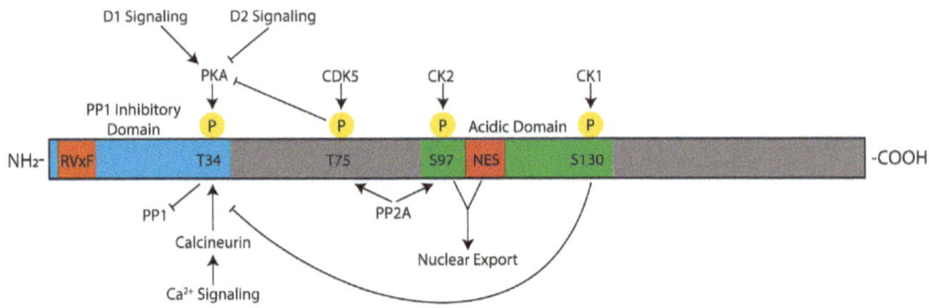

Fig. 2 DARPP-32 phosphorylation occurs at several residues with various effects on DA signaling. DA signaling through the D1 receptor activates PKA, whereas D2 receptor signaling inhibits PKA. PKA phosphorylates Thr34, leading to potent inhibition of PP1. Activation of calcineurin through Ca^{2+} signaling dephosphorylates Thr34. CDK5 phosphorylates Thr75, resulting in inhibition of PKA. Phosphorylation of Ser97 by CK2 reveals a nuclear export sequence (NES), facilitating the export of DARPP-32 to the cytoplasm. Both Thr75 and Ser97 can be dephosphorylated by PP2A-B56δ. Ser130 is phosphorylated by CK1 and prevents calcineurin-mediated dephosphorylation of Thr34.

context in which DARPP-32 exists also determines its downstream effects (Fig. 2). Phosphorylation of Thr34 and three other residues on DARPP-32 (Thr75, Ser97, and Ser130 in rat DARPP-32) modulate changes in the function, sub-cellular localization, and interacting partners (Engmann et al., 2015; Walaas et al., 2011). The interplay between these sites is thus crucial in the regulation of DARPP-32 and integration of signaling stimuli.

DARPP-32 inhibits PKA when phosphorylated at Thr75 by Cdk5. Cdk5 is basally active; therefore Thr75 is basally phosphorylated and a subset of PKA inhibited (Bibb et al., 1999). Through DA-mediated activation of D1 receptors, Thr75 phosphorylation is reduced through a cAMP/PKA/PP2A-B56δ pathway (Nishi et al., 2000). As a result, PKA is disinhibited and this contributes to greater phosphorylation of Thr34 and inhibition of PP1 signaling. Additionally, Ser97 and Ser130 of DARPP-32 are phosphorylated to a high level *in vivo* by casein kinase (CK) 2 and CK1, respectively (Desdouits et al., 1995; Girault, Hemmings, Williams, Nairn, & Greengard, 1989). Phosphorylation/dephosphorylation of Ser97 regulates shutting of DARPP-32 between the cytoplasm and nucleus. Phosphorylation of Ser97 promotes export into the cytoplasm in conjunction with a strong nuclear export motif, whereas dephosphorylation by PP2A-B56δ promotes the nuclear accumulation of DARPP-32 (Girault, 2012; Stipanovich et al., 2008). Nuclear DARPP-32 is involved in regulation of epigenetic pathways, and can promote the inhibition of nuclear

PP1, the phosphorylation of Histone H3, and transcriptional activation (Stipanovich et al., 2008). Ser130 phosphorylation protects Thr34 from being dephosphorylated by calcineurin (PP2B), a phosphatase activated via Ca^{2+} ion influx through NMDA and AMPA receptors as a result of glutamate signaling (Hemmings, Nairn, Aswad, & Greengard, 1984; King et al., 1984; Nishi, Snyder, & Greengard, 1997; Nishi et al., 2005).

This complicated ensemble of kinases and phosphatases acting on DARPP-32 implies a converging and modulatory function of DARPP-32 on several signaling cascades from neurotransmitter receptors to translational changes. Many studies employing a variety of model systems, including *in vitro* biochemistry experiments, DARPP-32 knockout mice, and DARPP-32 "knock-in" mice that express mutant forms of the four phosphorylation sites, have together provided extensive evidence that regulation of DARPP-32 by DA in conjunction with other neurotransmitter inputs results in long-term changes in neuronal function, plasticity, and behavior (Bertran-Gonzalez et al., 2009; Borgkvist, Usiello, Greengard, & Fisone, 2007; Fienberg et al., 1998; Stipanovich et al., 2008; Svenningsson et al., 2003, 2004, 2005; Valjent et al., 2005; Zachariou et al., 2006; Zhang et al., 2006). Therefore, one central tenet of DARPP-32-dependent signaling in direct pathway MSNs is to amplify DA/cAMP/PKA through D1 receptors. However, DARPP-32 phosphorylation at multiple sites allows it to integrate DA signaling with signaling by other neurotransmitters such as glutamate acting at NMDA and AMPA ionotropic receptors or metabotropic receptors in MSNs (Girault, 2012; Greengard, 2001). Moreover, these regulatory signaling pathways can function in reverse via D2 receptors and inhibition of cAMP/PKA in indirect MSNs, thus playing a critical role in the balanced output of the striatum as part of the basal ganglia.

This concept was demonstrated using transgenic mice expressing two tagged versions of DARPP-32: FLAG tagged DARPP-32 under the control of the D1R promoter and Myc-tagged DARPP-32 under the control of the D2R promoter (Bateup et al., 2008). These two forms express in D1 MSNs and D2 MSNs respectively without overlapping. Mice were exposed to acute cocaine treatment to block the DA transporter, thereby increasing DA signaling. D1 MSNs showed increased Thr34 phosphorylation and decreased Thr75 phosphorylation, whereas the opposite pattern presented in D2 MSNs (decreased Thr34 phosphorylation and increased Thr75 phosphorylation) (Bateup et al., 2008). Further experiments knocking out DARPP-32 selectively in D1 or D2 MSNs resulted in a similar observation of opposite effects. Mice with DARPP-32 knocked out in D1 MSNs displayed decreased locomotor activity and dyskinetic behaviors at baseline and when acutely treated with cocaine or L-DOPA, a common pharmacological therapy to treat Parkinson's disease. Mice with DARPP-32 knocked out in D2 MSNs showed the opposite, namely an increase in locomotor activity (Bateup et al., 2010). Taken together these studies illustrate the important biochemical differences between DARPP-32 regulation in D1 and D2 MSN populations and their roles in maintaining a balance between excitatory and inhibitory signaling in the striatum.

5. RCS function is mediated through PKA phosphorylation

RCS, also known as ARPP-21, is similar to DARPP-32 and ARPP-16 in that it is a small acid- and heat-stable protein that can be phosphorylated by PKA (Hemmings & Greengard, 1989). Analysis of the amino acid sequence of RCS revealed it to be acidic and unlikely to form secondary structure; therefore it is considered an intrinsically disordered protein like DARPP-32 and ARPP-16 (Williams, Hemmings, LoPresti, & Greengard, 1989). Immunohistochemistry studies showed RCS to be highly enriched in MSNs located in the striatum and nucleus accumbens, with a more moderate expression in the amygdala, indicating a probable role in regulation of DA signaling in postsynaptic neurons (Brene et al., 1994; Ouimet, Hemmings, & Greengard, 1989). Two phosphorylation sites exist in RCS. The most extensively studied phospho-site is Ser55, which is phosphorylated by PKA in response to activation of D1 receptors, and dephosphorylated via activation of D2 receptors (Caporaso et al., 2000; Hemmings & Greengard, 1989; Tsou, Girault, & Greengard, 1993). Treating mice with cocaine or methamphetamine also increases Ser55 phosphorylation (Caporaso et al., 2000). *In vitro*, dephosphorylation occurs through the action of both PP1 and PP2A, however, studies with DARPP-32 knockout mice suggest PP2A is the main RCS phosphatase *in vivo* (Caporaso et al., 2000; (Hemmings & Greengard, 1989)). The second phosphorylation site, Ser32, was recently identified using top-down proteomics in several mice strains (Davis et al., 2018). However, to date no studies have been performed investigating the function of Ser32 phosphorylation, which kinases and phosphatases act on Ser32, or whether it even is observed in humans.

Calmodulin (CaM), the namesake of RCS, is a ubiquitous Ca^{2+}-binding protein that regulates many proteins in a reversible manner through protein-protein interactions. Upon Ca^{2+} binding, CaM acts as a primary effector for

Ca^{2+} signaling (Chin & Means, 2000; Sharma & Parameswaran, 2018). RCS influences CaM's ability to interact with downstream targets by directly binding CaM (Rakhilin et al., 2004). Phosphorylation at Ser55 of RCS by PKA increases the binding affinity of RCS for CaM, resulting in sequestration of CaM and subsequent inhibition of, for example, calcineurin and CaM kinase I, a CaM-dependent protein phosphatase and protein kinase, respectively (Walaas et al., 2011). This RCS pathway and the DARPP-32 pathway described above converge through calcineurin activity, as calcineurin dephosphorylates Thr34 of DARPP-32. This interplay was confirmed by infusing striatal slices with D2-receptor agonists, leading to activation of calcineurin and dephosphorylation of Thr34 (Nishi, Snyder, Nairn, & Greengard, 1999). Additionally, treating striatal neurons from RCS knockout mice with the D2-receptor agonist quinpirole resulted in greater DARPP-32 Thr34 dephosphorylation when compared to striatal neurons from wild-type mice (Rakhilin et al., 2004). Therefore, increased RCS signaling leads to an increase of Thr34 DARPP-32 phosphorylation and inhibition of PP1, essentially amplifying D1-receptor signaling (Walaas et al., 2011).

6. The ARPP-16/19 family of phosphoproteins modulates PP2A activity in a cAMP-dependent manner

ARPP-16 and ARPP-19 (cAMP-regulated phosphoprotein, 16 and 19 kDa respectively) were discovered as acid-soluble PKA substrates in striatum shortly after DARPP-32 and RCS, and continue to be actively researched and characterized in numerous contexts (Andrade et al., 2017; Dulubova et al., 2001; Horiuchi et al., 1990; Leslie & Nairn, 2019; Musante et al., 2017). A related phosphoprotein, α-endosulfine (ENSA), was also discovered to contain a similar structure, amino acid sequence, and phosphorylation pattern as ARPP-16/19 (Dulubova et al., 2001; Heron et al., 1998). ARPP-16 and ARPP-19 arise from alternative splicing of the same gene (*ARPP19*) (Horiuchi et al., 1990) whereas ENSA is produced from a different gene (*ENSA*) (Peyrollier, Héron, Virsolvy-Vergine, Le Cam, & Bataille, 1996). The amino acid sequences of these proteins are remarkably similar; ARPP-19 contains 16 additional residues at its N-terminus than ARPP-16, whereas ENSA has a distinct N-terminus from ARPP-19 (Heron et al., 1998; Horiuchi et al., 1990). Additionally, these proteins are highly conserved across species, indicating an important evolutionary role in protein function (Dulubova et al., 2001). The expression patterns of the three phosphoproteins differs. ARPP-16 is solely expressed in the brain, with high enrichment in striatal MSNs but also expressed in forebrain structures (Brene et al., 1994; Girault, Horiuchi, Gustafson, Rosen, & Greengard, 1990). ARPP-19 is expressed throughout the body with a relatively low expression in the striatum (Dulubova et al., 2001). ENSA is more highly expressed in the striatum than ARPP-19 and is also found in other brain regions (Horiuchi et al., 1990).

A breakthrough in elucidating the function of the ARPP-16/19-related proteins resulted from studies of mitosis in *Xenopus* oocytes. Two groups independently found a critical role for ARPP-19 and ENSA in regulating the G2/M phase of the cell cycle (Gharbi-Ayachi et al., 2010; Mochida, Maslen, Skehel, & Hunt, 2010). These groups were searching for substrates of Greatwall kinase (Gwl), which was already established as a potential link between cyclin-dependent kinase 1 (Cdk1), a key regulatory protein of the cell cycle, and the inhibition of protein phosphatase 2A (PP2A), a ubiquitous protein phosphatase (Virshup & Kaldis, 2010). The two groups found that either ARPP-19 or ENSA were major targets of Gwl, and found that phosphorylation resulted in potent inhibition of PP2A (Gharbi-Ayachi et al., 2010; Mochida et al., 2010). Gwl phosphorylates Ser62 in ARPP-19 and ENSA (Ser46 in ARPP-16) located in a central, conserved amino acid sequence, KYFDSGDY. This phosphorylation event promotes the binding of ARPP-19/ENSA to PP2A, resulting in phosphatase inhibition (Gharbi-Ayachi et al., 2010; Mochida et al., 2010). Experiments in several model systems including *Drosophila melanogaster* and mammalian cell lines expanded these findings and conclusions of ARPP-19/ENSA function to the human cellular environment (Álvarez-Fernández et al., 2013; Burgess et al., 2010; Gharbi-Ayachi et al., 2010; Yu et al., 2004).

PP2A exists as a heterotrimer of an A scaffolding subunit, a catalytic C subunit, and a variable regulatory interacting B subunit (Janssens & Goris, 2001). The B subunits have a high degree of diversity, including four families with multiple isoforms, but only one can exist per heterotrimer complex (Mayer-Jaekel & Hemmings, 1994). Moreover, the B subunit subtype is thought to be responsible for directing intracellular localization and substrate specificity (Virshup & Shenolikar, 2009). PP2A-mediated dephosphorylation of substrates is a central process in numerous physiological pathways, and deficits of PP2A activity is linked with several human diseases including Alzheimer's disease, epilepsy, and cancer (Reynhout et al., 2019; Sangodkar et al., 2016; Sontag & Sontag, 2014). Subsequent studies of ARPP-16 have found that the efficacy of PP2A inhibition depends on the specific B subunit found in the heterotrimer. The mammalian homolog of Gwl is microtubule-associated serine/threonine protein kinase-like (MASTL) and is also important for regulating mitosis and the cell cycle (Voets & Wolthuis, 2010). In post-mitotic striatal neurons, experiments utilizing ARPP-16, the dominant ARPP-related protein in the striatum, identified the scaffolding A subunit of PP2A as an interacting partner, a result validated using recombinant proteins (Andrade et al., 2017). This led to the hypothesis that phosphorylation of ARPP-16 at the conserved Ser46 position is important for PP2A binding and inhibition. MAST3, the most abundant MAST kinase isoform related to MASTL and Gwl in the striatum (Garland, Quraishe, French, & O'Connor, 2008), phosphorylates ARPP-16 at Ser46 resulting in inhibition of PP2A complexes containing the Bα or B56δ subunits. Additionally, MAST3 is basally active and ARPP-16 is phosphorylated to a high stoichiometry in the striatum, suggesting that a significant fraction of PP2A is basally inhibited (Andrade et al., 2017).

As discussed earlier, postsynaptic DA signaling in MSNs leads to an increase in cAMP concentration and PKA activation. PKA phosphorylates both PP2A and the ARPP-related proteins, resulting in different downstream effects. PKA phosphorylates PP2A holoenzymes containing the B56δ subunit at multiple sites, with phosphorylation at Ser566 leading to activation of PP2A-B56δ (Ahn et al., 2007; Usui et al., 1998). Therefore, DA signaling through cAMP and PKA causes an increase in dephosphorylation of some PP2A substrates (Hertz et al., 2016). Important to note is that this is a specific effect of the B56δ-containing PP2A complex (Leslie & Nairn, 2019); Usui et al., 1998). Concurrently, PKA phosphorylates ARPP-16 at Ser88 and this also leads indirectly to activation of PP2A. Notably, Ser88 phosphorylation was found to possess a mutually antagonistic relationship with Ser46 phosphorylation, i.e. increased phosphorylation at one residue is associated with reduced phosphorylation at the other (Andrade et al., 2017; Musante et al., 2017) (Fig. 3). Biochemical characterization of this relationship revealed a switch-like mechanism of PP2A regulation. Increased PKA-mediated phosphorylation of ARPP 16 at Ser88 prevented MAST3 from phosphorylating Ser46, resulting in PP2A disinhibition (Musante et al., 2017). Furthermore, PKA can directly phosphorylate MAST3, leading to inhibition of the kinase and consequently increased PP2A activity. This potentially includes Thr75 of DARPP-32 thereby contributing to the ability of DARPP-32 to inhibit PP1 (Andrade et al., 2017; Walaas et al., 2011). Combined with phosphorylation at Ser88 of ARPP-16, PP2A takes on a "non-inhibitable" form, which could influence numerous downstream signaling cascades and physiological functions (Leslie & Nairn, 2019); Musante et al., 2017).

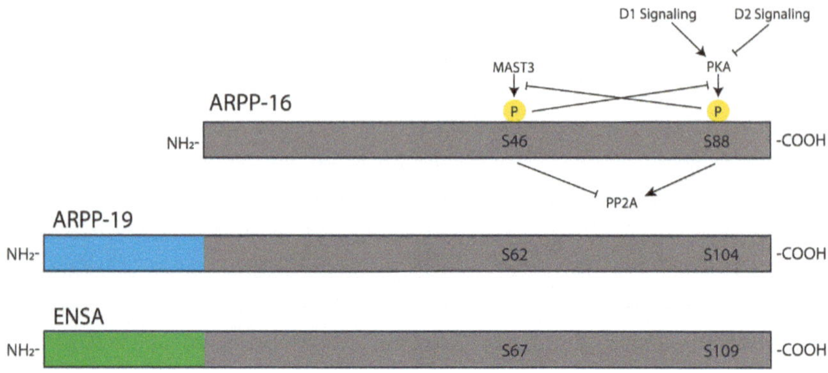

Fig. 3 ARPP proteins are phosphorylated by PKA and MAST3 to regulate PP2A activity. PKA phosphorylates ARPP-16 at Ser88 (Ser104 in ARPP-19 and Ser109 in ENSA), leading to activation of PP2A. MAST3 phosphorylates Ser46 in ARPP-16 (Ser62 in ARPP-19 and Ser67 in ENSA) and inhibits PP2A activity. These two phosphorylation sites act in a switch-like manner, where phosphorylation at one site inhibits the phosphorylation at the other.

Taken together, the DA/cAMP/PKA/MAST3/ARPP-16/PP2A signaling pathway in MSN neuronal transmission is tightly regulated to maintain a balance between kinase and phosphatase activities. Since these proteins have been implicated in several neurological disorders, including Alzheimer's disease, epilepsy, drug abuse, cancer, major depressive disorder, and several more, further studies aimed at elucidating this pathway as a molecular mechanism involved in disease has the potential to reveal profound insights into neurobiology and therapies (Houge et al., 2015; Loveday et al., 2015; O'Connor, Perl, Leonard, Sangodkar, & Narla, 2018; Reynhout et al., 2019; Sangodkar et al., 2016; Shang et al., 2016; Sontag & Sontag, 2014; Yu et al., 2004).

7. Conclusions

DA signaling in striatal MSNs is tightly regulated by several interrelated signaling cascades. These pathways converge on targets of PKA, most notably in regulating PP1 and PP2A phosphatase activity. Studies pioneered by Paul Greengard and his many colleagues established slow synaptic transmission as a fascinatingly complex network of numerous proteins with downstream effects on all aspects of cellular function. However, the proper balance between these components is paramount, as shifting the homeostasis to favor one pathway or another has been implicated in several neurological conditions. Several tools exist to investigate specific cellular subtypes present in the striatum and basal ganglia circuitry (Wilson & Nairn, 2018), including tagged proteins expressed under control of brain region-specific promoters in transgenic mice (Bateup et al., 2008), animal models that express fluorescently tagged proteins of interest whose cells can be isolated through fluorescence-activated cell sorting (Lobo, Karsten, Gray, Geschwind, & Yang, 2006) or laser capture microdissection (García-Berrocoso et al., 2018; Hondius et al., 2018). Additionally, epigenetic changes and other nuclear modifications in specific cell types can be studied through fluorescently-tagged proteins and molecules to easily and robustly identify subsets of neurons in a heterogenous population (Jordi et al., 2013).

Importantly, investigating these signaling pathways regulated by DA and other neurotransmitters has initiated the development of several pharmaceutical therapies, such as levodopa for Parkinson's disease, olanzapine and other D2 receptor antagonists for schizophrenia, and bupropion for nicotine addiction, among many others (Hornykiewicz, 2010; Potenza, Sofuoglu, Carroll, & Rounsaville, 2011; Rampino et al., 2019). Continuing to explore, investigate, and understand neuronal intracellular signaling pathways and mechanisms of signal transduction in the brain will hopefully provide incalculable benefits for society in the form of further therapies and treatments.

Acknowledgments

We dedicate this chapter to Paul Greengard, who one of us (ACN) had the privilege of working with for almost 40 years. We also thank the many members of the Greengard laboratory who contributed to the work reviewed here, especially Drs. Ivar Walaas, Hugh Hemmings Jr, Jean-Antoine Girault, and Atsuko Horiuchi. Research in the laboratory of ACN is supported by the National Institutes of Health (NIH) (AG047270, AG062306, AG066508, DA018343) and the State of Connecticut Department of Mental Health and Addiction Services.

Conflict of interest statement

The authors declare no conflicts of interest.

References

Ahn, J. H., McAvoy, T., Rakhilin, S. V., Nishi, A., Greengard, P., & Nairn, A. C. (2007). Protein kinase A activates protein phosphatase 2A by phosphorylation of the B56delta subunit. *Proceedings of the National Academy of Sciences of the United States of America*, *104*(8), 2979–2984. https://doi.org/10.1073/pnas.0611532104.

Álvarez-Fernández, M., Sánchez-Martínez, R., Sanz-Castillo, B., Gan, P. P., Sanz-Flores, M., Trakala, M., et al. (2013). Greatwall is essential to prevent mitotic collapse after nuclear envelope breakdown in mammals. *Proceedings of the National Academy of Sciences of the United States of America*, *110*(43), 17374–17379. https://doi.org/10.1073/pnas.1310745110.

Andén, N. E., Fuxe, K., Hamberger, B., & Hökfelt, T. (1966). A quantitative study on the nigro-neostriatal dopamine neuron system in the rat. *Acta Physiologica Scandinavica*, *67*(3), 306–312. https://doi.org/10.1111/j.1748-1716.1966.tb03317.x.

Andrade, E. C., Musante, V., Horiuchi, A., Matsuzaki, H., Brody, A. H., Wu, T., et al. (2017). ARPP-16 is a striatal-enriched inhibitor of protein phosphatase 2A regulated by microtubule-associated serine/threonine kinase 3 (mast 3 kinase). *The Journal of Neuroscience : The Official Journal of the Society for Neuroscience*, *37*(10), 2709–2722. https://doi.org/10.1523/jneurosci.4559-15.2017.

Aswad, D. W., & Greengard, P. (1981a). A specific substrate from rabbit cerebellum for guanosine 3':5'-monophosphate-dependent protein kinase. I. Purification and characterization. *Journal of Biological Chemistry*, *256*(7), 3487–3493.

Aswad, D. W., & Greengard, P. (1981b). A specific substrate from rabbit cerebellum for guanosine 3':5'-monophosphate-dependent protein kinase. II. Kinetic studies on its phosphorylation by guanosine 3':5'-monophosphate-dependent and adenosine 3':5'-monophosphate-dependent protein kinases. *Journal of Biological Chemistry*, *256*(7), 3494–3500.

Azevedo, F. A., Carvalho, L. R., Grinberg, L. T., Farfel, J. M., Ferretti, R. E., Leite, R. E., et al. (2009). Equal numbers of neuronal and nonneuronal cells make the human brain an isometrically scaled-up primate brain. *The Journal of Comparative Neurology*, *513*(5), 532–541. https://doi.org/10.1002/cne.21974.

Bateup, H. S., Santini, E., Shen, W., Birnbaum, S., Valjent, E., Surmeier, D. J., et al. (2010). Distinct subclasses of medium spiny neurons differentially regulate striatal motor behaviors. *Proceedings of the National Academy of Sciences of the United States of America*, *107*(33), 14845–14850. https://doi.org/10.1073/pnas.1009874107.

Bateup, H. S., Svenningsson, P., Kuroiwa, M., Gong, S., Nishi, A., Heintz, N., et al. (2008). Cell type-specific regulation of DARPP-32 phosphorylation by psychostimulant and antipsychotic drugs. *Nature Neuroscience*, *11*(8), 932–939. https://doi.org/10.1038/nn.2153.

Beaulieu, J. M., & Gainetdinov, R. R. (2011). The physiology, signaling, and pharmacology of dopamine receptors. *Pharmacological Reviews*, *63*(1), 182–217. https://doi.org/10.1124/pr.110.002642.

Berger, B., Febvret, A., Greengard, P., & Goldman-Rakic, P. S. (1990). DARPP-32, a phosphoprotein enriched in dopaminoceptive neurons bearing dopamine D1 receptors: Distribution in the cerebral cortex of the newborn and adult rhesus monkey. *The Journal of Comparative Neurology*, *299*(3), 327–348. https://doi.org/10.1002/cne.902990306.

Berthet, J., Rall, T. W., & Sutherland, E. W. (1957). The relationship of epinephrine and glucagon to liver phosphorylase. IV. Effect of epinephrine and glucagon on the reactivation of phosphorylase in liver homogenates. *The Journal of Biological Chemistry*, *224*(1), 463–475.

Bertran-Gonzalez, J., Håkansson, K., Borgkvist, A., Irinopoulou, T., Brami-Cherrier, K., Usiello, A., et al. (2009). Histone H3 phosphorylation is under the opposite tonic control of dopamine D2 and adenosine A2A receptors in striatopallidal neurons. *Neuropsychopharmacology*, *34*(7), 1710–1720. https://doi.org/10.1038/npp.2008.228.

Bibb, J. A., Snyder, G. L., Nishi, A., Yan, Z., Meijer, L., Fienberg, A. A., et al. (1999). Phosphorylation of DARPP-32 by Cdk5 modulates dopamine signalling in neurons. *Nature*, *402*(6762), 669–671. https://doi.org/10.1038/45251.

Björklund, A., & Dunnett, S. B. (2007). Dopamine neuron systems in the brain: An update. *Trends in Neurosciences*, *30*(5), 194–202. https://doi.org/10.1016/j.tins.2007.03.006.

Bollen, M., Peti, W., Ragusa, M. J., & Beullens, M. (2010). The extended PP1 toolkit: Designed to create specificity. *Trends in Biochemical Sciences*, *35*(8), 450–458. https://doi.org/10.1016/j.tibs.2010.03.002.

Borgkvist, A., Usiello, A., Greengard, P., & Fisone, G. (2007). Activation of the cAMP/PKA/DARPP-32 signaling pathway is required for morphine psychomotor stimulation but not for morphine reward. *Neuropsychopharmacology*, *32*(9), 1995–2003. https://doi.org/10.1038/sj.npp.1301321.

Bostan, A. C., Dum, R. P., & Strick, P. L. (2018). Functional anatomy of basal ganglia circuits with the cerebral cortex and the cerebellum. *Progress in Neurological Surgery*, *33*, 50–61. https://doi.org/10.1159/000480748.

Brene, S., Lindefors, N., Ehrlich, M., Taubes, T., Horiuchi, A., Kopp, J., et al. (1994). Expression of mRNAs encoding ARPP-16/19, ARPP-21, and DARPP-32 in human brain tissue. *The Journal of Neuroscience*, *14*(3), 985–998. Pt. 1.

Brunenberg, E. J., Moeskops, P., Backes, W. H., Pollo, C., Cammoun, L., Vilanova, A., et al. (2012). Structural and resting state functional connectivity of the subthalamic nucleus: Identification of motor STN parts and the hyperdirect pathway. *PLoS One*, *7*(6), e39061. https://doi.org/10.1371/journal.pone.0039061.

Burgess, A., Vigneron, S., Brioudes, E., Labbé, J. C., Lorca, T., & Castro, A. (2010). Loss of human Greatwall results in G2 arrest and multiple mitotic defects due to deregulation of the cyclin B-Cdc2/PP2A balance. *Proceedings of the National Academy of Sciences of the United States of America*, *107*(28), 12564–12569. https://doi.org/10.1073/pnas.0914191107.

Caporaso, G. L., Bibb, J. A., Snyder, G. L., Valle, C., Rakhilin, S., Fienberg, A. A., et al. (2000). Drugs of abuse modulate the phosphorylation of ARPP-21, a cyclic AMP-regulated phosphoprotein enriched in the basal ganglia. *Neuropharmacology*, *39*(9), 1637–1644. https://doi.org/10.1016/s0028-3908(99)00230-0.

Carlsson, A. (2001). A half-century of neurotransmitter research: impact on neurology and psychiatry. Nobel lecture. *Bioscience Reports*, *21*(6), 691–710. https://doi.org/10.1023/a:1015556204669.

Chin, D., & Means, A. R. (2000). Calmodulin: A prototypical calcium sensor. *Trends in Cell Biology*, *10*(8), 322–328. https://doi.org/10.1016/s0962-8924(00)01800-6.

Clarke, R., & Adermark, L. (2015). Dopaminergic regulation of striatal interneurons in reward and addiction: Focus on alcohol. *Neural Plasticity*, *2015*. https://doi.org/10.1155/2015/814567.

Clement-Cormier, Y. C., Kebabian, J. W., Petzold, G. L., & Greengard, P. (1974). Dopamine-sensitive adenylate cyclase in mammalian brain: A possible site of action of antipsychotic drugs. *Proceedings of the National Academy of Sciences of the United States of America*, *71*(4), 1113–1117. https://doi.org/10.1073/pnas.71.4.1113.

Cohen, P. T. (2002). Protein phosphatase 1—Targeted in many directions. *Journal of Cell Science*, *115*, 241–256. Pt. 2.

Connors, B. W., & Long, M. A. (2004). Electrical synapses in the mammalian brain. *Annual Review of Neuroscience*, *27*, 393–418. https://doi.org/10.1146/annurev.neuro.26.041002.131128.

da Cruz e Silva, E. F., Fox, C. A., Ouimet, C. C., Gustafson, E., Watson, S. J., & Greengard, P. (1995). Differential expression of protein phosphatase 1 isoforms in mammalian brain. *Journal of Neuroscience*, *15*(5), 3375–3389. https://doi.org/10.1523/jneurosci.15-05-03375.1995. Pt. 1.

Davis, R. G., Park, H. M., Kim, K., Greer, J. B., Fellers, R. T., LeDuc, R. D., et al. (2018). Top-down proteomics enables comparative analysis of brain proteoforms between mouse strains. *Analytical Chemistry*, *90*(6), 3802–3810. https://doi.org/10.1021/acs.analchem.7b04108.

De Camilli, P., Benfenati, F., Valtorta, F., & Greengard, P. (1990). The synapsins. *Annual Review of Cell Biology*, *6*, 433–460. https://doi.org/10.1146/annurev.cb.06.110190.002245.

Desdouits, F., Cheetham, J. J., Huang, H. B., Kwon, Y. G., da Cruz e Silva, E. F., Denefle, P., et al. (1995). Mechanism of inhibition of protein phosphatase 1 by DARPP-32: Studies with recombinant DARPP-32 and synthetic peptides. *Biochemical and Biophysical Research Communications*, *206*(2), 652–658. https://doi.org/10.1006/bbrc.1995.1092.

Dulubova, I., Horiuchi, A., Snyder, G. L., Girault, J. A., Czernik, A. J., Shao, L., et al. (2001). ARPP-16/ARPP-19: A highly conserved family of cAMP-regulated phosphoproteins. *Journal of Neurochemistry*, 77(1), 229–238.

Egloff, M. P., Johnson, D. F., Moorhead, G., Cohen, P. T., Cohen, P., & Barford, D. (1997). Structural basis for the recognition of regulatory subunits by the catalytic subunit of protein phosphatase 1. *The EMBO Journal*, *16*(8), 1876–1887. https://doi.org/10.1093/emboj/16.8.1876.

Engmann, O., Giralt, A., Gervasi, N., Marion-Poll, L., Gasmi, L., Filhol, O., et al. (2015). DARPP-32 interaction with adducin may mediate rapid environmental effects on striatal neurons. *Nature Communications*, *6*, 10099. https://doi.org/10.1038/ncomms10099.

Enjalbert, A., & Bockaert, J. (1983). Pharmacological characterization of the D2 dopamine receptor negatively coupled with adenylate cyclase in rat anterior pituitary. *Molecular Pharmacology*, *23*(3), 576–584.

Fardilha, M., Esteves, S. L., Korrodi-Gregório, L., da Cruz e Silva, O. A., & da Cruz e Silva, F. F. (2010). The physiological relevance of protein phosphatase 1 and its interacting proteins to health and disease. *Current Medicinal Chemistry*, *17*(33), 3996–4017. https://doi.org/10.2174/092986710793205363.

Farsad, K., & De Camilli, P. (2002). Neurotransmission and the synaptic vesicle cycle. *The Yale Journal of Biology and Medicine*, *75*(5-6), 261–284.

Fienberg, A. A., Hiroi, N., Mermelstein, P. G., Song, W., Snyder, G. L., Nishi, A., et al. (1998). DARPP-32: Regulator of the efficacy of dopaminergic neurotransmission. *Science*, *281*(5378), 838–842. https://doi.org/10.1126/science.281.5378.838.

García-Berrocoso, T., Llombart, V., Colàs-Campàs, L., Hainard, A., Licker, V., Penalba, A., et al. (2018). Single cell immuno-laser microdissection coupled to label-free proteomics to reveal the proteotypes of human brain cells after ischemia. *Molecular & Cellular Proteomics*, *17*(1), 175–189. https://doi.org/10.1074/mcp.RA117.000419.

Garland, P., Quraishe, S., French, P., & O'Connor, V. (2008). Expression of the MAST family of serine/threonine kinases. *Brain Research*, *1195*, 12–19. https://doi.org/10.1016/j.brainres.2007.12.027.

Gharbi-Ayachi, A., Labbé, J. C., Burgess, A., Vigneron, S., Strub, J. M., Brioudes, E., et al. (2010). The substrate of Greatwall kinase, Arpp19, controls mitosis by inhibiting protein phosphatase 2A. *Science*, *330*(6011), 1673–1677. https://doi.org/10.1126/science.1197048.

Gibbons, J. A., Kozubowski, L., Tatchell, K., & Shenolikar, S. (2007). Expression of human protein phosphatase-1 in Saccharomyces cerevisiae highlights the role of phosphatase isoforms in regulating eukaryotic functions. *Journal of Biological Chemistry*, *282*(30), 21838–21847. https://doi.org/10.1074/jbc.M701272200.

Girault, J. A. (2012). Integrating neurotransmission in striatal medium spiny neurons. *Advances in Experimental Medicine and Biology*, *970*, 407–429. https://doi.org/10.1007/978-3-7091-0932-8_18.

Girault, J. A., Hemmings, H. C., Jr., Williams, K. R., Nairn, A. C., & Greengard, P. (1989). Phosphorylation of DARPP-32, a dopamine- and cAMP-regulated phosphoprotein, by casein kinase II. *The Journal of Biological Chemistry*, *264*(36), 21748–21759.

Girault, J. A., Horiuchi, A., Gustafson, E. L., Rosen, N. L., & Greengard, P. (1990). Differential expression of ARPP-16 and ARPP-19, two highly related cAMP-regulated phosphoproteins, one of which is specifically associated with dopamine-innervated brain regions. *The Journal of Neuroscience*, *10*(4), 1124–1133.

Glausier, J. R., Maddox, M., Hemmings, H. C., Jr., Nairn, A. C., Greengard, P., & Muly, E. C. (2010). Localization of dopamine- and cAMP-regulated phosphoprotein-32 and inhibitor-1 in area 9 of Macaca mulatta prefrontal cortex. *Neuroscience, 167*(2), 428–438. https://doi.org/10.1016/j.neuroscience.2010.02.014.

Goldberg, J., Huang, H. B., Kwon, Y. G., Greengard, P., Nairn, A. C., & Kuriyan, J. (1995). Three-dimensional structure of the catalytic subunit of protein serine/threonine phosphatase-1. *Nature, 376*(6543), 745–753. https://doi.org/10.1038/376745a0.

Graves, J. D., & Krebs, E. G. (1999). Protein phosphorylation and signal transduction. *Pharmacology & Therapeutics, 82*(2-3), 111–121. https://doi.org/10.1016/s0163-7258(98)00056-4.

Greengard, P. (1978). Phosphorylated proteins as physiological effectors. *Science, 199*(4325), 146–152. https://doi.org/10.1126/science.22932.

Greengard, P. (2001). The neurobiology of slow synaptic transmission. *Science, 294*(5544), 1024–1030. https://doi.org/10.1126/science.294.5544.1024.

Greengard, P., Valtorta, F., Czernik, A. J., & Benfenati, F. (1993). Synaptic vesicle phosphoproteins and regulation of synaptic function. *Science, 259*(5096), 780–785. https://doi.org/10.1126/science.8430330.

Hemmings, H. C., Jr., & Greengard, P. (1989). ARPP-21, a cyclic AMP-regulated phosphoprotein enriched in dopamine-innervated brain regions. I. Purification and characterization of the protein from bovine caudate nucleus. *The Journal of Neuroscience, 9*(3), 851–864. https://doi.org/10.1523/jneurosci.09-03-00851.1989.

Hemmings, H. C., Jr., Greengard, P., Tung, H. Y., & Cohen, P. (1984). DARPP-32, a dopamine-regulated neuronal phosphoprotein, is a potent inhibitor of protein phosphatase-1. *Nature, 310*(5977), 503–505. https://doi.org/10.1038/310503a0.

Hemmings, H. C., Jr., Nairn, A. C., Aswad, D. W., & Greengard, P. (1984). DARPP-32, a dopamine- and adenosine 3':5'-monophosphate-regulated phosphoprotein enriched in dopamine-innervated brain regions. II. Purification and characterization of the phosphoprotein from bovine caudate nucleus. *The Journal of Neuroscience, 4*(1), 99–110. https://doi.org/10.1523/jneurosci.04-01-00099.1984.

Hemmings, H. C., Jr., Nairn, A. C., & Greengard, P. (1984). DARPP-32, a dopamine- and adenosine 3':5'-monophosphate-regulated neuronal phosphoprotein. II. Comparison of the kinetics of phosphorylation of DARPP-32 and phosphatase inhibitor 1. *Journal of Biological Chemistry, 259*(23), 14491–14497.

Hendrickx, A., Beullens, M., Ceulemans, H., Den Abt, T., Van Eynde, A., Nicolaescu, E., et al. (2009). Docking motif-guided mapping of the interactome of protein phosphatase-1. *Chemistry & Biology, 16*(4), 365–371. https://doi.org/10.1016/j.chembiol.2009.02.012.

Hendry, S. H., Schwark, H. D., Jones, E. G., & Yan, J. (1987). Numbers and proportions of GABA-immunoreactive neurons in different areas of monkey cerebral cortex. *The Journal of Neuroscience, 7*(5), 1503–1519. https://doi.org/10.1523/jneurosci.07-05-01503.1987.

Heron, L., Virsolvy, A., Peyrollier, K., Cribble, F. M., Le Cam, A., Ashcroft, F. M., et al. (1998). Human alpha-endosulfine, a possible regulator of sulfonylurea-sensitive KATP channel: Molecular cloning, expression and biological properties. *Proceedings of the National Academy of Sciences of the United States of America, 95*(14), 8387–8391. https://doi.org/10.1073/pnas.95.14.8387.

Hertz, E. P. T., Kruse, T., Davey, N. E., López-Méndez, B., Sigurðsson, J. O., Montoya, G., et al. (2016). A conserved motif provides binding specificity to the PP2A-B56 phosphatase. *Molecular Cell, 63*(4), 686–695. https://doi.org/10.1016/j.molcel.2016.06.024.

Hondius, D. C., Eigenhuis, K. N., Morrema, T. H. J., van der Schors, R. C., van Nierop, P., Bugiani, M., et al. (2018). Proteomics analysis identifies new markers associated with capillary cerebral amyloid angiopathy in Alzheimer's disease. *Acta Neuropathologica Communications, 6*(1), 46. https://doi.org/10.1186/s40478-018-0540-2.

Horiuchi, A., Williams, K. R., Kurihara, T., Nairn, A. C., & Greengard, P. (1990). Purification and cDNA cloning of ARPP-16, a cAMP-regulated phosphoprotein enriched in basal ganglia, and of a related phosphoprotein, ARPP-19. *The Journal of Biological Chemistry*, *265*(16), 9476–9484.

Hornykiewicz, O. (2010). A brief history of levodopa. *Journal of Neurology*, *257*(Suppl. 2), S249–S252. https://doi.org/10.1007/s00415-010-5741-y.

Houge, G., Haesen, D., Vissers, L. E., Mehta, S., Parker, M. J., Wright, M., et al. (2015). B56δ-related protein phosphatase 2A dysfunction identified in patients with intellectual disability. *The Journal of Clinical Investigation*, *125*(8), 3051–3062. https://doi.org/10.1172/jci79860.

Huang, H. B., Horiuchi, A., Watanabe, T., Shih, S. R., Tsay, H. J., Li, H. C., et al. (1999). Characterization of the inhibition of protein phosphatase-1 by DARPP-32 and inhibitor-2. *The Journal of Biological Chemistry*, *274*(12), 7870–7878. https://doi.org/10.1074/jbc.274.12.7870.

Janssens, V., & Goris, J. (2001). Protein phosphatase 2A: A highly regulated family of serine/threonine phosphatases implicated in cell growth and signalling. *Biochemical Journal*, *353*, 417–439. https://doi.org/10.1042/0264-6021:3530417. Pt. 3.

Jordi, E., Heiman, M., Marion-Poll, L., Guermonprez, P., Cheng, S. K., Nairn, A. C., et al. (2013). Differential effects of cocaine on histone posttranslational modifications in identified populations of striatal neurons. *Proceedings of the National Academy of Sciences of the United States of America*, *110*(23), 9511–9516. https://doi.org/10.1073/pnas.1307116110.

Kebabian, J. W., & Calne, D. B. (1979). Multiple receptors for dopamine. *Nature*, *277*(5692), 93–96. https://doi.org/10.1038/277093a0.

Kebabian, J. W., & Greengard, P. (1971). Dopamine-sensitive adenyl cyclase: possible role in synaptic transmission. *Science*, *174*(4016), 1346–1349. https://doi.org/10.1126/science.174.4016.1346.

Kebabian, J. W., Petzold, G. L., & Greengard, P. (1972). Dopamine-sensitive adenylate cyclase in caudate nucleus of rat brain, and its similarity to the "dopamine receptor". *Proceedings of the National Academy of Sciences of the United States of America*, *69*(8), 2145–2149. https://doi.org/10.1073/pnas.69.8.2145.

Kelly, P. T., Cotman, C. W., & Largen, M. (1979). Cyclic AMP-stimulated protein kinases at brain synaptic junctions. *The Journal of Biological Chemistry*, *254*(5), 1564–1575.

King, M. M., Huang, C. Y., Chock, P. B., Nairn, A. C., Hemmings, H. C., Jr., Chan, K. F., et al. (1984). Mammalian brain phosphoproteins as substrates for calcineurin. *The Journal of Biological Chemistry*, *259*(13), 8080–8083.

Kitagawa, Y., Sasaki, K., Shima, H., Shibuya, M., Sugimura, T., & Nagao, M. (1990). Protein phosphatases possibly involved in rat spermatogenesis. *Biochemical and Biophysical Research Communications*, *171*(1), 230–235. https://doi.org/10.1016/0006-291x(90)91381-2.

Korrodi-Gregório, L., Esteves, S. L., & Fardilha, M. (2014). Protein phosphatase 1 catalytic isoforms: Specificity toward interacting proteins. *Translational Research*, *164*(5), 366–391. https://doi.org/10.1016/j.trsl.2014.07.001.

Kuo, J. F., & Greengard, P. (1969). Cyclic nucleotide-dependent protein kinases. IV. Widespread occurrence of adenosine 3',5'-monophosphate-dependent protein kinase in various tissues and phyla of the animal kingdom. *Proceedings of the National Academy of Sciences of the United States of America*, *64*(4), 1349–1355. https://doi.org/10.1073/pnas.64.4.1349.

Kwon, Y. G., Huang, H. B., Desdouits, F., Girault, J. A., Greengard, P., & Nairn, A. C. (1997). Characterization of the interaction between DARPP-32 and protein phosphatase 1 (PP-1): DARPP-32 peptides antagonize the interaction of PP-1 with binding proteins. *Proceedings of the National Academy of Sciences of the United States of America*, *94*(8), 3536–3541. https://doi.org/10.1073/pnas.94.8.3536.

Leslie, S. N., & Nairn, A. C. (2019). cAMP regulation of protein phosphatases PP1 and PP2A in brain. *Biochimica et Biophysica Acta. Molecular Cell Research, 1866*(1), 64–73. https://doi.org/10.1016/j.bbamcr.2018.09.006.

Lobo, M. K., Karsten, S. L., Gray, M., Geschwind, D. H., & Yang, X. W. (2006). FACS-array profiling of striatal projection neuron subtypes in juvenile and adult mouse brains. *Nature Neuroscience, 9*(3), 443–452. https://doi.org/10.1038/nn1654.

Loveday, C., Tatton-Brown, K., Clarke, M., Westwood, I., Renwick, A., Ramsay, E., et al. (2015). Mutations in the PP2A regulatory subunit B family genes PPP2R5B, PPP2R5C and PPP2R5D cause human overgrowth. *Human Molecular Genetics, 24*(17), 4775–4779. https://doi.org/10.1093/hmg/ddv182.

Maeno, H., Johnson, E. M., & Greengard, P. (1971). Subcellular distribution of adenosine 3',5'-monophosphate-dependent protein kinase in rat brain. *The Journal of Biological Chemistry, 246*(1), 134–142.

Mayer-Jaekel, R. E., & Hemmings, B. A. (1994). Protein phosphatase 2A—A 'menage a trois'. *Trends in Cell Biology, 4*(8), 287–291.

McAfee, D. A., Schorderet, M., & Greengard, P. (1971). Adenosine 3',5'-monophosphate in nervous tissue: Increase associated with synaptic transmission. *Science, 171*(3976), 1156–1158. https://doi.org/10.1126/science.171.3976.1156.

Meiselbach, H., Sticht, H., & Enz, R. (2006). Structural analysis of the protein phosphatase 1 docking motif: molecular description of binding specificities identifies interacting proteins. *Chemistry & Biology, 13*(1), 49–59. https://doi.org/10.1016/j.chembiol.2005.10.009.

Miyamoto, E., Kuo, J. F., & Greengard, P. (1969). Adenosine 3',5'-monophosphate-dependent protein kinase from brain. *Science, 165*(3888), 63–65. https://doi.org/10.1126/science.165.3888.63.

Mochida, S., Maslen, S. L., Skehel, M., & Hunt, T. (2010). Greatwall phosphorylates an inhibitor of protein phosphatase 2A that is essential for mitosis. *Science, 330*(6011), 1670–1673. https://doi.org/10.1126/science.1195689.

Musante, V., Li, L., Kanyo, J., Lam, T. T., Colangelo, C. M., Cheng, S. K., et al. (2017). Reciprocal regulation of ARPP-16 by PKA and MAST3 kinases provides a cAMP-regulated switch in protein phosphatase 2A inhibition. *eLife, 6*. https://doi.org/10.7554/eLife.24998.

Nairn, A. C., Hemmings, H. C., Jr., & Greengard, P. (1985). Protein kinases in the brain. *Annual Review of Biochemistry, 54*, 931–976. https://doi.org/10.1146/annurev.bi.54.070185.004435.

Nairn, A. C., Svenningsson, P., Nishi, A., Fisone, G., Girault, J. A., & Greengard, P. (2004). The role of DARPP-32 in the actions of drugs of abuse. *Neuropharmacology, 47*(Suppl. 1), 14–23. https://doi.org/10.1016/j.neuropharm.2004.05.010.

Nambu, A. (2004). A new dynamic model of the cortico-basal ganglia loop. *Progress in Brain Research, 143*, 461–466. https://doi.org/10.1016/s0079-6123(03)43043-4.

Nambu, A., Tokuno, H., Hamada, I., Kita, H., Imanishi, M., Akazawa, T., et al. (2000). Excitatory cortical inputs to pallidal neurons via the subthalamic nucleus in the monkey. *Journal of Neurophysiology, 84*(1), 289–300. https://doi.org/10.1152/jn.2000.84.1.289.

Nambu, A., Tokuno, H., & Takada, M. (2002). Functional significance of the cortico-subthalamo-pallidal 'hyperdirect' pathway. *Neuroscience Research, 43*(2), 111–117. https://doi.org/10.1016/s0168-0102(02)00027-5.

Nestler, E. J., Walaas, S. I., & Greengard, P. (1984). Neuronal phosphoproteins: Physiological and clinical implications. *Science, 225*(4668), 1357–1364. https://doi.org/10.1126/science.6474180.

Nishi, A., Bibb, J. A., Snyder, G. L., Higashi, H., Nairn, A. C., & Greengard, P. (2000). Amplification of dopaminergic signaling by a positive feedback loop. *Proceedings of the National Academy of Sciences of the United States of America, 97*(23), 12840–12845. https://doi.org/10.1073/pnas.220410397.

Nishi, A., Snyder, G. L., & Greengard, P. (1997). Bidirectional regulation of DARPP-32 phosphorylation by dopamine. *The Journal of Neuroscience*, *17*(21), 8147–8155. https://doi.org/10.1523/jneurosci.17-21-08147.1997.

Nishi, A., Snyder, G. L., Nairn, A. C., & Greengard, P. (1999). Role of calcineurin and protein phosphatase-2A in the regulation of DARPP-32 dephosphorylation in neostriatal neurons. *Journal of Neurochemistry*, *72*(5), 2015–2021. https://doi.org/10.1046/j.1471-4159.1999.0722015.x.

Nishi, A., Watanabe, Y., Higashi, H., Tanaka, M., Nairn, A. C., & Greengard, P. (2005). Glutamate regulation of DARPP-32 phosphorylation in neostriatal neurons involves activation of multiple signaling cascades. *Proceedings of the National Academy of Sciences of the United States of America*, *102*(4), 1199–1204. https://doi.org/10.1073/pnas.0409138102.

O'Connor, C. M., Perl, A., Leonard, D., Sangodkar, J., & Narla, G. (2018). Therapeutic targeting of PP2A. *The International Journal of Biochemistry & Cell Biology*, *96*, 182–193. https://doi.org/10.1016/j.biocel.2017.10.008.

Ouimet, C. C., da Cruz e Silva, E. F., & Greengard, P. (1995). The alpha and gamma 1 isoforms of protein phosphatase 1 are highly and specifically concentrated in dendritic spines. *Proceedings of the National Academy of Sciences of the United States of America*, *92*(8), 3396–3400. https://doi.org/10.1073/pnas.92.8.3396.

Ouimet, C. C., & Greengard, P. (1990). Distribution of DARPP-32 in the basal ganglia: An electron microscopic study. *Journal of Neurocytology*, *19*(1), 39–52. https://doi.org/10.1007/bf01188438.

Ouimet, C. C., Hemmings, H. C., Jr., & Greengard, P. (1989). ARPP-21, a cyclic AMP-regulated phosphoprotein enriched in dopamine-innervated brain regions. II. Immunocytochemical localization in rat brain. *Journal of Neuroscience*, *9*(3), 865–875. https://doi.org/10.1523/jneurosci.09-03-00865.1989.

Ouimet, C. C., LaMantia, A. S., Goldman-Rakic, P., Rakic, P., & Greengard, P. (1992). Immunocytochemical localization of DARPP-32, a dopamine and cyclic-AMP-regulated phosphoprotein, in the primate brain. *The Journal of Comparative Neurology*, *323*(2), 209–218. https://doi.org/10.1002/cne.903230206.

Ouimet, C. C., Langley-Gullion, K. C., & Greengard, P. (1998). Quantitative immunocytochemistry of DARPP-32-expressing neurons in the rat caudatoputamen. *Brain Research*, *808*(1), 8–12. https://doi.org/10.1016/s0006-8993(98)00724-0.

Ouimet, C. C., Miller, P. E., Hemmings, H. C., Jr., Walaas, S. I., & Greengard, P. (1984). DARPP-32, a dopamine- and adenosine 3':5'-monophosphate-regulated phosphoprotein enriched in dopamine-innervated brain regions. III. Immunocytochemical localization. *The Journal of Neuroscience*, *4*(1), 111–124. https://doi.org/10.1523/jneurosci.04-01-00111.1984.

Peyrollier, K., Héron, L., Virsolvy-Vergine, A., Le Cam, A., & Bataille, D. (1996). Alpha endosulfine is a novel molecule, structurally related to a family of phosphoproteins. *Biochemical and Biophysical Research Communications*, *223*(3), 583–586. https://doi.org/10.1006/bbrc.1996.0938.

Potenza, M. N., Sofuoglu, M., Carroll, K. M., & Rounsaville, B. J. (2011). Neuroscience of behavioral and pharmacological treatments for addictions. *Neuron*, *69*(4), 695–712. https://doi.org/10.1016/j.neuron.2011.02.009.

Quartarone, A., Cacciola, A., Milardi, D., Ghilardi, M. F., Calamuneri, A., Chillemi, G., et al. (2020). New insights into cortico-basal-cerebellar connectome: Clinical and physiological considerations. *Brain*, *143*(2), 396–406. https://doi.org/10.1093/brain/awz310.

Rakhilin, S. V., Olson, P. A., Nishi, A., Starkova, N. N., Fienberg, A. A., Nairn, A. C., et al. (2004). A network of control mediated by regulator of calcium/calmodulin-dependent signaling. *Science*, *306*(5696), 698–701. https://doi.org/10.1126/science.1099961.

Rampino, A., Marakhovskaia, A., Soares-Silva, T., Torretta, S., Veneziani, F., & Beaulieu, J. M. (2019). Antipsychotic drug responsiveness and dopamine receptor signaling; old players and new prospects. *Frontiers in Psychiatry, 9*, 702. https://doi.org/10.3389/fpsyt.2018.00702.

Redgrave, P., Rodriguez, M., Smith, Y., Rodriguez-Oroz, M. C., Lehericy, S., Bergman, H., et al. (2010). Goal-directed and habitual control in the basal ganglia: Implications for Parkinson's disease. *Nature Reviews. Neuroscience, 11*(11), 760–772. https://doi.org/10.1038/nrn2915.

Reynhout, S., Jansen, S., Haesen, D., van Belle, S., de Munnik, S. A., Bongers, E., et al. (2019). De novo mutations affecting the catalytic calpha subunit of PP2A, PPP2CA, cause syndromic intellectual disability resembling other PP2A-related neurodevelopmental disorders. *American Journal of Human Genetics, 104*(2), 357. https://doi.org/10.1016/j.ajhg.2019.01.003.

Sangodkar, J., Farrington, C. C., McClinch, K., Galsky, M. D., Kastrinsky, D. B., & Narla, G. (2016). All roads lead to PP2A: Exploiting the therapeutic potential of this phosphatase. *The FEBS Journal, 283*(6), 1004–1024. https://doi.org/10.1111/febs.13573.

Sano, H., Chiken, S., Hikida, T., Kobayashi, K., & Nambu, A. (2013). Signals through the striatopallidal indirect pathway stop movements by phasic excitation in the substantia nigra. *The Journal of Neuroscience, 33*(17), 7583–7594. https://doi.org/10.1523/jneurosci.4932-12.2013.

Shang, L., Henderson, L. B., Cho, M. T., Petrey, D. S., Fong, C. T., Haude, K. M., et al. (2016). De novo missense variants in PPP2R5D are associated with intellectual disability, macrocephaly, hypotonia, and autism. *Neurogenetics, 17*(1), 43–49. https://doi.org/10.1007/s10048-015-0466-9.

Sharma, R. K., & Parameswaran, S. (2018). Calmodulin-binding proteins: A journey of 40 years. *Cell Calcium, 75*, 89–100. https://doi.org/10.1016/j.ceca.2018.09.002.

Shima, H., Haneji, T., Hatano, Y., Kasugai, I., Sugimura, T., & Nagao, M. (1993). Protein phosphatase 1 gamma 2 is associated with nuclei of meiotic cells in rat testis. *Biochemical and Biophysical Research Communications, 194*(2), 930–937. https://doi.org/10.1006/bbrc.1993.1910.

Sontag, J. M., & Sontag, E. (2014). Protein phosphatase 2A dysfunction in Alzheimer's disease. *Frontiers in Molecular Neuroscience, 7*, 16. https://doi.org/10.3389/fnmol.2014.00016.

Stipanovich, A., Valjent, E., Matamales, M., Nishi, A., Ahn, J. H., Maroteaux, M., et al. (2008). A phosphatase cascade by which rewarding stimuli control nucleosomal response. *Nature, 453*(7197), 879–884. https://doi.org/10.1038/nature06994.

Straub, C., Saulnier, J. L., Bègue, A., Feng, D. D., Huang, K. W., & Sabatini, B. L. (2016). Principles of synaptic organization of GABAergic interneurons in the striatum. *Neuron, 92*(1), 84–92. https://doi.org/10.1016/j.neuron.2016.09.007.

Sutherland, E. W. (1972). Studies on the mechanism of hormone action. *Science, 177*(4047), 401–408. https://doi.org/10.1126/science.177.4047.401.

Sutherland, E. W., & Rall, T. W. (1958). Fractionation and characterization of a cyclic adenine ribonucleotide formed by tissue particles. *The Journal of Biological Chemistry, 232*(2), 1077–1091.

Svenningsson, P., Nairn, A. C., & Greengard, P. (2005). DARPP-32 mediates the actions of multiple drugs of abuse. *The AAPS Journal, 7*(2), E353–E360. https://doi.org/10.1208/aapsj070235.

Svenningsson, P., Nishi, A., Fisone, G., Girault, J. A., Nairn, A. C., & Greengard, P. (2004). DARPP-32: An integrator of neurotransmission. *Annual Review of Pharmacology and Toxicology, 44*, 269–296. https://doi.org/10.1146/annurev.pharmtox.44.101802.121415.

Svenningsson, P., Tzavara, E. T., Carruthers, R., Rachleff, I., Wattler, S., Nehls, M., et al. (2003). Diverse psychotomimetics act through a common signaling pathway. *Science*, *302*(5649), 1412–1415. https://doi.org/10.1126/science.1089681.

Tsou, K., Girault, J. A., & Greengard, P. (1993). Dopamine D1 agonist SKF 38393 increases the state of phosphorylation of ARPP-21 in substantia nigra. *Journal of Neurochemistry*, *60*(3), 1043–1046. https://doi.org/10.1111/j.1471-4159.1993.tb03252.x.

Ueda, T., Greengard, P., Berzins, K., Cohen, R. S., Blomberg, F., Grab, D. J., et al. (1979). Subcellular distribution in cerebral cortex of two proteins phosphorylated by a cAMP-dependent protein kinase. *The Journal of Cell Biology*, *83*(2), 308–319. https://doi.org/10.1083/jcb.83.2.308. Pt 1.

Usui, H., Inoue, R., Tanabe, O., Nishito, Y., Shimizu, M., Hayashi, H., et al. (1998). Activation of protein phosphatase 2A by cAMP-dependent protein kinase-catalyzed phosphorylation of the 74-kDa B″ (δ) regulatory subunit in vitro and identification of the phosphorylation sites. *FEBS Letters*, *430*(3), 312–316. https://doi.org/10.1016/s0014-5793(98)00684-x.

Valjent, E., Pascoli, V., Svenningsson, P., Paul, S., Enslen, H., Corvol, J. C., et al. (2005). Regulation of a protein phosphatase cascade allows convergent dopamine and glutamate signals to activate ERK in the striatum. *Proceedings of the National Academy of Sciences of the United States of America*, *102*(2), 491–496. https://doi.org/10.1073/pnas.0408305102.

Virshup, D. M., & Kaldis, P. (2010). Cell biology. enforcing the greatwall in mitosis. *Science*, *330*(6011), 1638–1639. https://doi.org/10.1126/science.1199898.

Virshup, D. M., & Shenolikar, S. (2009). From promiscuity to precision: Protein phosphatases get a makeover. *Molecular Cell*, *33*(5), 537–545. https://doi.org/10.1016/j.molcel.2009.02.015.

Voets, E., & Wolthuis, R. M. (2010). MASTL is the human orthologue of Greatwall kinase that facilitates mitotic entry, anaphase and cytokinesis. *Cell Cycle*, *9*(17), 3591–3601. https://doi.org/10.4161/cc.9.17.12832.

Wakula, P., Beullens, M., Ceulemans, H., Stalmans, W., & Bollen, M. (2003). Degeneracy and function of the ubiquitous RVXF motif that mediates binding to protein phosphatase-1. *The Journal of Biological Chemistry*, *278*(21), 18817–18823. https://doi.org/10.1074/jbc.M300175200.

Walaas, S. I., Aswad, D. W., & Greengard, P. (1983). A dopamine- and cyclic AMP-regulated phosphoprotein enriched in dopamine-innervated brain regions. *Nature*, *301*(5895), 69–71. https://doi.org/10.1038/301069a0.

Walaas, S. I., & Greengard, P. (1984). DARPP-32, a dopamine- and adenosine 3':5'-monophosphate-regulated phosphoprotein enriched in dopamine-innervated brain regions. I. Regional and cellular distribution in the rat brain. *The Journal of Neuroscience*, *4*(1), 84–98. https://doi.org/10.1523/jneurosci.04-01-00084.1984.

Walaas, S. I., Hemmings, H. C., Jr., Greengard, P., & Nairn, A. C. (2011). Beyond the dopamine receptor: regulation and roles of serine/threonine protein phosphatases. *Frontiers in Neuroanatomy*, *5*, 50. https://doi.org/10.3389/fnana.2011.00050.

Walaas, S. I., Nairn, A. C., & Greengard, P. (1983a). Regional distribution of calcium- and cyclic adenosine 3':5'-monophosphate-regulated protein phosphorylation systems in mammalian brain. I. Particulate systems. *The Journal of Neuroscience*, *3*(2), 291–301. https://doi.org/10.1523/jneurosci.03-02-00291.1983.

Walaas, S. I., Nairn, A. C., & Greengard, P. (1983b). Regional distribution of calcium- and cyclic adenosine 3':5'-monophosphate-regulated protein phosphorylation systems in mammalian brain. II. Soluble systems. *The Journal of Neuroscience*, *3*(2), 302–311. https://doi.org/10.1523/jneurosci.03-02-00302.1983.

Walaas, S. I., & Ouimet, C. C. (1989). The ventral striatopallidal complex: An immunocytochemical analysis of medium-sized striatal neurons and striatopallidal fibers in the basal forebrain of the rat. *Neuroscience*, *28*(3), 663–672. https://doi.org/10.1016/0306-4522(89)90013-4.

Walsh, D. A., Perkins, J. P., & Krebs, E. G. (1968). An adenosine 3',5'-monophosphate-dependant protein kinase from rabbit skeletal muscle. *The Journal of Biological Chemistry*, *243*(13), 3763–3765.

Walter, U., Kanof, P., Schulman, H., & Greengard, P. (1978). Adenosine 3':5'-monophosphate receptor proteins in mammalian brain. *The Journal of Biological Chemistry*, *253*(17), 6275–6280.

Watkins, J. C. (2000). l-glutamate as a central neurotransmitter: Looking back. *Biochemical Society Transactions*, *28*(4), 297–309.

Weller, M., & Morgan, I. G. (1976). Localization in the synaptic junction of the cyclic AMP stimulated intrinsic protein kinase activity of synaptosomal plasma membranes. *Biochimica et Biophysica Acta*, *433*(1), 223–227. https://doi.org/10.1016/0005-2736(76)90190-5.

Williams, K. R., Hemmings, H. C., Jr., LoPresti, M. B., & Greengard, P. (1989). ARPP-21, a cyclic AMP-regulated phosphoprotein enriched in dopamine-innervated brain regions. I. Amino acid sequence of ARPP-21B from bovine caudate nucleus. *The Journal of Neuroscience*, *9*(10), 3631–3637. https://doi.org/10.1523/jneurosci.09-10-03631.1989.

Wilson, R. S., & Nairn, A. C. (2018). Cell-type-specific proteomics: A neuroscience perspective. *Proteome*, *6*(4). https://doi.org/10.3390/proteomes6040051.

Yu, J., Fleming, S. L., Williams, B., Williams, E. V., Li, Z., Somma, P., et al. (2004). Greatwall kinase: a nuclear protein required for proper chromosome condensation and mitotic progression in Drosophila. *The Journal of Cell Biology*, *164*(4), 487–492. https://doi.org/10.1083/jcb.200310059.

Zachariou, V., Sgambato-Faure, V., Sasaki, T., Svenningsson, P., Berton, O., Fienberg, A. A., et al. (2006). Phosphorylation of DARPP-32 at Threonine-34 is required for cocaine action. *Neuropsychopharmacology*, *31*(3), 555–562. https://doi.org/10.1038/sj.npp.1300832.

Zhai, S., Tanimura, A., Graves, S. M., Shen, W., & Surmeier, D. J. (2018). Striatal synapses, circuits, and Parkinson's disease. *Current Opinion in Neurobiology*, *48*, 9–16. https://doi.org/10.1016/j.conb.2017.08.004.

Zhang, Y., Svenningsson, P., Picetti, R., Schlussman, S. D., Nairn, A. C., Ho, A., et al. (2006). Cocaine self-administration in mice is inversely related to phosphorylation at Thr34 (protein kinase A site) and Ser130 (kinase CK1 site) of DARPP-32. *The Journal of Neuroscience*, *26*(10), 2645–2651. https://doi.org/10.1523/jneurosci.3923 05.2006.

CHAPTER FOUR

DARPP-32 40 years later

Jean-Antoine Girault[a,b,c,*] and Angus C. Nairn[d]
[a]Inserm UMR-S 1270, Paris, France
[b]Sorbonne Université, Faculty of Science and Engineering, Paris, France
[c]Institut du Fer à Moulin, Paris, France
[d]Department of Psychiatry, Yale School of Medicine, Connecticut Mental Health Center, New Haven, CT, United States
*Corresponding author: e-mail address: jean-antoine.girault@inserm.fr

Contents

Abstract

DARPP-32 (dopamine- and cAMP-regulated phosphoprotein with an apparent Mr of 32,000), now also known as phosphoprotein phosphatase 1 regulatory subunit 1B (PPP1R1B), is a potent inhibitor of protein phosphatase 1 (PP1, also known as PPP1) when phosphorylated at Thr34 by cAMP-dependent protein kinase (PKA). DARPP-32 exhibits a remarkable regional distribution in brain, roughly similar to that of dopamine innervation. Its discovery was a culmination of the long-standing effort of Paul Greengard to understand the mechanisms through which neurotransmitters such as dopamine exert their effects on target neurons. DARPP-32 is particularly enriched in striatal projection neurons where it is regulated by numerous signals through which it integrates and amplifies responses to many stimuli. Molecular studies of DARPP-32 have revealed that its regulation and function are more complex than anticipated. It is phosphorylated on multiple sites by several protein kinases that modulate

Advances in Pharmacology, Volume 90
ISSN 1054-3589
https://doi.org/10.1016/bs.apha.2020.09.004

DARPP-32 properties. Primarily, when phosphorylated at Thr34 DARPP-32 is a potent inhibitor of PP1, whereas when phosphorylated at Thr75 by Cdk5 it inhibits PKA. Phosphorylation at serine residues by CK1 and CK2 modulates its intracellular localization and its sensitivity to kinases or phosphatases. Modeling studies provide evidence that the signaling pathways including DARPP-32 are endowed of strong robustness and bistable properties favoring switch-like responses. Thus DARPP-32 combined with a set of other distinct signaling molecules enriched in striatal projection neurons plays a key role in the characteristic properties and physiological function of these neurons.

Abbreviations

Cdk5	cyclin-dependent protein kinase 5
CK1	casein kinase 1
CK2	casein kinase 2
D1	D1 dopamine receptor (a.k.a. Drd1)
D2	D2 dopamine receptor (a.k.a. Drd2)
DARPP-32	dopamine- and cAMP-regulated phosphoprotein with an apparent Mr of 32,000 (a.k.a. PPP1R1B)
ERK	extracellular signal-regulated kinase
GWAS	genome-wide association study
I1	inhibitor 1 (a.k.a. PPP1R1A)
KIQF	Lys-Ile-Gln-Phe consensus motif binding
L-DOPA	L-dihydroxyphenylalanine
LID	L-DOPA-induced dyskinesia
LTD	long-term depression
LTP	long-term potentiation
MSN	medium-size spiny neuron (a.k.a. SPN)
NES	nuclear export signal
NMDA	*N*-methyl-D-aspartate
PKA	cAMP-dependent protein kinase
PKG	cGMP-dependent protein kinase
PP1	protein phosphatase 1 (a.k.a. PPP1)
PP2A	protein phosphatase 2A (a.k.a. PPP2)
PP2B	protein phosphatase 2B (a.k.a. PPP3, calcineurin)
PPP1	phosphoprotein phosphatase 1 (a.k.a. PP1)
PPP1R1A	phosphoprotein phosphatase 1 regulatory subunit 1A (a.k.a. inhibitor 1, I1)
PPP1R1B	phosphoprotein phosphatase 1 regulatory subunit 1B (a.k.a. DARPP-32)
PPP1R1C	phosphoprotein phosphatase 1 regulatory subunit 1C
PPP2	phosphoprotein phosphatase 2 (a.k.a. PP2A)
PPP2R3A	phosphoprotein phosphatase 2 regulatory subunit (a.k.a. PR72, Ca^{2+}-sensitive regulatory subunit)
PPP2R5D	phosphoprotein phosphatase 2 regulatory subunit 5D (a.k.a. B56δ)
PPP3	calcineurin (a.k.a. protein phosphatase 2B, PP2B)
PPM	phosphoprotein phosphatase requiring Mg^{2+}/Mn^{2+} (a.k.a. PP2C)
PR72	72-kDa regulatory protein of PP2A (a.k.a. PPP2R3A)
SPN	striatal projection neuron (a.k.a. MSN)
tDARPP	truncated DARPP-32

1. Introduction

DARPP-32 stands for dopamine- and cAMP-regulated phosphoprotein with an apparent Mr of 32,000 on polyacrylamide gel electrophoresis. Now, it is also known as PPP1R1B, phosphoprotein phosphatase 1 regulatory subunit 1B, based on its major biochemical property, which is to inhibit phosphoprotein phosphatase 1 (PPP1, previously known as PP1) when DARPP-32 is phosphorylated on Thr-34 (see below). DARPP-32 is arguably one of the most prototypical proteins discovered in Paul Greengard's laboratory and certainly one of the most iconic (its name appears in more than 1200 Pubmed references and 236,000 hits in Google). Since its discovery 40 years ago, it has been the subject of intense study and has been key to understanding the complexity of signal transduction in neurons, especially in striatal projection neurons in which DARPP-32 is particularly abundant. Three related proteins with sequence similarities to DARPP-32 are found in vertebrates encoded by the *PPP1R1A*, *PPP1R1B*, and *PPP1R1C* genes, but only the first two are highly expressed in neurons. PPP1R1B/DARPP-32 has a number of unique features that distinguish it from the two other paralogues. This review summarizes what we have discovered about DARPP-32 over the past 40 years, focusing on the contributions of the laboratories of Paul Greengard and his close collaborators and placing them in the perspective of current knowledge of neuronal signaling mechanisms.

2. The discovery of DARPP-32

In the 1970s, Greengard and his colleagues identified mechanisms by which neurotransmitters exert many of their effects, through second messenger systems and activation of protein kinases (Greengard, 1978). In doing so they extended and generalized findings initially done in the study of glycogen metabolism in the liver and skeletal muscle (Krebs, 1997). These studies provided a basis for elucidating the molecular mechanisms of complex synaptic properties such as neuromodulation and synaptic plasticity. In the course of this work several novel second messenger-regulated protein kinases were identified and their actions investigated in neurons. In the late 1970s and early 1980s a major question was the identity of the substrates of these protein kinases, the "third messengers" that were ultimately responsible for the action of neurotransmitters and other intercellular messengers (Nestler & Greengard, 1983). In an attempt to identify these substrates and to determine whether they were the same in different neuronal cell types, new approaches were explored to compare potential substrates for various protein kinases in different brain regions. Notably, this was more than 10 years before the word proteome was coined and tools became available to explore it. Walaas, Nairn, and Greengard in 1983 published two papers describing many brain-region-specific proteins whose phosphorylation was enhanced by activation of diverse second messengers (Walaas, Nairn, & Greengard, 1983a, 1983b).

A few of these proteins attracted particular attention because they were detected in only one or a few of the brain regions investigated. Among these, a protein in the "soluble fraction" phosphorylated in response to cAMP stimulation was rapidly scrutinized because of its enrichment in the striatum, a region densely innervated by dopamine, which was known from previous work to act, at least in part, through stimulation of cAMP production (Kebabian & Greengard, 1971). Walaas and colleagues showed the phosphorylation of this protein was increased by cAMP and dopamine in striatal slices and named it "DARPP-32" for that reason (Walaas, Aswad, & Greengard, 1983). Attempts to purify DARPP-32 were rapidly successful and the first information obtained about its properties showed it resembled a molecule known as protein phosphatase 1 inhibitor-1 (I1) (Hemmings, Nairn, Aswad, & Greengard, 1984). I1 had been discovered in the lab of Philip Cohen in Dundee, a leader in the description of phosphatases, and shown to inhibit one of them, PP1. Sensitivity to phosphorylated I1 was in fact one of the key operational criteria used to classify protein phosphatases, at a time when their sequences were not known (Ingebritsen & Cohen, 1983). Hugh Hemmings Jr., the graduate student who had purified DARPP-32 in Paul Greengard's laboratory, went for a few weeks to Philip Cohen's laboratory and showed that DARPP-32 was a very potent PP1 inhibitor when it was phosphorylated by cAMP-dependent protein kinase (PKA) (Hemmings, Greengard, Tung, & Cohen, 1984). These discoveries were major steps in the early deciphering of how dopamine is acting in the striatum. It opened up a broad perspective for understanding of the mechanisms of neuromodulation by dopamine since phosphatase inhibition was potentially capable to have numerous regulatory effects on target cells by reinforcing the effects of diverse signaling pathways, including, but not limited to, cAMP.

Detailed immunohistofluorescence studies showed that DARPP-32 was highly enriched in all striatal projection neurons (SPNs, a.k.a. medium-size spiny neurons or MSNs), as well as in a number of other cells in dopaminoceptive regions such as the cerebral cortex and beyond, for instance in Purkinje cells in the cerebellum or in non-neuronal cells in the hypothalamus (Ouimet, Miller, Hemmings, Walaas, & Greengard, 1984). Further studies of DARPP-32 revealed that it had a wider distribution and more complex properties and functions than initially thought. First, DARPP-32 is expressed in many neurons and a few other cell types including some that do not receive dopamine innervation. For example, DARPP-32 is present at high levels in choroid plexus where it is regulated by serotonin (Snyder et al., 1992). Outside of the CNS, DARPP-32 is found, for example, in kidney (Aperia et al., 1990) or parathyroid (Meister, Askergren, Tunevall, Hemmings, & Greengard, 1991). Even in the main target of dopamine neurons, the striatum, it was apparent that the SPNs are divided in two populations, striatonigral and striatopallidal, with only the first being enriched in D1 dopamine receptors which activate adenylyl cyclase (Gerfen et al., 1990). Therefore the link between DARPP-32 and dopamine was not obligatory and turned out to be more complex than originally thought (Svenningsson et al., 2004). Part of this complexity is related to the multiple mechanisms of regulation of DARPP-32 by phosphorylation which we briefly discuss (for in-depth reviews see Svenningsson et al., 2004; Walaas, Hemmings, Greengard, & Nairn, 2011; Yger & Girault, 2011).

3. Regulation of DARPP-32 by phosphorylation of Thr34

DARPP-32 was discovered as a protein phosphorylated by PKA with a notable distribution in brain regions that generally overlapped with dopamine innervation (Walaas, Aswad, & Greengard, 1983). The first biochemical studies showed that DARPP-32 is a protein with little or no stable 3-D structure, making it resistant to acidic pH and heat (Hemmings, Nairn, Aswad, et al., 1984), corresponding to a typical intrinsically unstructured protein (Dancheck, Nairn, & Peti, 2008). The key sequences for PPP1 inhibition include the phosphorylated Thr34 and a conserved motif found in many proteins interacting with PPP1 (Lys-Ile-Gln-Phe or KIQF) (Kwon et al., 1997). It is likely that the combination of these two binding sites is responsible for the very low IC50 of pThr34-DARPP-32 on PPP1 activity (Desdouits, Cheetham, et al., 1995; Kwon et al., 1997).

Thr34 is phosphorylated by PKA and also by cGMP-dependent protein kinase, *in vitro* (Hemmings, Nairn, & Greengard, 1984) and in cells (Snyder et al., 1992; Tsou, Snyder, & Greengard, 1993). It is dephosphorylated by protein phosphatases 2A (PP2A, now PPP2) (Hemmings, Greengard, et al., 1984) and 2B (PP2B, now PPP3, a.k.a. calcineurin), a Ca^{2+}-activated phosphatase (King et al., 1984). This latter property provides, among others, an interesting cross-talk between cAMP and stimuli that raise intracellular free Ca^{2+}, including glutamate acting on NMDA receptors which can have opposing effects on DARPP-32 Thr34 phosphorylation (Halpain, Girault, & Greengard, 1990). Over the years a large number of extracellular signals increasing cAMP, or sometimes cGMP, levels have been shown to enhance DARPP-32 Thr34 phosphorylation (Svenningsson et al., 2004). Conversely various stimuli increasing intracellular free Ca^{2+} trigger its dephosphorylation, thereby finely tuning PPP1 activity (Nishi, Snyder, Nairn, & Greengard, 1999). Importantly the regulation and function of Thr34 in DARPP-32 is similar to that of the homologous threonine residue in I1 (PPP1R1A), which is also abundant in the striatum but has a much broader distribution throughout brain (Hemmings, Girault, Nairn, Bertuzzi, & Greengard, 1992). This raises the question of why DARPP-32 was selected throughout evolution to exhibit its unique expression pattern. The answer may come from additional properties of DARPP-32, which were discovered through the thorough investigation of its other phosphorylation sites (see Fig. 1).

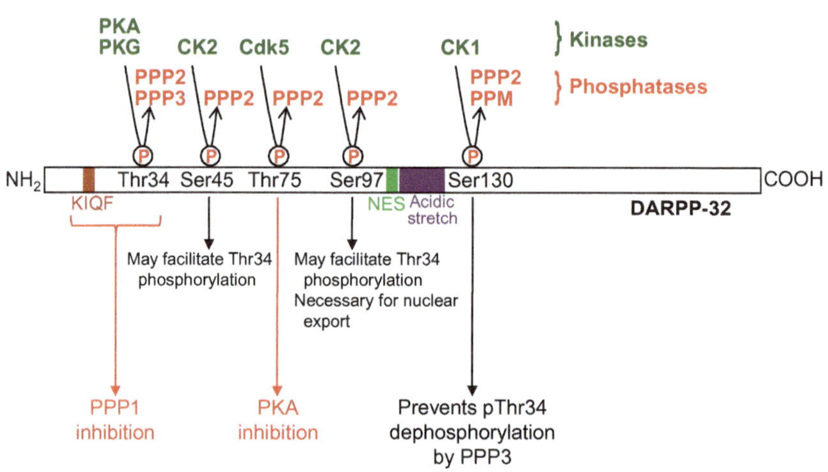

Fig. 1 Schematic representation of DARPP-32 main features. The main phosphorylated amino acid residues are indicated with the kinases that phosphorylate them (green) and the phosphatases that remove phosphates from these residues (red). Some additional features are indicated: KIQF, consensus motif (Lys-Ile-Gln-Phe) that binds PPP1 and contributes to its inhibition with phosphoThr34, the nuclear export sequence (NES) and the acidic stretch characteristic of DARPP-32. Other abbreviations: CK1, casein kinase 1; CK2, casein kinase 2; Cdk5, cyclin-dependent protein kinase 5; PKA, cAMP-dependent protein kinase; PKG, cGMP-dependent protein kinase; PPP1, protein phosphatase 1 (a.k.a. PP1); PPP2, protein phosphatase 2A (PP2A); PPP3, calcineurin (a.k.a. protein phosphatase 2B, PP2B, calcineurin); PPM, phosphoprotein phosphatase requiring Mg^{2+}/Mn^{2+} (a.k.a. PP2C).

4. Regulation of DARPP-32 by phosphorylation of multiple residues

When labeled with ^{32}P in living striatal slices, DARPP-32 is mostly phosphorylated on serine (Girault, Hemmings, Williams, Nairn, & Greengard, 1989; Halpain et al., 1990). Study of these site(s) first led to the discovery that DARPP-32 is a substrate for "casein kinase II," now referred to as protein kinase CK2, which is broadly expressed and highly active in the brain (Girault, Hemmings, Zorn, Gustafson, & Greengard, 1990). Mutant mice lacking CK2α in D1-expressing neurons have a strong phenotype including novelty-induced hyperlocomotion and exploratory behavior as well as defective motor control and motor learning, presumably resulting from enhanced D1 signaling (Rebholz, Zhou, Nairn, Greengard, & Flajolet, 2013). CK2 phosphorylates Ser45 and Ser97 (in mouse sequence numbering, Ser102 in rat) (Girault, Hemmings, et al., 1989). Although phosphorylation at these site(s) appears to facilitate DARPP-32 phosphorylation by PKA (Girault, Hemmings, et al., 1989), the phosphorylation of Thr34 was increased in CK2α KO mice (Rebholz et al., 2013), suggesting that this direct effect was overcome by indirect mechanisms *in vivo*. In agreement with this hypothesis, CK2 has a strong negative effect on $G\alpha_s$ and $G\alpha_{olf}$ (Rebholz et al., 2009), the latter being the G protein that activates adenylyl cyclase in SPNs (Corvol, Studler, Schonn, Girault, & Herve, 2001).

Importantly, phosphorylation of Ser97 regulates intracellular localization of DARPP-32, facilitating its nuclear export (Stipanovich et al., 2008). Dephosphorylation of Ser97 is catalyzed by PPP2 (Girault, Hemmings, et al., 1989). This dephosphorylation can be stimulated by phosphorylation of PPP2 regulatory subunit B56δ (PPP2R5D), triggering nuclear accumulation of pThr34-DARPP-32, thus facilitating inhibition of nuclear PPP1 and enhancing phosphorylation of histone H3 (Stipanovich et al., 2008). Conversely, dephosphorylation of Ser97 by PPP2 associated with a Ca^{2+}-sensitive regulatory subunit, PR72 (PPP2R3A) in response to glutamate stimulation favors nuclear accumulation of dephospho-Thr34-DARPP-32 and reduces PKA-dependent DARPP-32 signaling (Nishi et al., 2017).

DARPP-32 is also phosphorylated by casein kinase I (protein kinase CK1) on Ser130 (in mouse sequence, Ser137 in rat sequence) (Desdouits, Cohen, Nairn, Greengard, & Girault, 1995). This phosphorylation takes place at the C-terminus of a long stretch of acidic residue present in DARPP-32 from many species. It partly corrects the aberrant mobility of DARPP-32 in SDS/PAGE, which has a mobility of a 30–32-kDa protein whereas its real molecular mass is about 22kDa, an observation which led to the identification of this phosphorylation site (Desdouits, Cohen, et al., 1995). Phosphorylation of DARPP-32 by CK1 renders phospho-Thr34 resistant to the action of PPP3 (Desdouits, Siciliano, Greengard, & Girault, 1995) and is enhanced by stimulation of metabotropic glutamate receptors (Liu et al., 2001). Phospho-Ser130 is dephosphorylated by PPP2 and, especially *in vivo*, by PP2C (phosphoprotein phosphatase requiring Mg^{2+}/Mn^{2+}, PPM) (Desdouits, Siciliano, Nairn, Greengard, & Girault, 1998).

Finally, DARPP-32 Thr75 is a substrate of Cdk5 and when DARPP-32 is phosphorylated on that site it becomes an inhibitor of PKA catalytic subunit (Bibb et al., 1999). Thus, DARPP-32 can switch from mediating cAMP-induced PPP1 inhibition to inhibiting PKA in response to phosphorylation by Cdk5. The switch-like property is enhanced by the fact that PKA can activate PPP2 associated with B56δ (PPP2R5D), which dephosphorylates Thr-75 and amplifies cAMP signaling (Nishi et al., 2000).

Recent work has identified protein partners of DARPP-32 and emphasizes the importance of localized regulation of PKA activity by DARPP-32. DARPP-32 can interact with adducins (Engmann et al., 2015), which are important linkers between the actin/spectrin cytoskeleton and the plasma membrane. Phospho-Thr75-DARPP-32 facilitates phosphorylation of β-adducin at Ser713 through inhibition of a cAMP-dependent protein kinase/phosphatase-2A cascade thereby facilitating the depolymerization of the cortical cytoskeleton (Engmann et al., 2015). Behavioral evidence suggests that this regulatory mechanism is implicated in the effects of enriched environment on the properties of SPNs and their responsiveness to cocaine (Engmann et al., 2015). Dysregulation of this mechanism may be implicated in the depressive phenotype of a mouse model of Huntington's disease (Brito et al., 2019). Thr75 phosphorylation is enhanced by caffeine and may contribute to its psychostimulatory effects (Lindskog et al., 2002). Thr75 is also implicated in the interaction of DARPP-32 with the CLOCK protein, which prevents the binding of CLOCK to BMAL and its transcriptional effects, suggesting a possible link with caffeine-induced effects on mood (Trautmann, Burek, Hubner, Girault, & Engmann, 2020).

These regulations by multiple phosphorylation sites distinguish DARPP-32 from the other related inhibitors of PPP1, PPP1R1A and PPP1R1C. Experimental evidence suggests these sites are implicated in the fine regulation of DARPP-32 function. However, the resulting imbrication of these various regulatory mechanisms and the multiple potential positive and negative feedback interactions make it challenging to make simple predictions about their contribution to regulatory processes. Therefore it has been of great interest to use the power of computer modeling to dissect the potential regulation and roles of DARPP-32 in a more integrated context.

5. Computational modeling of DARPP-32 phosphorylation and activity

The positioning of DARPP-32 at the crossroad of signaling by important neurotransmitters with a strong importance in the control of basal ganglia functions and in several pathological conditions has attracted the attention of several computationally-oriented groups. A first attempt showed that DARPP-32 is a robust signal integrator, whose response depends on the delay between cAMP and Ca^{2+} signals (Fernandez, Schiappa, Girault, & Le Novere, 2006), providing a mechanism for tuning physiological responses to the timing of inputs to SPNs. Moreover, a non-intuitive convergent synergism of cAMP- and Ca^{2+}-dependent pathways on DARPP-32 phosphorylation was disclosed by a different study (Lindskog, Kim, Wikstrom, Blackwell, & Kotaleski, 2006). A collaborative effort between Paul Greengard's lab and his son, who is mathematician, used an approach of dimensionality reduction to provide evidence that the network in which DARPP-32 participates has particularly robust features in the presence of noise (Barbano et al., 2007). A model including additional steps identified a positive feedback loop consisting of PKA, PPP2, and phospho-Thr-75 DARPP-32 serving as a major switch for inducing LTD and LTP (Nakano, Doi, Yoshimoto, & Doya, 2010). Calcium input modulates this loop through the PPP3-CK1-Cdk5-Thr75 pathway and PPP2, whereas Ca^{2+} and dopamine inputs together activate the loop *via* PKA. Interestingly this positive feedback loop displayed robust bistable responses. A recent study also provided experimental and computational evidence for a switch-like PKA response in the nucleus of SPNs that requires a positive feedback through a phosphatase inhibitor like DARPP-32 (Yapo, Nair, Hellgren Kotaleski, Vincent, & Castro, 2018).

A different approach, investigating DARPP-32 as an index of signaling from synapses to the nucleus, revealed the importance of dendrite diameter in the cellular responses (Li, Gervasi, & Girault, 2015). Model predictions of nuclear DARPP-32 phosphorylation as a readout of cAMP signaling pointed to the particular efficiency of synapses on secondary dendrites to activate nuclear PKA, which was confirmed by live imaging (Li et al., 2015). Taken together these modeling approaches have shown that the complex regulatory steps in which DARPP-32 plays a central role have important properties including robustness to noise and bistability. They also led to the discovery of the importance of dendritic tree geometry on synapse-to-nucleus signaling. It is important to emphasize that the regulation of protein phosphatases by DARPP-32 is only one aspect of regulatory signaling networks in SPNs which also include several other regulatory proteins and phosphatase inhibitors (see chapter "cAMP-regulated phosphoproteins DARPP-32, ARPP16/19, and RCS modulate striatal signal transduction through protein kinases and phosphatases" by Christensen and Nairn, in this issue) that shape the particular responses of SPNs.

6. Role of DARPP-32 in the physiology of the basal ganglia

Since DARPP-32 is a phosphorylation-controlled phosphatase/kinase inhibitor, with the complex regulations emphasized above, it has been difficult to ascribe to it a simple function. Depending on its state of phosphorylation, its intracellular localization, and its interaction with partners, it can modulate a variety of targets. To try and address the functional implications of these signaling regulations, mutant mice lacking DARPP-32 either completely (Fienberg et al., 1998) or in specific cell types (Bateup et al., 2010) have been used. In addition, the consequences of point mutation of the various phosphorylation sites have been investigated in some detail (Svenningsson et al., 2003). The first conclusion from these studies was that, in laboratory housing conditions, mice do perfectly well without DARPP-32 (Fienberg et al., 1998). They breed and reproduce as their wild-type littermates. However, the consequences of the absence of the protein become apparent when mice are challenged. The initial studies revealed that a variety of direct or indirect responses to dopamine or other neurotransmitters are altered (Fienberg et al., 1998; Hiroi et al., 1999). In most instances these effects are not completely lost but require stronger stimuli to occur; in other words the dose-response curves are shifted to the right. However, in particular experimental conditions, the responses can be lost. For example, it is striking that in striatal slices, in the absence of DARPP-32, specific forms of long-term potentiation and depression (LTP and LTD) at corticostriatal synapses disappeared and were restored by bath application of a cell-permeant phosphatase inhibitor (Calabresi et al., 2000). An elegant study compared the consequences of a conditional loss of DARPP-32 in either of the two populations of SPNs (Bateup et al., 2010). The loss of DARPP-32 in striatonigral neurons decreased basal and cocaine-induced locomotion. Conversely, the loss of DARPP-32 in striatopallidal neurons produced a robust increase in locomotor activity and strongly reduced cataleptic response to the antipsychotic drug haloperidol. Point mutation of the main phosphorylation sites in knock-in mice (Svenningsson et al., 2003) allowed a dissection of their contribution *in vivo* and was helpful to address the role of DARPP-32 in pathology.

What is the role of DARPP-32 in the brain in physiological conditions? It is probably over simplistic to look for a straightforward correlation between a signaling molecule with complex regulatory functions and a "simple" functional output at the behavioral level. Several studies, however, implicate DARPP-32 in the processing of natural rewards. In rats it was shown that the phosphorylation pattern of DARPP-32 undergoes specific modifications in the nucleus accumbens in response to exposure to food reward, in line with the important role of dopamine in this context (see Scheggi, De Montis, & Gambarana, 2018 for a review). Mutation of DARPP-32 does not grossly impair food intake and DARPP-32 KO mice learn to nose-poke for food in the same way as wild-type controls (Heyser, Fienberg, Greengard, & Gold, 2000). However, the mice lacking DARPP-32 are impaired when the rewarded hole is reversed (Heyser et al., 2000). Moreover, motivation for food reward is decreased in Ser97Ala mutant mice (Stipanovich et al., 2008), providing evidence for a role of DARPP-32 in tuning food related behaviors. DARPP-32 also plays a role in some aspects of sexual behavior both in female (Mani et al., 2000; Meredith et al., 1998) and male (McHenry, Bell, Parrish, & Hull, 2012) rodents. These effects appear to indicate a role of DARPP-32 in hypothalamic nuclei, and, at least in females, its contribution to actions of progesterone. These results suggest that DARPP-32 is implicated at various levels in the correct processing of natural rewards and their consequences on behavior, possibly improving complex adaptive responses.

7. DARPP-32 in pathological conditions

The possible role of DARPP-32 in various pathological conditions has been investigated both in humans, using postmortem tissues and genetic approaches, and in animal models. Notably, besides its role in neurons, DARPP-32 and its shorter splice variant that lacks the N-terminal moiety including Thr34 and termed "truncated DARPP-32" (tDarpp), have been implicated in several cancers (see Avanes, Lenz, & Momand, 2019 for a recent review). These important findings are not discussed here and we focus on neurological and psychiatric conditions.

7.1 Drugs of abuse and addiction

Given the enrichment of DARPP-32 in SPNs, which are the major target of dopamine, and since drugs of abuse all share the ability to increase extracellular dopamine in the striatum, particularly in its ventral component, the nucleus accumbens (Di Chiara, 1999), it is not surprising that many drugs of abuse act *via* DARPP-32. Drugs of abuse alter DARPP-32 phosphorylation and their effects are modified in DARPP-32 KO mice (see Nairn et al., 2004 for a review). For example, DARPP-32 participates in the signaling mechanisms that promote ERK phosphorylation in response to cocaine (Valjent et al., 2005), an important step in the long-term responses of striatal neurons (Girault, Valjent, Caboche, & Herve, 2007). The use of point mutant mice pinpointed the importance of diverse components of DARPP-32 signaling. Mice bearing the Thr34Ala point mutation display a decreased locomotor sensitization in response to cocaine (Valjent et al., 2005) or morphine (Valjent et al., 2010) administration in a 2-injection protocol. Cocaine-induced conditioned place preference was also decreased in DARPP-32 KO (Zachariou et al., 2002) and Thr34Ala mutant mice (Zachariou et al., 2006). Acquisition of stable cocaine self-administration was delayed in Thr34Ala mice but both Thr34Ala and Ser130Ala DARPP-32 mutant mice self-administered more cocaine than their respective wild-type controls (Zhang et al., 2006). Interestingly it appears that acute injection and chronic self-administration of cocaine have different effects on Thr34 phosphorylation, which is increased in the first case (Bateup et al., 2008; Nishi et al., 2000) and decreased in the second (Zhang et al., 2006). Accordingly, induction of Cdk5 by chronic cocaine and the resulting phosphorylation of DARPP-32 at Thr75, may act as a negative feedback homeostatic mechanism with respect to the behavioral effects of cocaine (Bibb et al., 2001). In conclusion, although DARPP-32 is not necessary for the appearance of addiction-like behavior, it plays a dual modulatory role in animal models of cocaine addiction, with positive and negative effects on different aspects.

7.2 Movement disorders

The treatment of Parkinsonian patients with L-DOPA corresponds to another condition in which there is a strong pharmacological stimulation of dopamine signaling in SPNs. Converging evidence shows that this intermittent stimulation, beyond its initial symptomatic efficacy, contributes to the appearance of the abnormal movements triggered by L-DOPA that complicate treatment of Parkinson's disease after several years. These movements are designated as L-DOPA-induced dyskinesia or LID. Intermittent L-DOPA treatment alternates with periods of lack of dopamine stimulation, a situation that presents some similarity with what is observed in addiction when the self-administration of drugs triggers irregular and intense stimulation of dopaminergic neurotransmission. Although its striatal levels are not altered in Parkinsonian patients (Girault, Raisman-Vozari, Agid, & Greengard, 1989; Raisman-Vozari et al., 1990), DARPP-32 contributes to the generation of LID. In rats with lesioned dopamine neurons that display LID following L-DOPA treatment, the lack of synaptic depotentiation is accompanied by high levels of phospho-Thr34 DARPP-32 (Picconi et al., 2003). LID are attenuated in DARPP-32 KO mice as well as following treatment with a compound that prevents activation of the ERK pathway (Santini et al., 2007). Thr34Ala mutation diminishes LID and ERK activation (Santini et al., 2012) suggesting some similarities in the consequences of L-DOPA treatment and cocaine administration (Valjent et al., 2005). In the case of L-DOPA, however, ERK activation is not completely dependent on DARPP-32 (Alcacer et al., 2012; Gerfen, Paletzki, & Worley, 2008). Strikingly, conditional KO of DARPP-32 in striatonigral neurons abolishes LID (Bateup et al., 2010). These results indicate that DARPP-32 is an important component of the signaling pathways that result in LID, and may be involved in the induction or in the expression of these abnormal movements or in both.

7.3 Psychiatric disorders

Because of DARPP-32's role in mediating dopamine actions and the implication of dopamine in schizophrenia, several studies have been carried out in animal models and in humans to address the possible involvement of DARPP-32 in this disease or group of diseases. In mice various psychotomimetic drugs change DARPP-32 phosphorylation and their effects are altered by selective mutation of DARPP-32 phosphorylation sites (Svenningsson et al., 2003). These results supported the role of DARPP-32 in the signaling mechanisms activated by these drugs, but evidence for a possible role in human patients required the investigation of human brain samples. A first postmortem study found that DARPP-32 protein levels were decreased in the prefrontal cortex of schizophrenic patients as compared with matched controls (Albert et al., 2002). Similar observations were then reported in patients with schizophrenia or bipolar disorder (Ishikawa, Mizukami, Iwakiri, & Asada, 2007), in schizophrenic patients dead from suicide (Feldcamp, Souza, Romano-Silva, Kennedy, & Wong, 2008) and in schizophrenic patients (Kunii et al., 2019). A frequent 7-single nucleotide polymorphism (7-SNP) haplotype in DARPP-32 gene (*PPP1R1B*) predicting the expression levels of its isoforms in postmortem human brain, was associated with enhanced performance on cognitive tests depending on frontostriatal function (Meyer-Lindenberg et al., 2007). Although preliminary evidence suggested that this haplotype could be associated with risk of schizophrenia (Meyer-Lindenberg et al., 2007), the association of *PPP1R1B* locus with increased risk for major psychiatric was not found in other small scale studies or in major GWAS. However, relationships between genetic variants and expression levels have been confirmed. In a study including a large number of cases, tDarpp was found to be increased in the dorsolateral prefrontal cortex of patients with schizophrenia and bipolar disorder, and was strongly associated with *PPP1R1B* genotypes (Kunii et al., 2014). Some evidence even suggested that genetic variants associated with higher tDarpp expression predict worse cognitive performance (Kunii et al., 2014). Taken together these studies support the existence of a decrease in DARPP-32 associated with an increased expression of tDarpp in the prefrontal cortex of patients with schizophrenia and possibly bipolar disorder. Since tDarpp may oppose cAMP-regulated functions of DARPP-32, this combination suggests an overall decreased function of DARPP-32 in these conditions. How these observations are related with the disease mechanisms remains to be determined. One obvious link could be through the consequences of chronic treatment with antipsychotics, but, in rats, prolonged administration of dopamine antagonists or antipsychotics does not alter DARPP-32 or tDARPP levels (Grebb, Girault, Ehrlich, & Greengard, 1990; Kunii et al., 2014). It is therefore possible that the observed changes reflect primary cellular alterations in patients which warrant further exploration. Given the reported alterations of DARPP-32 in both bipolar disorder and schizophrenia and the heterogeneity of the latter condition, it is possible that changes in DARPP-32 are more pronounced in specific subgroups of patients. Whether this corresponds to particular clinical features or response to treatment is an intriguing question. However, the current impossibility to non-invasively evaluate DARPP-32 levels in living subjects makes it very difficult to address.

8. Conclusion

Throughout his academic career Paul Greengard provided major discoveries related to the mechanisms of action of neurotransmitters in general, but especially to the details of dopamine signaling. After the initial discovery that dopamine activated the production of cAMP in the striatum in the early 1970s, he pioneered the elucidation of the mechanisms by which cAMP acts in striatal neurons. This demonstrated the paramount importance of intracellular protein phosphorylation pathways, an idea that Greengard put forward early on. In-depth exploration of the regulation and properties of DARPP-32 in striatal neurons led to the discovery of a variety of mechanisms whose importance, or even existence, in brain was previously not known. They include the role of several protein kinases such as CK1, CK2, and Cdk5 as well as the importance and intricacy in neurons of the regulation of major protein phosphatases, PPP1, PPP2, PPP3, and PPM. Given that DARPP-32 is a regulatory protein with multiple functions at the crossroads of several signaling pathways, it is not surprising that its role cannot be restricted to a simple functional output. The use of computer modeling revealed that it provides robustness to intracellular signaling pathways and endows them with a bistable activity, switching between states of strong and weak cAMP signaling. As a result we can hypothesize that DARPP-32 enhances the contrast in the responses of the striatal network to stimulation, and increases the overall signal to noise ratio. A characteristic of the regulatory networks in which DARPP-32 participates is their high degree of redundancy, which makes them difficult to fully evaluate *in vivo*, since altering any single component has only relatively mild consequences. However the properties of these multiple intricate signaling networks, including their redundancy, are likely to be essential for the fine and adapted control of action and movement as well as its adaptation over time through reward-controlled procedural learning that characterizes the integrated function of striatal projection neurons.

Acknowledgments

The authors dedicate this review to the memory of Paul Greengard who was a visionary scientist, an extraordinary mentor, and a wonderful friend.

Research in the laboratory of J.-A.G. is currently supported by Inserm and *Sorbonne Université* and grants from *Agence Nationale de la Recherche* (ANR-16-CE16-0018,

ANR-19-CE16-0020), Laboratory of Excellence Bio-Psy (*Investissements d'Avenir*, ANR-11-IDEX-0004-02), and *Fondation pour la Recherche Médicale*. Research in the laboratory of A.C.N. is supported by the National Institutes of Health (NIH) (AG047270, AG062306, AG066508, DA018343) and the State of Connecticut Department of Mental Health and Addiction Services.

Conflict of interest statement

The authors have no conflicts of interest.

References

Albert, K. A., Hemmings, H. C., Jr., Adamo, A. I., Potkin, S. G., Akbarian, S., Sandman, C. A., et al. (2002). Evidence for decreased DARPP-32 in the prefrontal cortex of patients with schizophrenia. *Archives of General Psychiatry*, *59*, 705–712.

Alcacer, C., Santini, E., Valjent, E., Gaven, F., Girault, J. A., & Herve, D. (2012). Galpha(olf) mutation allows parsing the role of cAMP-dependent and extracellular signal-regulated kinase-dependent signaling in L-3,4-dihydroxyphenylalanine-induced dyskinesia. *The Journal of Neuroscience*, *32*, 5900–5910.

Aperia, A., Hökfelt, T., Meister, B., Bertorello, A., Fryckstedt, J., Holtbäck, U., et al. (1990). The significance of L-amino acid decarboxylase and DARPP-32 in the kidney. *American Journal of Hypertension*, (Suppl. 3), 11S–13S.

Avanes, A., Lenz, G., & Momand, J. (2019). Darpp-32 and t-Darpp protein products of PPP1R1B: Old dogs with new tricks. *Biochemical Pharmacology*, *160*, 71–79.

Barbano, P. E., Spivak, M., Flajolet, M., Nairn, A. C., Greengard, P., & Greengard, L. (2007). A mathematical tool for exploring the dynamics of biological networks. *Proceedings of the National Academy of Sciences of the United States of America*, *104*, 19169–19174.

Bateup, H. S., Santini, E., Shen, W., Birnbaum, S., Valjent, E., Surmeier, D. J., et al. (2010). Distinct subclasses of medium spiny neurons differentially regulate striatal motor behaviors. *Proceedings of the National Academy of Sciences of the United States of America*, *107*, 14845–14850.

Bateup, H. S., Svenningsson, P., Kuroiwa, M., Gong, S., Nishi, A., Heintz, N., et al. (2008). Cell type-specific regulation of DARPP-32 phosphorylation by psychostimulant and antipsychotic drugs. *Nature Neuroscience*, *11*, 932–939.

Bibb, J. A., Chen, J., Taylor, J. R., Svenningsson, P., Nishi, A., Snyder, G. L., et al. (2001). Effects of chronic exposure to cocaine are regulated by the neuronal protein Cdk5. *Nature*, *410*, 376–380.

Bibb, J. A., Snyder, G. L., Nishi, A., Yan, Z., Meijer, L., Fienberg, A. A., et al. (1999). Phosphorylation of DARPP-32 by Cdk5 modulates dopamine signalling in neurons. *Nature*, *402*, 669–671.

Brito, V., Giralt, A., Masana, M., Royes, A., Espina, M., Sieiro, E., et al. (2019). Cyclin-dependent kinase 5 dysfunction contributes to depressive-like behaviors in Huntington's disease by altering the DARPP-32 phosphorylation status in the nucleus accumbens. *Biological Psychiatry*, *86*, 196–207.

Calabresi, P., Gubellini, P., Centonze, D., Picconi, B., Bernardi, G., Chergui, K., et al. (2000). Dopamine and cAMP-regulated phosphoprotein 32 kDa controls both striatal long-term depression and long-term potentiation, opposing forms of synaptic plasticity. *The Journal of Neuroscience*, *20*, 8443–8451.

Corvol, J. C., Studler, J. M., Schonn, J. S., Girault, J. A., & Herve, D. (2001). Galpha(olf) is necessary for coupling D1 and A2a receptors to adenylyl cyclase in the striatum. *Journal of Neurochemistry*, *76*, 1585–1588.

Dancheck, B., Nairn, A. C., & Peti, W. (2008). Detailed structural characterization of unbound protein phosphatase 1 inhibitors. *Biochemistry*, *47*, 12346–12356.

Desdouits, F., Cheetham, J. J., Huang, H. B., Kwon, Y. G., Silva, E. F. D. E., Denefle, P., et al. (1995). Mechanism of inhibition of protein phosphatase 1 by DARPP-32: Studies with recombinant DARPP-32 and synthetic peptides. *Biochemical and Biophysical Research Communications*, *206*, 652–658.

Desdouits, F., Cohen, D., Nairn, A. C., Greengard, P., & Girault, J. A. (1995). Phosphorylation of DARPP-32, a dopamine-and cAMP-regulated phosphoprotein, by casein kinase I in vitro and in vivo. *The Journal of Biological Chemistry*, *270*, 8772–8778.

Desdouits, F., Siciliano, J. C., Greengard, P., & Girault, J. A. (1995). Dopamine- and cAMP-regulated phosphoprotein DARPP-32: Phosphorylation of Ser-137 by casein kinase I inhibits dephosphorylation of Thr-34 by calcineurin. *Proceedings of the National Academy of Sciences of the United States of America*, *92*, 2682–2685.

Desdouits, F., Siciliano, J. C., Nairn, A. C., Greengard, P., & Girault, J. A. (1998). Dephosphorylation of Ser-137 in DARPP-32 by protein phosphatases 2A and 2C: Different roles *in vitro* and in striatonigral neurons. *The Biochemical Journal*, *330*, 211–216.

Di Chiara, G. (1999). Drug addiction as dopamine-dependent associative learning disorder. *European Journal of Pharmacology*, *375*, 13–30.

Engmann, O., Giralt, A., Gervasi, N., Marion-Poll, L., Gasmi, L., Filhol, O., et al. (2015). DARPP-32 interaction with adducin may mediate rapid environmental effects on striatal neurons. *Nature Communications*, *6*, 10099.

Feldcamp, L. A., Souza, R. P., Romano-Silva, M., Kennedy, J. L., & Wong, A. H. (2008). Reduced prefrontal cortex DARPP-32 mRNA in completed suicide victims with schizophrenia. *Schizophrenia Research*, *103*, 192–200.

Fernandez, E., Schiappa, R., Girault, J. A., & Le Novere, N. (2006). DARPP-32 is a robust integrator of dopamine and glutamate signals. *PLoS Computational Biology*, *2*, e176.

Fienberg, A. A., Hiroi, N., Mermelstein, P. G., Song, W. J., Snyder, G. L., Nishi, A., et al. (1998). DARPP-32: Regulator of the efficacy of dopaminergic neurotransmission. *Science*, *281*, 838–839.

Gerfen, C. R., Engber, T. M., Mahan, L. C., Susel, Z., Chase, T. N., Monsma, F. J., Jr., et al. (1990). D_1 and D_2 dopamine receptor-regulated gene expression of striatonigral and striatopallidal neurons. *Science*, *250*, 1429–1432.

Gerfen, C. R., Paletzki, R., & Worley, P. (2008). Differences between dorsal and ventral striatum in Drd1a dopamine receptor coupling of dopamine- and cAMP-regulated phosphoprotein-32 to activation of extracellular signal-regulated kinase. *The Journal of Neuroscience*, *28*, 7113–7120.

Girault, J. A., Hemmings, H. C., Jr., Williams, K. R., Nairn, A. C., & Greengard, P. (1989). Phosphorylation of DARPP-32, a dopamine- and cAMP-regulated phosphoprotein, by casein kinase II. *The Journal of Biological Chemistry*, *264*, 21748–21759.

Girault, J. A., Hemmings, H. C., Jr., Zorn, S. H., Gustafson, E. L., & Greengard, P. (1990). Characterization in mammalian brain of a DARPP-32 serine kinase identical to casein kinase II. *Journal of Neurochemistry*, *55*, 1772–1783.

Girault, J. A., Raisman-Vozari, R., Agid, Y., & Greengard, P. (1989). Striatal phosphoproteins in Parkinson disease and progressive supranuclear palsy. *Proceedings of the National Academy of Sciences of the United States of America*, *86*, 2493–2497.

Girault, J. A., Valjent, E., Caboche, J., & Herve, D. (2007). ERK2: A logical AND gate critical for drug-induced plasticity? *Current Opinion in Pharmacology*, *7*, 77–85.

Grebb, J. A., Girault, J. A., Ehrlich, M., & Greengard, P. (1990). Chronic treatment of rats with SCH-23390 or raclopride does not affect the concentrations of DARPP-32 or its mRNA in dopamine-innervated brain regions. *Journal of Neurochemistry*, *55*, 204–207.

Greengard, P. (1978). Phosphorylated proteins as physiological effectors. *Science*, *199*, 146–152.

Halpain, S., Girault, J. A., & Greengard, P. (1990). Activation of NMDA receptors induces dephosphorylation of DARPP-32 in rat striatal slices. *Nature*, *343*, 369–372.

Hemmings, H. C., Jr., Girault, J. A., Nairn, A. C., Bertuzzi, G., & Greengard, P. (1992). The distribution of protein phosphatase inhibitor-1 in brain and peripheral tissues of various species: Comparison with DARPP-32. *Journal of Neurochemistry*, *59*, 1053–1061.

Hemmings, H. C., Jr., Greengard, P., Tung, H. Y. L., & Cohen, P. (1984). DARPP-32, a dopamine-regulated neuronal phosphoprotein, is a potent inhibitor of protein phosphatase-1. *Nature*, *310*, 503–505.

Hemmings, H. C., Jr., Nairn, A. C., Aswad, D. W., & Greengard, P. (1984). DARPP-32, a dopamine- and adenosine 3′:5′-monophosphate-regulated phosphoprotein enriched in dopamine-innervated brain regions. II Purification and characterization of the phosphoprotein from bovine caudate nucleus. *The Journal of Neuroscience*, *4*, 99–110.

Hemmings, H. C., Jr., Nairn, A. C., & Greengard, P. (1984). DARPP-32, a dopamine- and adenosine 3′:5′-monophosphate-regulated neuronal phosphoprotein. II. Comparison of the kinetics of phosphorylation of DARPP-32 and phosphatase inhibitor 1. *The Journal of Biological Chemistry*, *259*, 14491–14497.

Heyser, C. J., Fienberg, A. A., Greengard, P., & Gold, L. H. (2000). DARPP-32 knockout mice exhibit impaired reversal learning in a discriminated operant task. *Brain Research*, *867*, 122–130.

Hiroi, N., Fienberg, A. A., Haile, C. N., Alburges, M., Hanson, G. R., Greengard, P., et al. (1999). Neuronal and behavioural abnormalities in striatal function in DARPP-32-mutant mice. *European Journal of Neuroscience*, *11*, 1114–1118.

Ingebritsen, T. S., & Cohen, P. (1983). The protein phosphatases involved in cellular regulation. 1 Classification and substrate specificities. *European Journal of Biochemistry*, *132*, 255–261.

Ishikawa, M., Mizukami, K., Iwakiri, M., & Asada, T. (2007). Immunohistochemical and immunoblot analysis of dopamine and cyclic AMP-regulated phosphoprotein, relative molecular mass 32,000 (DARPP-32) in the prefrontal cortex of subjects with schizophrenia and bipolar disorder. *Progress in Neuro-Psychopharmacology & Biological Psychiatry*, *31*, 1177–1181.

Kebabian, J. W., & Greengard, P. (1971). Dopamine-sensitive adenyl cyclase: Possible role in synaptic transmission. *Science*, *174*, 1346–1349.

King, M. M., Huang, C. Y., Chock, P. B., Nairn, A. C., Hemmings, H. C., Jr., Chan, K. F., et al. (1984). Mammalian brain phosphoproteins as substrates for calcineurin. *The Journal of Biological Chemistry*, *259*, 8080–8083.

Krebs, E. G. (1997). Protein phosphorylation and cellular regulation. In N. Ringertz (Ed.), *Nobel Lectures, Physiology or Medicine 1991–1995* (pp. 72–89). Singapore: World Scientific Publishing Co.

Kunii, Y., Hino, M., Matsumoto, J., Nagaoka, A., Nawa, H., Kakita, A., et al. (2019). Differential protein expression of DARPP-32 versus calcineurin in the prefrontal cortex and nucleus accumbens in schizophrenia and bipolar disorder. *Scientific Reports*, *9*, 14877.

Kunii, Y., Hyde, T. M., Ye, T., Li, C., Kolachana, B., Dickinson, D., et al. (2014). Revisiting DARPP-32 in postmortem human brain: Changes in schizophrenia and bipolar disorder and genetic associations with t-DARPP-32 expression. *Molecular Psychiatry*, *19*, 192–199.

Kwon, Y. G., Huang, H. B., Desdouits, F., Girault, J. A., Greengard, P., & Nairn, A. C. (1997). Characterization of the interaction between DARPP-32 and protein phosphatase 1 (PP-1): DARPP-32 peptides antagonize the interaction of PP-1 with binding proteins. *Proceedings of the National Academy of Sciences of the United States of America*, *94*, 3536–3541.

Li, L., Gervasi, N., & Girault, J. A. (2015). Dendritic geometry shapes neuronal cAMP signalling to the nucleus. *Nature Communications*, *6*(6319), 1–15.

Lindskog, M., Kim, M., Wikstrom, M. A., Blackwell, K. T., & Kotaleski, J. H. (2006). Transient calcium and dopamine increase PKA activity and DARPP-32 phosphorylation. *PLoS Computational Biology*, *2*, e119.

Lindskog, M., Svenningsson, P., Pozzi, L., Kim, Y., Fienberg, A. A., Bibb, J. A., et al. (2002). Involvement of DARPP-32 phosphorylation in the stimulant action of caffeine. *Nature*, *418*, 774–778.

Liu, F., Ma, X. H., Ule, J., Bibb, J. A., Nishi, A., DeMaggio, A. J., et al. (2001). Regulation of cyclin-dependent kinase 5 and casein kinase 1 by metabotropic glutamate receptors. *Proceedings of the National Academy of Sciences of the United States of America*, *98*, 11062–11068.

Mani, S. K., Fienberg, A. A., O'Callaghan, J. P., Snyder, G. L., Allen, P. B., Dash, P. K., et al. (2000). Requirement for DARPP-32 in progesterone-facilitated sexual receptivity in female rats and mice. *Science*, *287*, 1053–1056.

McHenry, J. A., Bell, G. A., Parrish, B. P., & Hull, E. M. (2012). Dopamine D1 receptors and phosphorylation of dopamine- and cyclic AMP-regulated phosphoprotein-32 in the medial preoptic area are involved in experience-induced enhancement of male sexual behavior in rats. *Behavioral Neuroscience*, *126*, 523–529.

Meister, B., Askergren, J., Tunevall, G., Hemmings, H. C., Jr., & Greengard, P. (1991). Identification of a dopamine- and 3′,5′-cyclic adenosine monophosphate-regulated phosphoprotein of 32 kDa (DARPP-32) in parathyroid hormone-producing cells of the human parathyroid gland. *Journal of Endocrinological Investigation*, *14*, 655–661.

Meredith, J. M., Moffatt, C. A., Auger, A. P., Snyder, G. L., Greengard, P., & Blaustein, J. D. (1998). Mating-related stimulation induces phosphorylation of dopamine- and cyclic AMP-regulated phosphoprotein-32 in progestin receptor-containing areas in the female rat brain. *Journal of Neuroscience*, *18*, 10189–10195.

Meyer-Lindenberg, A., Straub, R. E., Lipska, B. K., Verchinski, B. A., Goldberg, T., Callicott, J. H., et al. (2007). Genetic evidence implicating DARPP-32 in human frontostriatal structure, function, and cognition. *The Journal of Clinical Investigation*, *117*, 672–682.

Nairn, A. C., Svenningsson, P., Nishi, A., Fisone, G., Girault, J. A., & Greengard, P. (2004). The role of DARPP-32 in the actions of drugs of abuse. *Neuropharmacology*, *47*(Suppl. 1), 14–23.

Nakano, T., Doi, T., Yoshimoto, J., & Doya, K. (2010). A kinetic model of dopamine- and calcium-dependent striatal synaptic plasticity. *PLoS Computational Biology*, *6*, e1000670.

Nestler, E. J., & Greengard, P. (1983). Protein phosphorylation in the brain. *Nature*, *305*, 583–588.

Nishi, A., Bibb, J. A., Snyder, G. L., Higashi, H., Nairn, A. C., & Greengard, P. (2000). Amplification of dopaminergic signaling by a positive feedback loop. *Proceedings of the National Academy of Sciences of the United States of America*, *97*, 12840–12845.

Nishi, A., Matamales, M., Musante, V., Valjent, E., Kuroiwa, M., Kitahara, Y., et al. (2017). Glutamate counteracts dopamine/PKA signaling via dephosphorylation of DARPP-32 Ser-97 and alteration of its cytonuclear distribution. *The Journal of Biological Chemistry*, *292*, 1462–1476.

Nishi, A., Snyder, G. L., Nairn, A. C., & Greengard, P. (1999). Role of calcineurin and protein phosphatase-2A in the regulation of DARPP-32 dephosphorylation in neostriatal neurons. *Journal of Neurochemistry*, *72*, 2015–2021.

Ouimet, C. C., Miller, P. E., Hemmings, H. C., Jr., Walaas, S. I., & Greengard, P. (1984). DARPP-32, a dopamine- and adenosine 3′:5′-monophosphate-regulated phosphoprotein enriched in dopamine-innervated brain regions. III Immunocytochemical localization. *The Journal of Neuroscience*, *4*, 111–124.

Picconi, B., Centonze, D., Hakansson, K., Bernardi, G., Greengard, P., Fisone, G., et al. (2003). Loss of bidirectional striatal synaptic plasticity in L-DOPA-induced dyskinesia. *Nature Neuroscience*, *6*, 501–506.

Raisman-Vozari, R., Girault, J. A., Moussaoui, S., Feuerstein, C., Jenner, P., Marsden, C. D., et al. (1990). Lack of change in striatal DARPP-32 levels following nigrostriatal dopaminergic lesions in animals and in parkinsonian syndromes in man. *Brain Research*, *507*, 45–50.

Rebholz, H., Nishi, A., Liebscher, S., Nairn, A. C., Flajolet, M., & Greengard, P. (2009). CK2 negatively regulates Galphas signaling. *Proceedings of the National Academy of Sciences of the United States of America*, *106*, 14096–14101.

Rebholz, H., Zhou, M., Nairn, A. C., Greengard, P., & Flajolet, M. (2013). Selective knock-out of the casein kinase 2 in d1 medium spiny neurons controls dopaminergic function. *Biological Psychiatry*, *74*, 113–121.

Santini, E., Feyder, M., Gangarossa, G., Bateup, H. S., Greengard, P., & Fisone, G. (2012). Dopamine- and cAMP-regulated phosphoprotein of 32-kDa (DARPP-32)-dependent activation of extracellular signal-regulated kinase (ERK) and mammalian target of rapamycin complex 1 (mTORC1) signaling in experimental parkinsonism. *The Journal of Biological Chemistry*, *287*, 27806–27812.

Santini, E., Valjent, E., Usiello, A., Carta, M., Borgkvist, A., Girault, J. A., et al. (2007). Critical involvement of cAMP/DARPP-32 and extracellular signal-regulated protein kinase signaling in L-DOPA-induced dyskinesia. *The Journal of Neuroscience*, *27*, 6995–7005.

Scheggi, S., De Montis, M. G., & Gambarana, C. (2018). DARPP-32 in the orchestration of responses to positive natural stimuli. *Journal of Neurochemistry*, *147*, 439–453.

Snyder, G. L., Girault, J. A., Chen, J. Y. C., Czernik, A. J., Kebabian, J., Nathanson, J. A., et al. (1992). Phosphorylation of DARPP-32 and protein phosphatase inhibitor-1 in rat choroid plexus: Regulation by factors other than dopamine. *The Journal of Neuroscience*, *12*, 3071–3083.

Stipanovich, A., Valjent, E., Matamales, M., Nishi, A., Ahn, J. H., Maroteaux, M., et al. (2008). A phosphatase cascade by which rewarding stimuli control nucleosomal response. *Nature*, *453*, 879–884.

Svenningsson, P., Nishi, A., Fisone, G., Girault, J. A., Nairn, A. C., & Greengard, P. (2004). DARPP-32: An integrator of neurotransmission. *Annual Review of Pharmacology and Toxicology*, *44*, 269–296.

Svenningsson, P., Tzavara, E., Carruthers, R., Rachleff, I., Wattler, S., Nehls, M., et al. (2003). Diverse psychotomimetics act through a common signaling pathway. *Science*, *302*, 1412–1415.

Trautmann, C., Burek, D., Hubner, C. A., Girault, J. A., & Engmann, O. (2020). A regulatory pathway linking caffeine action, mood and the diurnal clock. *Neuropharmacology*, *172*, 108133.

Tsou, K., Snyder, G. L., & Greengard, P. (1993). Nitric oxide/cGMP pathway stimulates phosphorylation of DARPP-32, a dopamine- and cAMP-regulated phosphoprotein, in the substantia nigra. *Proceedings of the National Academy of Sciences of the United States of America*, *90*, 3462–3465.

Valjent, E., Bertran-Gonzalez, J., Aubier, B., Greengard, P., Herve, D., & Girault, J. A. (2010). Mechanisms of locomotor sensitization to drugs of abuse in a two-injection protocol. *Neuropsychopharmacology*, *35*, 401–415.

Valjent, E., Pascoli, V., Svenningsson, P., Paul, S., Enslen, H., Corvol, J. C., et al. (2005). Regulation of a protein phosphatase cascade allows convergent dopamine and glutamate signals to activate ERK in the striatum. *Proceedings of the National Academy of Sciences of the United States of America*, *102*, 491–496.

Walaas, S. I., Aswad, D. W., & Greengard, P. (1983). A dopamine- and cyclic AMP-regulated phosphoprotein enriched in dopamine-innervated brain regions. *Nature*, *301*, 69–71.

Walaas, S. I., Hemmings, H. C., Jr., Greengard, P., & Nairn, A. C. (2011). Beyond the dopamine receptor: Regulation and roles of serine/threonine protein phosphatases. *Frontiers in Neuroanatomy*, *5*, 50.

Walaas, S. I., Nairn, A. C., & Greengard, P. (1983a). Regional distribution of calcium- and cyclic adenosine 3′:5′-monophosphate-regulated protein phosphorylation systems in mammalian brain. II. Soluble systems. *The Journal of Neuroscience*, *3*, 302–311.

Walaas, S. I., Nairn, A. C., & Greengard, P. (1983b). Regional distribution of calcium- and cyclic adenosine 3′:5′-monophosphate-regulated protein phosphorylation systems in mammalian brain. I. Particulate systems. *The Journal of Neuroscience*, *3*, 291–301.

Yapo, C., Nair, A. G., Hellgren Kotaleski, J., Vincent, P., & Castro, L. R. V. (2018). Switch-like PKA responses in the nucleus of striatal neurons. *Journal of Cell Science*, *131*, jcs216556. https://doi.org/10.1242/jcs.216556.

Yger, M., & Girault, J. A. (2011). DARPP-32, Jack of all trades… master of which? *Frontiers in Behavioral Neuroscience*, *5*, 56.

Zachariou, V., Benoit-Marand, M., Allen, P. B., Ingrassia, P., Fienberg, A. A., Gonon, F., et al. (2002). Reduction of cocaine place preference in mice lacking the protein phosphatase 1 inhibitors DARPP 32 or inhibitor 1. *Biological Psychiatry*, *51*, 612–620.

Zachariou, V., Sgambato-Faure, V., Sasaki, T., Svenningsson, P., Berton, O., Fienberg, A. A., et al. (2006). Phosphorylation of DARPP-32 at Threonine-34 is required for cocaine action. *Neuropsychopharmacology*, *31*, 555–562.

Zhang, Y., Svenningsson, P., Picetti, R., Schlussman, S. D., Nairn, A. C., Ho, A., et al. (2006). Cocaine self-administration in mice is inversely related to phosphorylation at Thr34 (protein kinase A site) and Ser130 (kinase CK1 site) of DARPP-32. *The Journal of Neuroscience*, *26*, 2645–2651.

CHAPTER FIVE

Effects of nicotine on DARPP-32 and CaMKII signaling relevant to addiction

Angela M. Lee[a,b] and Marina R. Picciotto[a,b,*]
[a]Department of Psychiatry, Yale University, New Haven, CT, United States
[b]Yale Interdepartmental Neuroscience Program, New Haven, CT, United States
[*]Corresponding author: e-mail address: marina.picciotto@yale.edu

Contents

Abstract

Paul Greengard brought to neuroscience the idea of, and evidence for, the role of second messenger systems in neuronal signaling. The fundamental nature of his contributions is evident in the far reach of his work, relevant to various subfields and topics in neuroscience. In this review, we discuss some of Greengard's work from the perspective of nicotinic acetylcholine receptors and their relevance to nicotine addiction. Specifically, we review the roles of dopamine- and cAMP-regulated phosphoprotein of 32 kDa (DARPP-32) and Ca^{2+}/calmodulin-dependent kinase II (CaMKII) in nicotine-dependent behaviors. For each protein, we discuss the historical context of their discovery and initial characterization, focusing on the extensive biochemical

Advances in Pharmacology, Volume 90
ISSN 1054-3589
https://doi.org/10.1016/bs.apha.2020.09.002

and immunohistochemical work conducted by Greengard and colleagues. We then briefly summarize contemporary understanding of each protein in key intracellular signaling cascades and evidence for the role of each protein with respect to systems and behaviors relevant to nicotine addiction.

Abbreviations

α-BTX α-bungarotoxin
CaM Ca^{2+}/calmodulin
CaMKII Ca^{2+}/calmodulin-dependent kinase II
Cdk5 cyclin-dependent kinase 5
CK1 casein kinase 1
CK2 casein kinase 2
CPP conditioned place preference
CREB cAMP response element binding protein
DA dopamine
DARPP-32 dopamine- and cAMP-regulated phosphoprotein of 32 kDa
ERK1/2 extracellular signal-regulated kinase 1/2
NAc nucleus accumbens
nAChRs nicotinic acetylcholine receptors
pCaMKIIα phosphorylated CaMKIIα
PKA protein kinase A
PP2A protein phosphatase 2A
VGCC voltage-gated calcium channels
VTA ventral tegmental area

1. Introduction

1.1 "Slow signaling": The role of second messengers and protein kinases in neural signaling

In 1971, Earl Sutherland received the Nobel Prize in Physiology or Medicine for his discovery of adenosine 3′:5′-monophosphate (cyclic AMP; cAMP) (Blumenthal, 2012). Research in the field of endocrinology was showing that hormones could raise cAMP levels in liver and muscle tissue (Blumenthal, 2012; Greengard & Nestler, 2013). Furthermore, it became clear that many of the effects of cAMP were mediated through a cAMP-dependent protein kinase, also known as protein kinase A (PKA). These discoveries inspired Greengard to investigate similar signaling pathways in neurons. However, contemporary thought in the nascent field of neuroscience was focused on the idea that neurons signal only through electrical impulses or changing postsynaptic membrane potentials, and Greengard's ideas were largely rejected at first (Greengard, 2000; Greengard & Nestler, 2013).

Nevertheless, Greengard pursued this line of research and ultimately built the foundation for understanding the role of second messengers and protein phosphorylation in neuronal signaling. Importantly, his work connected extracellular events to intracellular signaling cascades in neuronal tissues. He and his lab members demonstrated that the phosphorylation state of intracellular proteins could be regulated not only by depolarizing agents and electrical impulses, but also neurotransmitters such as dopamine (DA) and adrenergic receptor agonists (Alper, Palfrey, DeRiemer, & Greengard, 1980; Nestler & Greengard, 1980; Tsou & Greengard, 1982). From those early discoveries and through the following decades, Greengard's work was critical to understanding molecular mechanisms of neuronal signaling and their significance for neuropsychiatric illnesses.

1.2 Application to nicotine addiction

In this review, we discuss two signaling pathways centered around dopamine- and cAMP-regulated phosphoprotein of 32 kDa (DARPP-32) and Ca^{2+}/calmodulin-dependent kinase II (CaMKII). Both proteins were initially discovered and characterized by Greengard and colleagues, and have since come to be recognized as key signaling molecules with critical roles in a range of neuropsychiatric illnesses. Although much has been written about these proteins since their discoveries in the late 1970s and early 1980s, we discuss them here in the context of nicotine addiction, including a brief history of the early work on their characterization focusing on Greengard's contributions, a summary of our current understanding of protein function and significance, and finally an updated review of their roles in nicotine addiction.

2. Nicotine addiction

Tobacco smoking is a major public health problem worldwide and continues to be a leading cause of premature death in the United States (Carter et al., 2015). Nicotine is the primary psychoactive component in tobacco that drives addiction to smoking (Picciotto & Kenny, 2013). Nicotine addiction, similar to other drug addictions, progresses from initial drug exposure to chronic intake, which in susceptible individuals spirals into compulsive use and a vicious cycle of withdrawal and relapse (Cleck & Blendy, 2008; Koob & Volkow, 2016).

Nicotine acts through nicotinic acetylcholine receptors (nAChRs) in the mesocorticolimbic system to mediate the initial stages of nicotine addiction (Pistillo, Clementi, Zoli, & Gotti, 2015). The mesocorticolimbic system is generally regarded as an essential component of the brain circuits mediating reward and associative learning. These circuits are pathologically altered by drugs of abuse, contributing to addiction. Much research has focused on the system comprising dopaminergic projections from the ventral tegmental area (VTA) to its targets in the ventral striatum, especially the nucleus accumbens (NAc), and the prefrontal cortex (PFC), as well as GABAergic projections from the NAc back to the VTA and glutamatergic projections from the PFC to VTA and NAc (Kalivas & Volkow, 2005; Laviolette & van der Kooy, 2004). Although each drug of abuse acts at different receptors and has different acute effects, they commonly converge on mechanisms that increase DA release from the VTA to the NAc, and nicotine is no exception (Di Chiara & Imperato, 1988; Nestler, 2005).

nAChRs are pentameric ligand-gated cation channels stimulated by nicotine, or the endogenous ligand acetylcholine, to allow influx of cations, including calcium, into cells on which they are expressed. They are composed of a combination of α (α2–α10) and β (β2–β4) subunits in heteromeric receptors, or five α7 subunits in homomeric receptors (Gotti et al., 2007). The subunit composition of nAChRs can determine key aspects of nAChR function, such as localization, kinetics, ligand affinity and cation permeability (Dani, 2015; Fucile, 2004; Gotti et al., 2007).

In the VTA, nicotine causes sustained increases in DA release by increasing phasic burst firing of DA neurons which is critical to the transmission of reward-related information (Schultz, 2010; Zhang & Sulzer, 2004). Nicotine's actions at various nAChR subtypes in the VTA mediate this effect (Dani, 2015; Picciotto, Addy, Mineur, & Brunzell, 2008; Picciotto & Kenny, 2013). In particular, β2 subunit-containing nAChRs (β2* nAChRs, where * denotes other subunits in the pentamer) on VTA dopaminergic neurons are essential for initial nicotine reward (Picciotto et al., 1998; Pons et al., 2008). β2 subunits may partner with, among others, α4 and α6 subunits, which also play critical roles in nicotine's ability to activate VTA dopaminergic neurons and support self-administration (Gotti et al., 2010; Liu, Zhao-Shea, McIntosh, Gardner, & Tapper, 2012; Pons et al., 2008).

nAChRs exist in closed, open, and desensitized states. Low levels of nicotine, such as the levels attained in the plasma of smokers, desensitize nAChRs on midbrain dopaminergic neurons, especially the high-affinity α4β2* nAChRs, within seconds (Dani, 2015; Pidoplichko, DeBiasi, Williams, & Dani, 1997; Wooltorton, Pidoplichko, Broide, & Dani, 2003). Yet DA levels in the NAc are elevated on a more prolonged time scale (Benwell & Balfour, 1992; Di Chiara & Imperato, 1988; Schilström, Svensson, Svensson, & Nomikos, 1998). Nicotine acts on multiple receptor and cell types to elicit this sustained DA release, including α4α6* nAChRs on DA neurons (Liu et al., 2012), α4β2* nAChRs on GABAergic inputs to DA neurons (Mansvelder, Keath, & McGehee, 2002), and α7 nAChRs on glutamatergic terminals in the VTA (Jones & Wonnacott, 2004; Mansvelder & McGehee, 2000; Mao, Gallagher, & Mcgehee, 2011; Schilström et al., 1998). The net effect of differential desensitization of nAChR subtypes on different cell types is to shift the inhibitory/excitatory influence on dopaminergic neurons toward excitation (Picciotto & Kenny, 2013). Similarly, in the striatum and PFC, the cell type-specific distribution of distinct nAChR subtypes determines nicotine's effects on dopaminergic, as well as glutamatergic, GABAergic, and cholinergic signaling in these key brain regions (reviewed in Pistillo et al., 2015). However, in addition to intrinsic nAChR properties, the longer term ability of nicotine to induce prolonged signaling in mesocorticolimbic circuits relies on activation of intracellular signaling pathways that alter activity in these circuits in response to nicotine exposure, cues that predict delivery of the drug, or stress, all of which lead to relapse to nicotine seeking, even years after cessation.

3. DARPP-32

3.1 Discovery of DARPP-32

The engagement of the mesolimbic DA system as a key circuit in addiction suggests that key signaling events downstream of DA would be likely to contribute to behaviors relevant to nicotine addiction. Greengard's pursuit of slow signaling mechanisms in neurons led to the discovery that DA can stimulate or inhibit adenylyl cyclase by action at one of two classes of DA receptors, termed D-1 and D-2 (De Camilli, Macconi, & Spada, 1979; Kebabian & Calne, 1978; Kebabian & Greengard, 1971). Downstream of DA and cAMP activation in rat striatum, Walaas, Aswad and Greengard identified a DA and adenosine 3′:5′-monophosphate-regulated phosphoprotein with apparent molecular weight of 32 kDa, DARPP-32 (Ivar Walaas, Aswad, & Greengard, 1983). The protein was subsequently purified from bovine brain tissue (Hemmings, Nairn, Aswad, & Greengard, 1984), and the phosphoprotein's distribution, function, and regulation were described extensively (Hemmings, Nairn, et al., 1984; Ouimet, Miller, Hemmings, Walaas, & Greengard, 1984; Walaas & Greengard, 1984).

DARPP-32 is highly expressed in dopaminoceptive regions, including caudate putamen, NAc, olfactory tubercle, and parts of the extended amygdala (Girault, Walaas, Hemmings, & Greengard, 1990; Hemmings & Greengard, 1986; Ouimet, Hemmings, & Greengard, 1989; Ouimet, Lamantia, Goldman-Rakic, Rakic, & Greengard, 1992; Ouimet, Miller, et al., 1984; Walaas & Greengard, 1984). Puncta representing axon terminals were also observed in the projection areas of these dopaminoceptive neurons, including the globus pallidus, ventral pallidum, entopeduncular nucleus, and SN pars reticulata (Ouimet et al., 1989, 1992). A small number of DARPP-32-labeled fibers were observed in the VTA (Ouimet, Miller, et al., 1984).

3.2 DARPP-32 regulation

Work from the Greengard lab and others identified the key phosphorylation sites on DARPP-32, the kinases and phosphatases targeting these residues, and their effects on regulating DARPP-32 function and localization (Fig. 1). The complex interplay of kinases, phosphatases, and DARPP-32 phosphorylation states has been reviewed in detail elsewhere (Svenningsson et al., 2004; Walaas, Hemmings, Greengard, & Nairn, 2011; Yger & Girault, 2011) and will be summarized briefly here.

The four key phosphorylation sites on DARPP-32 are Thr34, Thr75, Ser97 and Ser130 (or Ser102 and Ser137, respectively, in rat). The two threonine sites determine DARPP-32's dual inhibitory effects. DARPP-32 was initially identified as a potent inhibitor of protein phosphatase-1 (PP1) when phosphorylated at Thr34 by PKA or protein kinase G (PKG), but not when dephosphorylated (Hemmings, Greengard, Tung, & Cohen, 1984; Hemmings, Williams, Konigsberg, & Greengard, 1984). Thr34 is dephosphorylated by protein phosphatase 2A (PP2A), and PP2B, but preferentially by PP2B, also known as calcineurin (Hemmings, Greengard, et al., 1984). Thr75, when phosphorylated by cyclin-dependent kinase 5 (Cdk5), inhibits PKA and can thus limit PKA-mediated phosphorylation of Thr34 (Bibb et al., 1999). PKA can also activate PP2A to dephosphorylate Thr75

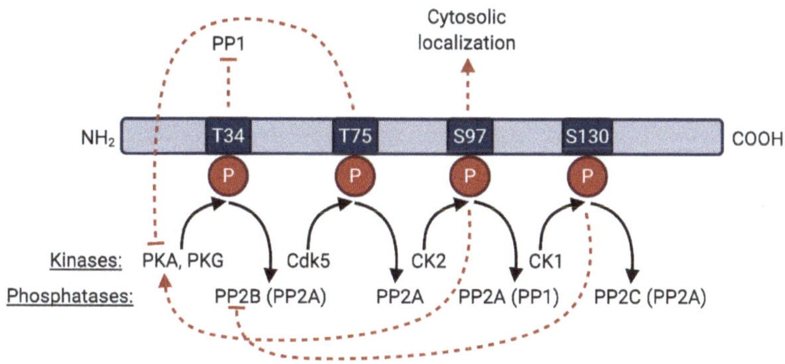

Fig. 1 DARPP-32 phosphorylation. The four main phosphorylation sites of DARPP-32, Thr34 (T34), Thr75(T75), Ser97(S97) and Ser130 (S130), are shown. Ser45 and Ser192 (not shown) are also phosphorylated, but their regulation and significance have not been concretely established. Solid lines with arrows indicate the kinases that phosphorylate, and phosphatases that dephosphorylate, each residue. Phosphatases in parentheses have been shown to dephosphorylate the respective residue, but are not the primary enzyme involved. Dashed red lines indicate the effect of the respective phosphorylated residue, where a flat-ended line indicates an inhibitory effect, and an arrow indicates an enhancing effect.

(Ahn et al., 2007). Thus, a single molecule, DARPP-32, regulates both a kinase and a phosphatase, each with significant effects on intracellular signaling (Bibb et al., 1999).

Two serine phosphorylation sites are also significant for DARPP-32 localization and function. Ser97 is phosphorylated by casein kinase 2 (CK2) and dephosphorylated primarily by PP2A but also by PP1 (Girault et al., 1989). Phosphorylation of Ser97 facilitates phosphorylation of Thr34 by PKA (Girault, Hemmings, Williams, Nairn, & Greengard, 1989). Further, Ser97 is positioned close to a nuclear export signal, and Ser97 phosphorylation induces cytosolic localization of DARPP-32, whereas Ser97 dephosphorylation increases nuclear localization (Stipanovich et al., 2008). Ser130 is phosphorylated by casein kinase 1 (CK1) and dephosphorylated by PP2A and PP2C, but preferentially by PP2C (Desdouits, Siciliano, Nairn, Greengard, & Girault, 1998). Phosphorylated Ser130 hinders calcineurin-mediated dephosphorylation of Thr34, thereby helping maintain Thr34 phosphorylation (Desdouits, Cohen, Nairn, Greengard, & Girault, 1995; Desdouits, Siciliano, Greengard, & Girault, 1995). Other phosphorylation sites, such as Ser45 and Ser192, have been identified but have unclear functional or physiologic relevance (Girault et al., 1989; Jin et al., 2005).

Importantly, the regulatory properties of DARPP-32 allow this molecule to serve as an integrative mechanism for the multiple signals that dopaminoceptive neurons receive (Svenningsson et al., 2004; Walaas et al., 2011). These signals include neurotransmitters and neuropeptides with receptors exposed to the extracellular space, like DA, serotonin, glutamate, GABA, adenosine, neurotensin, opioids, and cholecystokinin. DARPP-32 is also regulated by signaling molecules without extracellular receptors, such as nitric oxide and the steroid hormones estradiol and progesterone. Therapeutic drugs, in particular antipsychotics, antidepressants, and antiparkinsonian drugs, have also been linked to DARPP-32 signaling pathways (Svenningsson et al., 2004; Walaas et al., 2011; Yger & Girault, 2011). Of interest to the current review is how drugs of abuse affect DARPP-32. Nicotine, in addition to cocaine, amphetamine, ethanol, and even caffeine, can all regulate DARPP-32 phosphorylation (Nairn et al., 2004; Svenningsson, Nairn, & Greengard, 2008). The effects of this regulation have been demonstrated at both molecular and behavioral levels.

A key feature allowing diverse drugs of abuse and therapeutic agents to work through the same phosphoprotein is the differential regulation of DARPP-32 in striatonigral/direct pathway medium spiny neurons expressing D1-family receptors (D1R-MSNs) and striatopallidal/indirect pathway medium spiny neurons expressing D2-family receptors (D2R-MSNs) (Bateup et al., 2008; Nishi et al., 2000). One reason for differential regulation of DARPP-32 in direct and indirect pathways is that D1-family receptors are G_s-coupled, leading to increased cAMP, activation of PKA/PP2A, and subsequently, increased Thr34 and decreased Thr75 phosphorylation (Nishi et al., 2000; Nishi, Snyder, & Greengard, 1997). In contrast, D2-family receptors are G_i-coupled, inhibit cAMP generation and PKA/PP2A activity, and subsequently decrease Thr34 and increase Thr75 phosphorylation (Nishi et al., 2000, 1997). DA receptors are also targeted differentially by various pharmacologic agents. For example, cocaine inhibits DA reuptake and the increased DA levels alter Thr34 and Thr75 phosphorylation in both D1R-MSNs and D2R-MSNs in opposite directions based on DA receptor type (Bateup et al., 2008). Haloperidol, an antipsychotic drug, is a strong D2R antagonist and selectively increased Thr34 phosphorylation in D2R-MSNs, without affecting Thr34 or Thr75 phosphorylation in D1R-MSNs (Bateup et al., 2008). Clozapine is also an antipsychotic drug, but increases Thr34 phosphorylation in D2R-MSNs as well as phosphorylation of Thr75 in D2R-MSNs and Thr75 in D1R-MSNs, possibly by also acting at serotonergic receptors present on both MSN types

(Bateup et al., 2008). Thus DARPP-32 is differentially regulated in distinct MSN sub-populations, whose distinct output pathways can subsequently have different effects on behavior.

Furthermore, acute and chronic drug administration appear to have differential effects on DARPP-32 phosphorylation. For example, acute psychostimulant administration increases phospho-Thr34 and decreases phospho-Thr75 in striatal tissue, with differential regulation in D1R-MSNs and D2R-MSNs, but chronic administration decreases phospho-Thr34 and increases phospho-Thr75 (Bateup et al., 2008; Chen & Chen, 2005; Nishi & Shuto, 2017).

3.3 DARPP-32 and nicotine addiction

Studies in mouse neostriatal slices demonstrate a dose-dependent effect of nicotine on DARPP-32 phosphorylation (Table 1). At a low dose of 1 μM nicotine, Thr34 phosphorylation was decreased, likely through activation of α4β2 on dopaminergic terminals and subsequent activation of D2 receptors on striatopallidal/indirect pathway neurons. In contrast, at a high dose of 100 μM nicotine, Thr34 phosphorylation was increased transiently, likely through activation of α4β2 on dopaminergic terminals and α7 on glutamatergic terminals, stimulating more DA release and subsequent activation of lower affinity D1 receptors on striatonigral/direct pathway neurons (Hamada et al., 2004). The higher nicotine dose also decreased Thr75 phosphorylation and increased Ser97 and Ser130 phosphorylation, the cumulative effect of which would be to increase and stabilize Thr34 phosphorylation, thereby potentiating the D1 receptor-mediated signaling

Table 1 Nicotine-induced changes in DARPP-32 phosphorylation.

Nicotine conc/dose	T34	T75	S97	S130	Model and reference
1 mM	↓				Mouse striatal slices (Hamada, Higashi, Nairn, Greengard, & Nishi, 2004)
100 mM	↑	↓	↑	↑	Mouse striatal slices (Hamada et al., 2005, 2004)
0.8 mg/kg, sc	↑	↑			Female C57BL/6J mice (Zhu et al., 2005)
0.8 mg/kg, sc, 4 days	↑	↑			Female C57BL/6J mice (Zhu et al., 2005)

Sc = subcutaneously

pathway (Hamada et al., 2005). Of note, arterial nicotine concentrations in human smokers typically range from 20 to 60 ng/mL, or less than 0.5 μM (Benowitz, Hukkanen, & Jacob III, 2010). Nicotine's effects are highly dose-dependent and often exhibit an inverted U-shaped pattern of behavioral responses to increasing doses (Picciotto, 2003). Thus, it is important to consider *in vivo* effects.

Consistent with the ability of nicotine to increase release of DA in the striatum (Di Chiara & Imperato, 1988), both acute and subchronic nicotine exposure *in vivo* increased Thr34 and Thr75 phosphorylation in mouse striatum (combined dorsal and ventral) (Zhu et al., 2005). In the same study, DARPP-32 knock-out (KO) mice showed increased preference for, and intake of, oral nicotine solution and enhanced locomotor depression, suggesting either that nicotine-induced DARPP-32 phosphorylation *in vivo* normally serves an inhibitory role on nicotine's reinforcing effects, or that compensation for the lack of DARPP-32 in these animals reset a threshold for DA signaling in response to nicotine administration (Zhu et al., 2005). This contrasts with a decrease in behaviors related to cocaine reinforcement in DARPP-32 KO mice (Zachariou et al., 2002, 2006), and suggests that distinct circuit-level mechanisms are recruited by these two drugs with effects on the DA system. Given the differential effects of DA on DARPP-32 signaling in direct vs. indirect pathway MSNs, further research is needed on regulation of DARPP-32 by nicotine in specific cell types *in vivo*.

Outside of the striatum, nicotine self-administration followed by 7 days of abstinence increased DARPP-32 phosphorylation at Thr34 and Thr75 in the insular cortex of rats, but not in the mPFC or the NAc shell (Abdolahi, Acosta, Breslin, Hemby, & Lynch, 2010). At 1 day of abstinence, phospho-Thr75 was increased but not phospho-Thr34 in the insular cortex, and in the NAc core phospho-Thr75 was decreased at 7 days while phospho-Thr34 was unchanged. Importantly, reinstatement of nicotine self-administration was observed at 7 days of abstinence, but not 1-day abstinence. The regulation of intracellular signaling in the insular cortex is particularly interesting in light of the decrease in smoking observed in human subjects with damage to the insula (Naqvi, Rudrauf, Damasio, & Bechara, 2007). Further, the regulation of DARPP-32 following periods of abstinence suggests its role in the prolonged changes induced by nicotine that contribute to craving, withdrawal, and relapse in the absence of the drug.

In humans, one study examined single nucleotide polymorphisms (SNPs) in the DARPP-32 gene, *PPP1R1B*, and examined their association with smoking quantity and nicotine dependence. None of the six SNPs examined were significantly associated with smoking or nicotine dependence after correction for multiple comparisons. However, a haplotype of four SNPs was significantly associated with smoking quantity in the European-American cohort of the study (Beuten, Ma, Lou, Payne, & Li, 2007). This study appears to be the only genetic association between DARPP-32 and nicotine addiction in humans, although other studies have found associations between *PPP1R1B* haplotypes and cognitive function, schizophrenia (Meyer-Lindenberg et al., 2007), and personality traits (Li et al., 2011).

4. CaMKII

4.1 Discovery of CaMKII

While DA and cAMP signaling are central to the circuitry underlying addiction, a particular property of nAChRs that may contribute to plasticity in this and other systems is its permeability to calcium (Gotti et al., 2007). Thus, engagement of signaling molecules downstream of calcium entry is one likely mechanism contributing to the long-lasting behavioral changes that characterize nicotine addiction. CaMKII is one of many kinases in the calcium-calmodulin-dependent protein kinase family that are activated in response to calcium influx into neurons and other cell types. Other members of this family were discovered in skeletal muscle and liver tissues, and evidence for neuronal Ca^{2+}/calmodulin (CaM) kinases were discovered in independent labs concurrently (Colbran & Soderling, 1990; McGuinness, Lai, Greengard, Woodgett, & Cohen, 1983). Schulman and Greengard published a pair of papers in 1978 demonstrating the necessity of calcium and a cytosolic "calcium-dependent regulator" for calcium-dependent phosphorylation of rat and bovine cerebral cortex membrane proteins (Schulman & Greengard, 1978a, 1978b). Others determined the complete amino acid sequence of the calcium-dependent regulator, later termed calmodulin, from bovine brain tissue (Watterson, Sharief, & Vanaman, 1980). The CaM-dependent protein kinase was then purified by Kennedy and Greengard (1981). Immunohistochemistry, electron microscopy, and CaMKII activity assays showed that CaMKII was highly expressed in the brain, more prominently in somata, dendrites, and postsynaptic density than in axons and nerve terminals, and in hippocampus, lateral septum, cortex, neostriatum, and amygdala than in brainstem (Kennedy, Bennett, & Erondu, 1983; Kennedy & Greengard, 1981; Ouimet, McGuinness, & Greengard, 1984;

Walaas, Gorelick, & Greengard, 1989; Walaas, Nairn, & Greengard, 1983a, 1983b). Work in the Greengard lab also contributed to understanding how autophosphorylation of CaMKII produces a Ca^{2+}/calmodulin-independent form of the enzyme (Lai, Nairn, & Greengard, 1986), and to identifying Thr286 as the autophosphorylation site of CaMKIIα (Thiel, Czernik, Gorelick, Nairn, & Greengard, 1988).

4.2 Current views on CaMKII

CaMKII was hypothesized to be a "memory molecule" early on, with the discovery that autophosphorylation of CaMKII to a Ca^{2+}-independent form could produce persistent kinase activity extending beyond the initial post-synaptic Ca^{2+} influx (Colbran & Soderling, 1990). Since then, a wealth of evidence has identified the role of CaMKII in long-term potentiation and its interactions with key bindings partners, α-actinin and F-actin (reviewed in Coultrap & Bayer, 2012; Hell, 2014; Lisman, Schulman, & Cline, 2002). Emerging evidence also points to the role of CaMKII in long-term depression and in inhibitory synapses (Bayer & Schulman, 2019).

Abnormalities in CaMKII signaling are implicated in a variety of neuropsychiatric disorders, including mood disorders, schizophrenia, Alzheimer's disease, and drug addictions (Hell, 2014; Robison, 2014). Given its role in synaptic plasticity and its widespread distribution in the brain, it is not surprising that CaMKII in the mesocorticolimbic system is also involved in drug-induced neuronal and behavioral adaptations. A few examples of drugs of abuse linked to CaMKII include cocaine (Liu et al., 2014; Rich et al., 2016), alcohol (Easton et al., 2013), morphine (Wang et al., 2017), and amphetamine (Steinkellner et al., 2014). Below, we discuss the involvement of CaMKII in nicotine addiction in more detail.

4.3 CaMKII in nicotine addiction

4.3.1 CaMKII signaling downstream of nAChR activation

Nicotine-dependent activation of multiple nAChR subtypes can lead to increased calcium influx, after which several intracellular signaling cascades can be activated (Dajas-Bailador & Wonnacott, 2004; Pankratov & Lalo, 2014). Multiple lines of evidence have demonstrated that CaMKII is an important downstream mediator of acute and chronic nicotine exposure in both *in vitro* and *in vivo* experiments. In rat hippocampal cell culture, acute nicotine treatment increased levels of autophosphorylated CaMKIIα and CaMKIIβ proteins (Djemil et al., 2019). In mice, a single acute administration of nicotine (2 mg/kg, subcutaneously) increased CaMKII activity in the VTA, NAc, and amygdala (Jackson, Walters, & Damaj, 2009). After chronic nicotine exposure in mice, administered by subcutaneous osmotic minipumps for 14 days, phosphorylated CaMKIIα (pCaMKIIα) and total CaMKIIα protein levels were increased in the NAc (Jackson & Damaj, 2013). Calcium-dependent and calcium-independent CaMKII activity was elevated in the spinal cord after the same nicotine administration regimen (Damaj, 2005). Similarly, chronic nicotine administration resulting in a conditioned place preference (CPP) increased pCaMKIIα and pCaMKIIβ levels in the NAc and hippocampus CA1 of mice (Wilar, Shinoda, Sasaoka, & Fukunaga, 2019). An independent study also showed that nicotine CPP increased CaMKII activity in the VTA and NAc, but not PFC and hippocampus (Jackson, Muldoon, Walters, & Damaj, 2016). Taken together, these studies identify increases in CaMKII activity following a number of rewarding regimens of nicotine administration in rodents.

Evidence for manipulating CaMKII to alter nicotine reward-related behaviors has also been identified. CaMKII antagonists KN-62 and KN-93, but not the inactive analog KN-92, can block nicotine CPP in mice when administered intracerebroventricularly on the test day (Jackson et al., 2016). In the same study, heterozygous CaMKIIα$^{+/-}$ mice showed less nicotine CPP than their +/+ counterparts, although CPP was not completely abolished. Other nicotine-induced behaviors that may be mediated by CaMKII include nociception (Damaj, 2007a, 2007b), tolerance (Damaj, 2005), withdrawal (Jackson & Damaj, 2009; Jackson, Muldoon, De Biasi, & Damaj, 2015), and enhancement of cognitive functions (Wang et al., 2020).

Signaling molecules downstream of CaMKII are also necessary for behaviors relevant to nicotine addiction. Nicotine induces phosphorylation of extracellular signal-regulated kinase 1/2 (ERK1/2) in a CaMKII-dependent manner (Gubbins, Gopalakrishnan, & Li, 2010; Steiner, Heath, & Picciotto, 2007). Nicotine also increases phosphorylation of cAMP response element binding protein (CREB), a transcription factor, downstream of ERK and CaMKII activation (Hu, Liu, Chang, & Berg, 2002, Nakayama, Numakawa, Ikeuchi, & Hatanaka, 2001). Nicotine CPP can also increase levels of pCREB in key brain areas, including the NAc, VTA, PFC, dorsal striatum, hippocampus, and amygdala (Pascual, Pastor, & Bernabeu, 2009). Furthermore, CREB KO mice did not find nicotine rewarding (Walters, Cleck, Kuo, & Blendy, 2005). In the NAc shell, but not NAc core, nicotine

CPP increased pCREB levels, while CREB activity during CPP conditioning was necessary for nicotine CPP (Brunzell, Mineur, Neve, & Picciotto, 2009).

It is clear that a variety of nAChR subtypes are necessary for the development of nicotine addiction. While all nAChRs may allow calcium influx into cells on which they are expressed, homomeric α7 nAChRs are more selective for calcium flux compared to other subtypes (Fucile, 2004). These differences influence the downstream signaling pathways stimulated by nicotine's actions at different nAChRs (Fig. 2). For example, β2-mediated effects on pathways involving calcium signaling may depend on the opening of voltage-gated calcium channels (VGCC) (Dajas-Bailador, Mogg, & Wonnacott, 2002; Dajas-Bailador & Wonnacott, 2004; Damaj, 2007b). In contrast, VGCCs may be activated by α7 nAChRs, but they are not necessary for the sustained calcium signaling induced by α7 nAChR activation (Dajas-Bailador et al., 2002; Dajas-Bailador & Wonnacott, 2004; Tsuneki, Klink, Léna, Korn, & Changeux, 2000).

With respect to CaMKII signaling downstream of nAChR subtype-specific activation, there are mixed results. Studies in mice suggest that β2* nAChR-mediated calcium influx is primarily responsible for CaMKII activation. β2 KO mice or β2-selective antagonist DHβE in WT mice blocked acute and chronic nicotine-induced increases in CaMKII activity, pCaMKII, and pCREB in the VTA and NAc (Jackson & Damaj, 2013; Jackson et al., 2009). In these studies, α7 KO or treatment with α7-selective antagonist methyllycaconitine citrate (MLA) did not affect pCaMKII or pCREB levels. These results from *in vivo* experiments in key regions of the mesocorticolimbic circuit suggest that β2* nAChR-mediated CaMKII signaling contributes to nicotine reward.

In contrast, in other cell types, there appears to be an important role for α7 nAChRs in nicotine-induced CaMKII signaling. A study in PC12 cells, derived from rat adrenal medulla pheochromocytoma, used α7-specific agonists and antagonists to show that α7-mediated calcium transients were responsible for CaMKII activation as well as downstream phosphorylation of CREB and ERK1/2 (Gubbins et al., 2010). Electrophysiology studies in mouse brain slices suggest there may be a further distinction based on timing of the calcium transients. In mouse SN pars compacta slices from WT and β2 KO mice using the β2-selective antagonist DHβE, the authors suggest that β2* nAChRs are the major nAChR type responsible for nicotine-induced calcium transients (Tsuneki et al., 2000). However, there was a residual long-lasting calcium signal in β2 KO slices that was

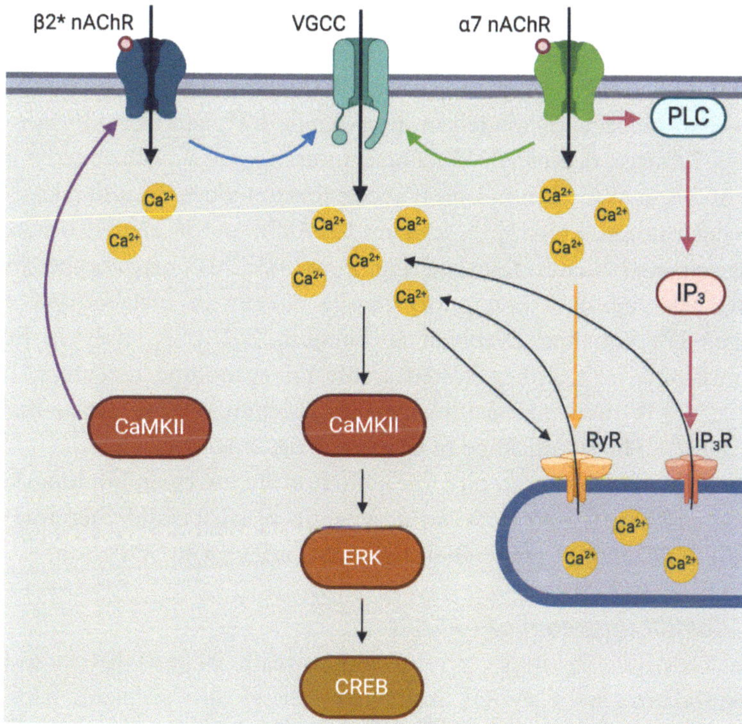

Fig. 2 nAChR subtype-dependent CaMKII signaling. Ca^{2+} permeability varies by nAChR subtype. In blue, β2* nAChRs allow influx of Na^+, K^+, and Ca^{2+} into cells on which they are expressed, but these nAChRs are less permeable to Ca^{2+} than α7 nAChRs. The majority of β2* nAChRs form heteromeric complexes with α4 subunits. The blue arrow emanating from the β2* nAChR indicates that cation influx through β2* nAChRs activates voltage-gated calcium channels (VGCC), which are necessary for β2* nAChR-mediated CaMKII activation and downstream ERK1/2 and CREB phosphorylation and activation. α7 nAChRs also allow Na^+, K^+, and Ca^{2+} to pass, but are more permeable to Ca^{2+} than β2* nAChRs. The green arrow emanating from the α7 nAChR indicates that depolarization from cation influx through α7 nAChRs can also activate VGCCs; however, this step is not necessary for α7-mediated calcium signaling. The yellow arrow from α7-mediated calcium influx to the ryanodine receptor (RyR) indicates that α7 nAChRs can activate RyRs directly to result in calcium-induced calcium release from intracellular stores, which can subsequently lead to CaMKII activation and downstream signaling. Pink arrows, leading from α7 nAChRs to PLC to IP_3 to IP_3 receptors, indicate that α7 nAChRs can also activate IP_3 receptors to induce calcium release from intracellular stores, again leading to CaMKII activation and downstream signaling. Finally, the leftmost purple arrow shows CaMKII interacting directly with β2* nAChRs; to date, there is no evidence of direct interaction of CaMKII with α7 nAChRs.

α7-dependent and blocked by α7-selective antagonists MLA and α-bungarotoxin (α-BTX). Similarly, in mouse ventral hippocampus-NAc synaptic co-cultures from WT or α7 KO mice, the sustained calcium response to nicotine depended on presynaptic α7*, but not β2*, nAChRs (Zhong, Talmage, & Role, 2013). These studies suggest a mechanism by which α7* nAChR activation stimulates IP_3 receptors to induce calcium release from intracellular stores, which then activates CaMKII, and pCaMKII is necessary for the sustained calcium response (Fig. 2). α7 nAChRs may also be coupled to $G\alpha_q$, allowing the receptor to engage directly in metabotropic PLC-mediated IP_3 signaling (Kabbani & Nichols, 2018). A study in human neuroblastoma cells also indicated a role for ryanodine receptors (RyR) in α7 nAChR-induced calcium-induced calcium release (Dajas-Bailador et al., 2002). The significance of these α7* nAChR-mediated calcium signaling pathways relevant to nicotine addiction are less clear, but long-lasting calcium signals may be critical for synaptic plasticity and therefore may contribute to nicotine-dependent behaviors relevant to addiction.

4.3.2 CaMKII upstream of nAChRs

While CaMKII signaling can be downstream of nAChR activation, phosphorylation by CaMKII and other kinases also regulates nAChRs. For example, phosphorylation by PKA or PKC and dephosphorylation by calcineurin can affect α4β2 nAChR assembly, stoichiometry, agonist sensitivity, and desensitization (Exley et al., 2006; Fenster et al., 1999; Pollock, Pastoor, Katnik, Cuevas, & Wecker, 2009; Wecker, Pollock, Pacheco, & Pastoor, 2010). At the neuromuscular junction, CaMKII is necessary for trafficking and recycling of internalized nAChRs (Martinez-Pena y Valenzuela, Mouslim, & Akaaboune, 2010), and αkap, a muscle-specific protein encoded within the *Camk2a* gene, can also regulate the degradation of nAChRs (Mouslim, Aittaleb, Hume, & Akaaboune, 2012).

A series of proteomic studies support a direct interaction between α4β2 nAChRs and CaMKIIα in the brain. Magnetic beads coupled to highly specific monoclonal antibodies against β2 nAChRs were used to pull down assembled α4β2* nAChRs and their interacting proteins in mouse forebrain tissue (Kabbani, Woll, Levenson, Lindstrom, & Changeux, 2007; McClure-Begley et al., 2013). In the 2013 study, different mouse genotypes, including WT, heterozygous and KO for either α4 or β2 nAChRs, generated gene dose-dependent variance in α4β2 nAChR abundance. The β2 interactome was then filtered to proteins with a significant and linear relationship to nAChR abundance. While CaMKIIα, β, δ, and γ were identified as proteins pulled down with α4β2 nAChRs, only CaMKIIα and γ levels correlated significantly with nAChR abundance. A follow-up study compared samples of mouse cortex after chronic nicotine administration and human cortex after tobacco exposure (McClure-Begley et al., 2016). Using stringent criteria, only eight proteins were identified as members of the β2 interactome that significantly correlated with β2 abundance in both mice and humans. Importantly, CaMKIIα was one of those eight proteins. Finally, a phosphoproteomic analysis of α4 and β2 nAChR subunits identified novel phosphorylation sites on the M3/M4 intracellular loop of the α4 subunit (Miller, Wilson, Lam, Nairn, & Picciotto, 2018). In HEK cells co-expressing nAChR subunits and protein kinases, CaMKIIα phosphorylated several serine residues on the α4 M3/M4 intracellular loop, some of which were distinct from sites phosphorylated by PKA. This study also provided the first demonstration of nAChR phosphorylation after acute nicotine exposure *in vivo* in mouse brain.

In contrast, two proteomics studies of the α7 nAChR interactome in mouse whole brain homogenates did not identify CaMKII isoforms as α7 nAChR binding partners (Mulcahy, Paulo, & Hawrot, 2018; Paulo, Brucker, & Hawrot, 2009). These studies used α-BTX to pull down α7 nAChRs and their interacting proteins. Interestingly, a study of simvastatin suggested that it could increase α7 nAChR activity and trafficking partly through NMDAR-mediated activation of CaMKII in mouse hippocampal slices (Chen et al., 2018).

5. Conclusion

Intracellular signaling pathways contribute to the neuronal plasticity that underlies long-lasting changes in behavior resulting in nicotine addiction. As reviewed briefly here, DARPP-32 regulation is a complex interplay between the four main phosphosites on the protein and the various regulatory signals that converge on DARPP-32. Importantly, these effects are specific to cell type, brain region, duration of drug administration, and drug dose. nAChRs are widely expressed across the brain, on soma and dendrites but particularly at presynaptic sites, where they modulate the release of various neurotransmitters that can subsequently affect DARPP-32 phosphorylation at their postsynaptic targets. Better understanding of DARPP-32 regulation in nicotine addiction will depend on diving into these specificities.

Compared to DARPP-32, there is more abundant evidence linking nAChR signaling to activation of CaMKII, and relatively good evidence for the role of CaMKII in mediating behaviors relevant to nicotine addiction. However, there is a lack of information on the role CaMKII plays in different stages of nicotine addiction, especially relapse. In addition, more work needs to be done to differentiate CaMKII and nAChR interactions in postsynaptic vs. presynaptic compartments. Finally, while proteomic studies have identified direct molecular interactions between CaMKII and nAChRs, more research is needed on how CaMKII is activated upstream of nAChRs, and on the contribution of CaMKII phosphorylation of nAChRs to long-term changes following nicotine exposure. There may be regional differences in different brain areas, and nAChR subtype-specific effects in this regulatory mechanism, as has been shown for effects of CaMKII downstream of nAChRs.

Finally, it is important to note, given the dedication Dr. Greengard had to promoting women in science as exemplified by the Pearl Meister Greengard Prize and the female scientists he trained in his lab, that the effects of sex on these signaling pathways have not been investigated. It is clear that sex hormones can alter DA dynamics, and it is therefore likely that there are sex differences in the intracellular signaling pathways downstream of nicotine-dependent DA signaling (Dluzen & Anderson, 1997; Zhang, Yang, Yang, Jin, & Zhen, 2008). Sex differences in nicotine addiction-related behaviors have been observed in both clinical and preclinical studies, underlining their importance (Flores, Pipkin, Uribe, Perez, & O'Dell, 2016; Lee, Calarco, McKee, Mineur, & Picciotto, 2020; Pogun & Yararbas, 2009; Smith, Bessette, Weinberger, Sheffer, & McKee, 2016). Future studies comparing tissue from male and female animals will be needed to elucidate any potential sex differences which would be essential for the development of specialized and more effective treatments for smoking, particularly in women.

Acknowledgments

Dr. Paul Greengard was MRP's graduate mentor and this article is a tribute to the influence his discoveries related to neuronal intracellular signaling have had on the work in our laboratory, as they have on the entire field of neuroscience. The idea that neurons are not just on-off switches, but instead, that second messenger signaling has long-lasting consequences on the information neurons can carry, is central to every experiment we have done in our laboratory. We thank Dr. Greengard for this and for his example as a mentor who was committed to training women in his laboratory.

This work was supported by National Institutes of Health grants DA050986, DA14241, MH077681, AA027989, T32 GM007205, and F30DA043943.

Figures were created using BioRender (BioRender.com).

Conflict of interest statement

The authors have no conflicts of interest to report.

References

Abdolahi, A., Acosta, G., Breslin, F. J., Hemby, S. E., & Lynch, W. J. (2010). Incubation of nicotine seeking is associated with enhanced protein kinase A-regulated signaling of dopamine- and cAMP-regulated phosphoprotein of 32 kDa in the insular cortex. *European Journal of Neuroscience*, *31*(4), 733–741.

Ahn, J. H., Jee, Y. S., McAvoy, T., Nishi, A., Janssens, V., Goris, J., et al. (2007). The B″/PR72 subunit mediates Ca2+-dependent dephosphorylation of DARPP-32 by protein phosphatase 2A. *Proceedings of the National Academy of Sciences of the United States of America*, *104*(23), 9876–9881.

Alper, S. L., Palfrey, H. C., DeRiemer, S. A., & Greengard, P. (1980). Hormonal control of protein phosphorylation in turkey erythrocytes. Phosphorylation by cAMP-dependent and Ca2+-dependent protein kinases of distinct sites in goblin, a high molecular weight protein of the plasma membrane. *The Journal of Biological Chemistry*, *255*(22), 11029–11039.

Batcup, H. S., Svenningsson, P., Kuroiwa, M., Gong, S., Nishi, A., Heintz, N., et al. (2008). Cell type-specific regulation of DARPP-32 phosphorylation by psychostimulant and antipsychotic drugs. *Nature Neuroscience*, *11*(8), 932–939.

Bayer, K. U., & Schulman, H. (2019). CaM kinase: Still inspiring at 40. *Neuron*, *103*(3), 380–394.

Benowitz, N., Hukkanen, J., & Jacob, P., III. (2010). Nicotine chemistry, metabolism and kinetics. *Handbook of Experimental Pharmacology*, *192*(192), 29–60.

Benwell, M. E. M., & Balfour, D. J. K. (1992). The effects of acute and repeated nicotine treatment on nucleus accumbens dopamine and locomotor activity. *British Journal of Pharmacology*, *105*(4), 849–856.

Beuten, J., Ma, J. Z., Lou, X. Y., Payne, T. J., & Li, M. D. (2007). Association analysis of the protein phosphatase 1 regulatory subunit 1B (PPP1R1B) gene with nicotine dependence in European- and African-American smokers. *American Journal of Medical Genetics, Part B: Neuropsychiatric Genetics*, *144*(3), 285–290.

Bibb, J. A., Snyder, G. L., Nishi, A., Yan, Z., Meijer, L., Flenberg, A. A., et al. (1999). Phosphorylation of DARPP-32 by Cdk5 modulates dopamine signalling in neurons. *Nature*, *402*(6762), 669–671.

Blumenthal, S. A. (2012). Earl sutherland and the discovery of cyclic AMP. *Perspectives in Biology and Medicine*, *55*(2), 236–249.

Brunzell, D. H., Mineur, Y. S., Neve, R. L., & Picciotto, M. R. (2009). Nucleus accumbens CREB activity is necessary for nicotine conditioned place preference. *Neuropsychopharmacology: Official Publication of the American College of Neuropsychopharmacology*, *34*, 1993–2001.

Carter, B. D., Abnet, C. C., Feskanich, D., Freedman, N. D., Hartge, P., Lewis, C. E., et al. (2015). Smoking and mortality—Beyond established causes. *New England Journal of Medicine*, *372*(7), 631–640.

Chen, P. C., & Chen, J. C. (2005). Enhanced Cdk5 activity and p35 translocation in the ventral striatum of acute and chronic methamphetamine-treated rats. *Neuropsychopharmacology*, *30*(3), 538–549.

Chen, T., Wang, Y., Zhang, T., Zhang, B., Chen, L., Zhao, L., et al. (2018). Simvastatin enhances activity and trafficking of α7 nicotinic acetylcholine receptor in hippocampal neurons through PKC and CaMKII signaling pathways. *Frontiers in Pharmacology*, *9*(APR), 1–12.

Cleck, J. N., & Blendy, J. A. (2008). Making a bad thing worse: Adverse effects of stress on drug addiction. *Journal of Clinical Investigation, 118*(2), 454–461.

Colbran, R. J., & Soderling, T. R. (1990). Calcium/calmodulin-dependent protein kinase II. *Current Topics in Cellular Regulation, 31*(C), 181–221.

Coultrap, S. J., & Bayer, K. U. (2012). CaMKII regulation in information processing and storage. *Trends in Neurosciences, 35*(10), 607–618.

Dajas-Bailador, F. A., Mogg, A. J., & Wonnacott, S. (2002). Intracellular Ca2+ signals evoked by stimulation of nicotinic acetylcholine receptors in SH-SY5Y cells: Contribution of voltage-operated Ca2+ channels and Ca2+ stores. *Journal of Neurochemistry, 81*(3), 606–614.

Dajas-Bailador, F. A., & Wonnacott, S. (2004). Nicotinic acetylcholine receptors and the regulation of neuronal signalling. *Trends in Pharmacological Sciences, 25*(6), 317–324.

Damaj, M. I. (2005). Calcium-acting drugs modulate expression and development of chronic tolerance to nicotine-induced antinociception in mice. *Journal of Pharmacology and Experimental Therapeutics, 315*(2), 959–964.

Damaj, M. I. (2007a). Behavioral modulation of neuronal calcium/calmodulin-dependent protein kinase II activity: Differential effects on nicotine-induced spinal and supraspinal antinociception in mice. *Biochemical Pharmacology, 74*(8), 1247–1252.

Damaj, M. I. (2007b). Nicotinic regulation of calcium/calmodulin-dependent protein kinase II activation in the spinal cord. *Journal of Pharmacology and Experimental Therapeutics, 320*(1), 244–249.

Dani, J. A. (2015). Neuronal nicotinic acetylcholine receptor structure and function and response to nicotine. In *Vol. 124. International review of neurobiology* (1st ed.).

De Camilli, P., Macconi, D., & Spada, A. (1979). Dopamine inhibits adenylate cyclase in human prolactin-secreting pituitary adenomas. *Nature, 278*(5701), 252–254.

Desdouits, F., Cohen, D., Nairn, A. C., Greengard, P., & Girault, J.-A. (1995). Phosphorylation of DARPP-32, a dopamine- and cAMP-regulated phosphoprotein, by casein kinase I in vitro and in vivo. *The Journal of Biological Chemistry, 270*(15), 8772–8778.

Desdouits, F., Siciliano, J. C., Greengard, P., & Girault, J. A. (1995). Dopamine- and cAMP-regulated phosphoprotein DARPP-32: Phosphorylation of Ser-137 by casein kinase I inhibits dephosphorylation of Thr-34 by calcineurin. *Proceedings of the National Academy of Sciences of the United States of America, 92*(7), 2682–2685.

Desdouits, F., Siciliano, J. C., Nairn, A. C., Greengard, P., & Girault, J. A. (1998). Dephosphorylation of Ser-137 in DARPP-32 by protein phosphatases 2A and 2C: Different roles in vitro and in striatonigral neurons. *Biochemical Journal, 330*(1), 211–216.

Di Chiara, G., & Imperato, A. (1988). Drugs abused by humans preferentially increase synaptic dopamine concentrations in the mesolimbic system of freely moving rats. *Proceedings of the National Academy of Sciences of the United States of America, 85*(14), 5274–5278.

Djemil, S., Chen, X., Zhang, Z., Lee, J., Rauf, M., Pak, D. T. S., et al. (2019). Activation of nicotinic acetylcholine receptors induces potentiation and synchronization within in vitro hippocampal networks. *Journal of Neurochemistry, 153*(4), 468–484.

Dluzen, D. E., & Anderson, L. I. (1997). Estrogen differentially modulates nicotine-evoked dopamine release from the striatum of male and female rats. *Neuroscience Letters, 230*(2), 140–142.

Easton, A. C., Lucchesi, W., Lourdusamy, A., Lenz, B., Solati, J., Golub, Y., et al. (2013). αcaMKII autophosphorylation controls the establishment of alcohol drinking behavior. *Neuropsychopharmacology, 38*(9), 1636–1647.

Exley, R., Moroni, M., Sasdelli, F., Houlihan, L. M., Lukas, R. J., Sher, E., et al. (2006). Chaperone protein 14-3-3 and protein kinase a increase the relative abundance of low agonist sensitivity human α4β2 nicotinic acetylcholine receptors in Xenopus oocytes. *Journal of Neurochemistry, 98*(3), 876–885.

Fenster, C. P., Beckman, M. L., Parker, J. C., Sheffield, E. B., Whitworth, T. L., Quick, M. W., et al. (1999). Regulation of α4β2 nicotinic receptor desensitization by calcium and protein kinase C. *Molecular Pharmacology*, *55*(3), 432–443.

Flores, R. J., Pipkin, J. A., Uribe, K. P., Perez, A., & O'Dell, L. E. (2016). Estradiol promotes the rewarding effects of nicotine in female rats. *Behavioural Brain Research*, *307*, 258–263.

Fucile, S. (2004). Ca2+ permeability of nicotinic acetylcholine receptors. *Cell Calcium*, *35*(1), 1–8.

Girault, J. A., Hemmings, H. C., Williams, K. R., Nairn, A. C., & Greengard, P. (1989). Phosphorylation of DARPP-32, a dopamine- and cAMP-regulated phosphoprotein, by casein kinase II. *The Journal of Biological Chemistry*, *264*(36), 21748–21759.

Girault, J. A., Walaas, S. I., Hemmings, H. C., & Greengard, P. (1990). ARPP-21, A cAMP-regulated phosphoprotein enriched in dopamine-innervated brain regions: Tissue distribution and regulation of phosphorylation in rat brain. *Neuroscience*, *37*(2), 317–325.

Gotti, C., Guiducci, S., Tedesco, V., Corbioli, S., Zanetti, L., Moretti, M., et al. (2010). Nicotinic acetylcholine receptors in the mesolimbic pathway: Primary role of ventral tegmental area α6β2* receptors in mediating systemic nicotine effects on dopamine release, locomotion, and reinforcement. *Journal of Neuroscience*, *30*(15), 5311–5325.

Gotti, C., Moretti, M., Gaimarri, A., Zanardi, A., Clementi, F., & Zoli, M. (2007). Heterogeneity and complexity of native brain nicotinic receptors. *Biochemical Pharmacology*, *74*(8), 1102–1111.

Greengard, P. (2000). The neurobiology of dopamine signaling. *Nobel Lectures, Physiology or Medicine 1996-2000* (pp. 1–20). Singapore: World Scientific Publishing Co.

Greengard, P., & Nestler, E. J. (2013). A conversation with Paul Greengard. *Annual Review of Pharmacology and Toxicology*, *53*(1), 1–16.

Gubbins, E. J., Gopalakrishnan, M., & Li, J. (2010). α7 nAChR-mediated activation of MAP kinase pathways in PC12 cells. *Brain Research*, *1328*, 1–11.

Hamada, M., Hendrick, J. P., Ryan, G. R., Kuroiwa, M., Higashi, H., Tanaka, M., et al. (2005). Nicotine regulates DARPP-32 (dopamine- and cAMP-regulated phosphoprotein of 32 kDa) phosphorylation at multiple sites in neostriatal neurons. *Journal of Pharmacology and Experimental Therapeutics*, *315*(2), 872–878.

Hamada, M., Higashi, H., Nairn, A. C., Greengard, P., & Nishi, A. (2004). Differential regulation of dopamine D1 and D2 signaling by nicotine in neostriatal neurons. *Journal of Neurochemistry*, *90*(5), 1094–1103.

Hell, J. W. (2014). CaMKII: Claiming center stage in postsynaptic function and organization. *Neuron*, *81*(2), 249–265.

Hemmings, H. C., & Greengard, P. (1986). DARPP-32, a dopamine- and adenosine 3':5'-monophosphate-regulated phosphoprotein: Regional tissue, and phylogenetic distribution. *Journal of Neuroscience*, *6*(5), 1469–1481.

Hemmings, H. C., Greengard, P., Tung, H. Y. L., & Cohen, P. (1984). DARPP-32, a dopamine-regulated neuronal phosphoprotein, is a potent inhibitor of protein phosphatase-1. *Nature*, *310*(5977), 503–505.

Hemmings, H. C., Nairn, A. C., Aswad, D. W., & Greengard, P. (1984). DARPP-32, a dopamine- and adenosine 3':5'-monophosphate-regulated phosphoprotein enriched in dopamine-innervated brain regions. II. Purification and characterization of the phosphoprotein from bovine caudate nucleus. *Journal of Neuroscience*, *4*(1), 99–110.

Hemmings, H. C., Williams, K. R., Konigsberg, W. H., & Greengard, P. (1984). DARPP-32, a dopamine- and adenosine 3':5'-monophosphate-regulated neuronal phosphoprotein. I. Amino acid sequence around the phosphorylated threonine. *The Journal of Biological Chemistry*, *259*(23), 14486–14490.

Hu, M., Liu, Q. S., Chang, K. T., & Berg, D. K. (2002). Nicotinic regulation of CREB activation in hippocampal neurons by glutamatergic and nonglutamatergic pathways. *Molecular and Cellular Neuroscience*, *21*(4), 616–625.

Ivar Walaas, S., Aswad, D. W., & Greengard, P. (1983). A dopamine- and cyclic AMP-regulated phosphoprotein enriched in dopamine-innervated brain regions. *Nature, 301*(5895), 69–71.

Jackson, K. J., & Damaj, M. I. (2009). L-type calcium channels and calcium/calmodulin-dependent kinase II differentially mediate behaviors associated with nicotine withdrawal in mice. *Journal of Pharmacology and Experimental Therapeutics, 330*(1), 152–161.

Jackson, K. J., & Damaj, M. I. (2013). Beta2-containing nicotinic acetylcholine receptors mediate calcium/calmodulin-dependent protein kinase-II and synapsin i protein levels in the nucleus accumbens after nicotine withdrawal in mice. *European Journal of Pharmacology, 701*(1–3), 1–6.

Jackson, K. J., Muldoon, P. P., De Biasi, M., & Damaj, M. I. (2015). New mechanisms and perspectives in nicotine withdrawal. *Neuropharmacology, 96*(PB), 223–234.

Jackson, K. J., Muldoon, P. P., Walters, C., & Damaj, M. I. (2016). Neuronal calcium/calmodulin-dependent protein kinase II mediates nicotine reward in the conditioned place preference test in mice. *Behavioural Pharmacology, 27*(1), 50–56.

Jackson, K. J., Walters, C. L., & Damaj, M. I. (2009). β2 Subunit-containing nicotinic receptors mediate acute nicotine-induced activation of calcium/calmodulin-dependent protein kinase II-dependent pathways in vivo. *Journal of Pharmacology and Experimental Therapeutics, 330*(2), 541–549.

Jin, M., Bateup, H., Padovan, J. C., Greengard, P., Nairn, A. C., & Chait, B. T. (2005). Quantitative analysis of protein phosphorylation in mouse brain by hypothesis-driven multistage mass spectrometry. *Analytical Chemistry*, 77(24), 7845–7851.

Jones, I. W., & Wonnacott, S. (2004). Precise localization of α7 nicotinic acetylcholine receptors on glutamatergic axon terminals in the rat ventral tegmental area. *Journal of Neuroscience, 24*(50), 11244–11252.

Kabbani, N., & Nichols, R. A. (2018). Beyond the channel: Metabotropic signaling by nicotinic receptors. *Trends in Pharmacological Sciences, 39*(4), 354–366.

Kabbani, N., Woll, M. P., Levenson, R., Lindstrom, J. M., & Changeux, J.-P. (2007). Intracellular complexes of the beta2 subunit of the nicotinic acetylcholine receptor in brain identified by proteomics. *Proceedings of the National Academy of Sciences of the United States of America, 104*(51), 20570–20575.

Kalivas, P. W., & Volkow, N. D. (2005). The neural basis of addiction: A pathology of motivation and choice. *The American Journal of Psychiatry, 162*(8), 1403–1413.

Kebabian, J. W., & Calne, D. B. (1978). Multiple receptors for brain dopamine. *Proceedings of the National Academy of Sciences of the United States of America, 75*(3), 1153–1156.

Kebabian, J. W., & Greengard, P. (1971). Dopamine-sensitive adenyl cyclase: Possible role in synaptic transmission. *Science, 174*(4016), 1346–1349.

Kennedy, M. B., Bennett, M. K., & Erondu, N. E. (1983). Biochemical and immunochemical evidence that the "major postsynaptic density protein" is a subunit of a calmodulin-dependent protein kinase. *Proceedings of the National Academy of Sciences of the United States of America, 80*(23 I), 7357–7361.

Kennedy, M. B., & Greengard, P. (1981). Two calcium/calmodulin-dependent protein kinases, which are highly concentrated in brain, phosphorylate protein I at distinct sites. *Proceedings of the National Academy of Sciences of the United States of America, 78*(2 II), 1293–1297.

Koob, G. F., & Volkow, N. D. (2016). Neurobiology of addiction: a neurocircuitry analysis. *Review Lancet Psychiatry, 3*(8), 760–773.

Lai, Y., Nairn, A. C., & Greengard, P. (1986). Autophosphorylation reversibly regulates the Ca2+/calmodulin-dependence of Ca2+/calmodulin-dependent protein kinase II. *Proceedings of the National Academy of Sciences of the United States of America, 83*(12), 4253–4257.

Laviolette, S. R., & van der Kooy, D. (2004). The neurobiology of nicotine addiction: Bridging the gap from molecules to behaviour. *Nature Reviews. Neuroscience*, *5*(1), 55–65.

Lee, A. M., Calarco, C. A., McKee, S. A., Mineur, Y. S., & Picciotto, M. R. (2020). Variability in nicotine conditioned place preference and stress-induced reinstatement in mice: Effects of sex, initial chamber preference, and guanfacine. *Genes, Brain and Behavior*, *19*(3), e12601.

Li, J., Ma, H., Zhou, H., Huang, Y., Wu, L., Li, J., et al. (2011). Association between DARPP-32 gene polymorphism and personality traits in healthy Chinese-Han subjects. *Journal of Molecular Neuroscience*, *44*(1), 48–52.

Lisman, J., Schulman, H., & Cline, H. (2002). The molecular basis of CaMKII function in synaptic and behavioural memory. *Nature Reviews. Neuroscience*, *3*(3), 175–190.

Liu, X., Liu, Y., Zhong, P., Wilkinson, B., Qi, J., Olsen, C. M., et al. (2014). CaMKII activity in the ventral tegmental area gates cocaine-induced synaptic plasticity in the nucleus accumbens. *Neuropsychopharmacology*, *39*(4), 989–999.

Liu, L., Zhao-Shea, R., McIntosh, J. M., Gardner, P. D., & Tapper, A. R. (2012). Nicotine persistently activates ventral tegmental area dopaminergic neurons via nicotinic acetylcholine receptors containing α4 and α6 subunits. *Molecular Pharmacology*, *81*(4), 541–548.

Mansvelder, H. D., Keath, J. R., & McGehee, D. S. (2002). Synaptic mechanisms underlie nicotine-induced excitability of brain reward areas. *Neuron*, *33*, 905–919.

Mansvelder, H. D., & McGehee, D. S. (2000). Long-term potentiation of excitatory inputs to brain reward areas by nicotine. *Neuron*, *27*(2), 349–357.

Mao, D., Gallagher, K., & Mcgehee, D. S. (2011). Nicotine potentiation of excitatory inputs to ventral tegmental area dopamine neurons. *Journal of Neuroscience*, *31*(18), 6710–6720.

Martinez-Pena y Valenzuela, I., Mouslim, C., & Akaaboune, M. (2010). Calcium/calmodulin kinase II-dependent acetylcholine receptor cycling at the mammalian neuromuscular junction in vivo. *Journal of Neuroscience*, *30*(37), 12455–12465.

McClure-Begley, T. D., Esterlis, I., Stone, K. L., Lam, T. T., Grady, S. R., Colangelo, C. M., et al. (2016). Evaluation of the nicotinic acetylcholine receptor-associated proteome at baseline and following nicotine exposure in human and mouse cortex. *ENeuro*, *3*(4), ENEURO.0166-16.2016.

McClure-Begley, T. D., Stone, K. L., Marks, M. J., Grady, S. R., Colangelo, C. M., Lindstrom, J. M., et al. (2013). Exploring the nicotinic acetylcholine receptor-associated proteome with iTRAQ and transgenic mice. *Genomics, Proteomics & Bioinformatics*, *11*(4), 207–218.

McGuinness, T. L., Lai, Y., Greengard, P., Woodgett, J. R., & Cohen, P. (1983). A multifunctional calmodulin-dependent protein kinase. Similarities between skeletal muscle glycogen synthase kinase and a brain synapsin I kinase. *FEBS Letters*, *163*(2), 329–334.

Meyer-Lindenberg, A., Straub, R. E., Lipska, B. K., Verchinski, B. A., Goldberg, T., Callicott, J. H., et al. (2007). Genetic evidence implicating DARPP-32 in human frontostriatal structure, function, and cognition. *Journal of Clinical Investigation*, *117*(3), 672–682.

Miller, M. B., Wilson, R. S., Lam, T. T., Nairn, A. C., & Picciotto, M. R. (2018). Evaluation of the phosphoproteome of mouse alpha 4/beta 2-containing nicotinic acetylcholine receptors in vitro and in vivo. *Proteomes*, *6*(4), 42.

Mouslim, C., Aittaleb, M., Hume, R. I., & Akaaboune, M. (2012). A role for the calmodulin kinase II-related anchoring protein (αkap) in maintaining the stability of nicotinic acetylcholine receptors. *Journal of Neuroscience*, *32*(15), 5177–5185.

Mulcahy, M. J., Paulo, J. A., & Hawrot, E. (2018). Proteomic investigation of murine neuronal α7-nicotinic acetylcholine receptor interacting proteins. *Journal of Proteome Research*, *17*(11), 3959–3975.

Nairn, A. C., Svenningsson, P., Nishi, A., Fisone, G., Girault, J. A., & Greengard, P. (2004). The role of DARPP-32 in the actions of drugs of abuse. *Neuropharmacology*, *47*(Suppl. 1), 14–23.

Nakayama, H., Numakawa, T., Ikeuchi, T., & Hatanaka, H. (2001). Nicotine-induced phosphorylation of extracellular signal-regulated protein kinase and CREB in PC12h cells. *Journal of Neurochemistry*, *79*(3), 489–498.

Naqvi, N. H., Rudrauf, D., Damasio, H., & Bechara, A. (2007). Damage to the insula disrupts addiction to cigarette smoking. *Science*, *315*(January), 531–534.

Nestler, E. J. (2005). Is there a common molecular pathway for addiction? *Nature Neuroscience*, *8*(11), 1445–1449.

Nestler, E. J., & Greengard, P. (1980). Dopamine and depolarizing agents regulate the state of phosphorylation of protein I in the mammalian superior cervical sympathetic ganglion. *Proceedings of the National Academy of Sciences of the United States of America*, 77(12 II), 7479–7483.

Nishi, A., Bibb, J. A., Snyder, G. L., Higashi, H., Nairn, A. C., & Greengard, P. (2000). Amplification of dopaminergic signaling by a positive feedback loop. *Proceedings of the National Academy of Sciences of the United States of America*, *97*(23), 12840–12845.

Nishi, A., & Shuto, T. (2017). Potential for targeting dopamine/DARPP-32 signaling in neuropsychiatric and neurodegenerative disorders. *Expert Opinion on Therapeutic Targets*, *21*(3), 259–272.

Nishi, A., Snyder, G. L., & Greengard, P. (1997). Bidirectional regulation of DARPP-32 phosphorylation by dopamine. *Journal of Neuroscience*, *17*(21), 8147–8155.

Ouimet, C. C., Hemmings, H. C., & Greengard, P. (1989). ARRP-21, a cyclic AMP-regulated phosphoprotein enriched in dopamine-innervated brain regions. II. Immunocytochemical localization in rat brain. *Journal of Neuroscience*, *9*(3), 865–875.

Ouimet, C. C., Lamantia, A. S., Goldman-Rakic, P., Rakic, P., & Greengard, P. (1992). Immunocytochemical localization of DARPP-32, a dopamine and cyclic- AMP-regulated phosphoprotein, in the primate brain. *The Journal of Comparative Neurology*, *323*(2), 209–218.

Ouimet, C. C., McGuinness, T. L., & Greengard, P. (1984). Immunocytochemical localization of calcium/calmodulin-dependent protein kinase II in rat brain. *Proceedings of the National Academy of Sciences of the United States of America*, *81*(17 I), 5604–5608.

Ouimet, C. C., Miller, P. E., Hemmings, H. C., Walaas, S. I., & Greengard, P. (1984). DARPP-32, a dopamine- and adenosine 3':5'-monophosphate-regulated phosphoprotein enriched in dopamine-innervated brain regions. III. Immunocytochemical localization. *Journal of Neuroscience*, *4*(1), 111–124.

Pankratov, Y., & Lalo, U. (2014). Calcium permeability of ligand-gated Ca2+ channels. *European Journal of Pharmacology*, *739*(C), 60–73.

Pascual, M. M., Pastor, V., & Bernabeu, R. O. (2009). Nicotine-conditioned place preference induced CREB phosphorylation and Fos expression in the adult rat brain. *Psychopharmacology*, *207*(1), 57–71.

Paulo, J. A., Brucker, W. J., & Hawrot, E. (2009). Proteomic analysis of an α7 nicotinic acetylcholine receptor interactome. *Journal of Proteome Research*, *8*(4), 1849–1858.

Picciotto, M. R. (2003). Nicotine as a modulator of behavior: Beyond the inverted U. *Trends in Pharmacological Sciences*, *24*(9), 493–499.

Picciotto, M. R., Addy, N. A., Mineur, Y. S., & Brunzell, D. H. (2008). It is not "either/or": Activation and desensitization of nicotinic acetylcholine receptors both contribute to behaviors related to nicotine addiction and mood. *Progress in Neurobiology*, *84*(4), 329–342.

Picciotto, M. R., & Kenny, P. J. (2013). Molecular mechanisms underlying behaviors related to nicotine addiction. *Cold Spring Harbor Perspectives in Medicine*, *3*(a012112).

Picciotto, M. R., Zoli, M., Rimondini, R., Léna, C., Marubio, L. M., Pich, E. M., et al. (1998). Acetylcholine receptors containing the β2 subunit are involved in the reinforcing properties of nicotine. *Nature, 391*(6663), 173–177.

Pidoplichko, V. I., DeBiasi, M., Williams, J. T., & Dani, J. A. (1997). Nicotine activates and desensitizes midbrain dopamine neurons. *Nature, 390*(6658), 401–404.

Pistillo, F., Clementi, F., Zoli, M., & Gotti, C. (2015). Nicotinic, glutamatergic and dopaminergic synaptic transmission and plasticity in the mesocorticolimbic system: Focus on nicotine effects. *Progress in Neurobiology, 124*, 1–27.

Pogun, S., & Yararbas, G. (2009). Sex differences in nicotine action. *Handbook of Experimental Pharmacology, 192*, 261–291.

Pollock, V. V., Pastoor, T., Katnik, C., Cuevas, J., & Wecker, L. (2009). Cyclic AMP-dependent protein kinase A and protein kinase C phosphorylate α4β2 nicotinic receptor subunits at distinct stages of receptor formation and maturation. *Neuroscience, 158*(4), 1311–1325.

Pons, S., Fattore, L., Cossu, G., Tolu, S., Porcu, E., McIntosh, J. M., et al. (2008). Crucial role of α4 and α6 nicotinic acetylcholine receptor subunits from ventral tegmental area in systemic nicotine self-administration. *Journal of Neuroscience, 28*(47), 12318–12327.

Rich, M. T., Abbott, T. B., Chung, L., Gulcicek, E. E., Stone, K. L., Colangelo, C. M., et al. (2016). Phosphoproteomic analysis reveals a novel mechanism of CaMKIIα regulation inversely induced by cocaine memory extinction versus reconsolidation. *Journal of Neuroscience, 36*(29), 7613–7627.

Robison, A. J. (2014). Emerging role of CaMKII in neuropsychiatric disease. *Trends in Neurosciences, 37*(11), 653–662.

Schilström, B., Svensson, H. M., Svensson, T. H., & Nomikos, G. G. (1998). Nicotine and food induced dopamine release in the nucleus accumbens of the rat putative role of α7 nicotinic receptors in the ventral tegmental area. *Neuroscience, 85*(4), 1005–1009.

Schulman, H., & Greengard, P. (1978a). Ca2+-dependent protein phosphorylation system in membranes from various tissues, and its activation by "calcium-dependent regulator". *Proceedings of the National Academy of Sciences of the United States of America, 75*(11), 5432–5436.

Schulman, H., & Greengard, P. (1978b). Stimulation of brain membrane protein phosphorylation by calcium and an endogenous heat-stable protein. *Nature, 271*(5644), 478–479.

Schultz, W. (2010). Dopamine signals for reward value and risk: Basic and recent data. *Behavioral and Brain Functions: BBF, 6*, 24.

Smith, P. H., Bessette, A. J., Weinberger, A. H., Sheffer, C. E., & McKee, S. A. (2016). Sex/gender differences in smoking cessation: A review. *Preventive Medicine, 92*, 135–140.

Steiner, R. C., Heath, C. J., & Picciotto, M. R. (2007). Nicotine-induced phosphorylation of ERK in mouse primary cortical neurons: Evidence for involvement of glutamatergic signaling and CaMKII. *Journal of Neurochemistry, 103*(2), 666–678.

Steinkellner, T., Mus, L., Eisenrauch, B., Constantinescu, A., Leo, D., Konrad, L., et al. (2014). In vivo amphetamine action is contingent on αCaMKII. *Neuropsychopharmacology, 39*(11), 2681–2693.

Stipanovich, A., Valjent, E., Matamales, M., Nishi, A., Ahn, J. H., Maroteaux, M., et al. (2008). A phosphatase cascade by which rewarding stimuli control nucleosomal response. *Nature, 453*(7197), 879–884.

Svenningsson, P., Nairn, A. C., & Greengard, P. (2008). DARPP-32 mediates the actions of multiple drugs of abuse. *Drug Addiction: From Basic Research to Therapy, 7*(2), 3–16.

Svenningsson, P., Nishi, A., Fisone, G., Girault, J.-A., Nairn, A. C., & Greengard, P. (2004). DARPP-32. An integrator of neurotransmission. *Annual Review of Pharmacology and Toxicology, 44*(1), 269–296.

Thiel, G., Czernik, A. J., Gorelick, F. S., Nairn, A. C., & Greengard, P. (1988). Ca2+/calmodulin-dependent protein kinase II: Identification of threonine-286 as the autophosphorylation site in the alpha subunit associated with the generation of Ca2+-independent activity. *Proceedings of the National Academy of Sciences of the United States of America, 85*(17), 6337–6341.

Tsou, K., & Greengard, P. (1982). Regulation of phosphorylation of proteins I, IIIa, and IIIb in rat neurohypophysis in vitro by electrical stimulation and by neuroactive agents. *Proceedings of the National Academy of Sciences of the United States of America, 79*(19 I), 6075–6079.

Tsuneki, H., Klink, R., Léna, C., Korn, H., & Changeux, J.-P. (2000). Calcium mobilization elicited by two types of nicotinic acetylcholine receptors in mouse substantia nigra pars compacta. *European Journal of Neuroscience, 12*(7), 2475–2485.

Walaas, S. I., Gorelick, F. S., & Greengard, P. (1989). Presence of calcium/calmodulin-dependent protein Kinase II in Nerve terminals of rat brain. *Synapse, 3*(4), 356–362.

Walaas, S. I., & Greengard, P. (1984). DARPP-32, a dopamine- and adenosine 3':5'-monophosphate-regulated phosphoprotein enriched in dopamine-innervated brain regions. I. Regional and cellular distribution in the rat brain. *Journal of Neuroscience, 4*(1), 84–98.

Walaas, S. I., Hemmings, H. C., Greengard, P., & Nairn, A. C. (2011). Beyond the dopamine receptor: Regulation and roles of serine/threonine protein phosphatases. *Frontiers in Neuroanatomy, 5*(AUG), 1–17.

Walaas, S. I., Nairn, A. C., & Greengard, P. (1983a). Regional distribution of calcium- and cyclic adenosine 3':5'-monophosphate-regulated protein phosphorylation systems in mammalian brain. I. Particulate systems. *The Journal of Neuroscience: The Official Journal of the Society for Neuroscience, 3*(2), 291–301.

Walaas, S. I., Nairn, A. C., & Greengard, P. (1983b). Regional distribution of calcium- and cyclic adenosine 3':5'-monophosphate-regulated protein phosphorylation systems in mammalian brain. II. Soluble systems. *Journal of Neuroscience, 3*(2), 302–311.

Walters, C. L., Cleck, J. N., Kuo, Y. C., & Blendy, J. A. (2005). μ-Opioid receptor and CREB activation are required for nicotine reward. *Neuron, 46*(6), 933–943.

Wang, X. L., Deng, Y. X., Gao, Y. M., Dong, Y. T., Wang, F., Guan, Z. Z., et al. (2020). Activation of α7 nAChR by PNU-282987 improves synaptic and cognitive functions through restoring the expression of synaptic-associated proteins and the CaM-CaMKII-CREB signaling pathway. *Aging, 12*(1), 543–570.

Wang, J., Li, M., Wang, P., Zha, Y., He, Z., & Li, Z. (2017). Inhibition of the lateral habenular CaMKII abolishes naloxone-precipitated conditioned place aversion in morphine-dependent mice. *Neuroscience Letters, 653*, 64–70.

Watterson, D. M., Sharief, F., & Vanaman, T. C. (1980). The complete amino acid sequence of the Ca2+-dependent modulator protein (calmodulin) of bovine brain. *The Journal of Biological Chemistry, 255*(3), 962–975.

Wecker, L., Pollock, V. V., Pacheco, M. A., & Pastoor, T. (2010). Nicotine-induced up regulation of α4β2 neuronal nicotinic receptors is mediated by the protein kinase c-dependent phosphorylation of α4 subunits. *Neuroscience, 171*(1), 12–22.

Wilar, G., Shinoda, Y., Sasaoka, T., & Fukunaga, K. (2019). Crucial role of dopamine D2 receptor signaling in nicotine-induced conditioned place preference. *Molecular Neurobiology, 56*(12), 7911–7928.

Wooltorton, J. R. A., Pidoplichko, V. I., Broide, R. S., & Dani, J. A. (2003). Differential desensitization and distribution of nicotinic acetylcholine receptor subtypes in midbrain dopamine areas. *Journal of Neuroscience, 23*(8), 3176–3185.

Yger, M., & Girault, J. A. (2011). DARPP-32, jack of all trades...master of which? *Frontiers in Behavioral Neuroscience, 5*(SEPTEMBER), 1–14.

Zachariou, V., Benoit-Marand, M., Allen, P. B., Ingrassia, P., Fienberg, A. A., Gonon, F., et al. (2002). Reduction of cocaine place preference in mice lacking the protein phosphatase 1 inhibitors DARPP 32 or inhibitor 1. *Biological Psychiatry*, *51*(8), 612–620.
Zachariou, V., Sgambato-Faure, V., Sasaki, T., Svenningsson, P., Berton, O., Fienberg, A. A., et al. (2006). Phosphorylation of DARPP-32 at threonine-34 is required for cocaine action. *Neuropsychopharmacology*, *31*(3), 555–562.
Zhang, H., & Sulzer, D. (2004). Frequency-dependent modulation of dopamine release by nicotine. *Nature Neuroscience*, 7(6), 581–582.
Zhang, D., Yang, S., Yang, C., Jin, G., & Zhen, X. (2008). Estrogen regulates responses of dopamine neurons in the ventral tegmental area to cocaine. *Psychopharmacology*, *199*(4), 625–635.
Zhong, C., Talmage, D. A., & Role, L. W. (2013). Nicotine elicits prolonged calcium signaling along ventral hippocampal axons. *PLoS ONE*, *8*(12), 1–14.
Zhu, H., Lee, M. S., Guan, F., Agatsuma, S., Scott, D., Fabrizio, K., et al. (2005). DARPP-32 phosphorylation opposes the behavioral effects of nicotine. *Biological Psychiatry*, *58*(12), 981–989.

CHAPTER SIX

Modulation of dendritic spines by protein phosphatase-1

Jimcy Platholi[a,b] and Hugh C. Hemmings Jr.[a,c,*]
[a]Department of Anesthesiology, Weill Cornell Medicine, New York, NY, United States
[b]Feil Family Brain and Mind Research Institute, Weill Cornell Medicine, New York, NY, United States
[c]Department of Pharmacology, Weill Cornell Medicine, New York, NY, United States
*Corresponding author: e-mail address: hchemmi@med.cornell.edu

Contents

Abstract

Protein phosphatase-1 (PP-1), a highly conserved multifunctional serine/threonine phosphatase, is enriched in dendritic spines where it plays a major role in modulating excitatory synaptic activity. In addition to established functions in spine maturation and development, multi-subunit holoenzyme forms of PP-1 modulate higher-order cognitive functions such learning and memory. Mechanisms involved in regulating PP-1 activity and localization in spines include interactions with neurabin and spinophilin, structurally related synaptic scaffolding proteins associated with the actin cytoskeleton. Since PP-1 is a critical element in synaptic development, signaling, and plasticity, alterations in PP-1 signaling in dendritic spines are implicated in various neurological and psychiatric disorders. The effects of PP-1 depend on its isoform-specific association with regulatory proteins and activation of downstream signaling pathways. Here we review the role of PP-1 and its binding proteins neurabin and spinophilin in both developing and established dendritic spines, as well as some of the disorders that result from its dysregulation.

Advances in Pharmacology, Volume 90
ISSN 1054-3589
https://doi.org/10.1016/bs.apha.2020.10.001

1. Introduction

A precisely regulated balance in the activities of protein kinases and phosphatases governs reversible phosphorylation states of key proteins essential for cellular function. Protein phosphatases, similar to protein kinases, include both protein serine-threonine phosphatases and protein tyrosine phosphatases based on the amino acid residues that they dephosphorylate. However, unlike the hundreds of kinases encoded by the human genome, protein phosphatases are relatively fewer in number. Their selectivity is conferred largely through formation of supramolecular complexes containing a variety of regulatory and targeting subunits that direct phosphatase catalytic subunits to specific subcellular locations and substrates.

Protein phosphatase-1 (PP-1) is a highly conserved serine/threonine phosphatase with multifunctional roles in diverse cellular processes. These multiple roles are mediated through interactions of the PP-1 catalytic subunit (PP-1c) with various regulatory subunits that regulate its activity and substrate specificity (Cohen, 2002). In addition, the PP-1c activity is modulated by the phosphorylation state of a number of regulatory or targeting subunits including inhibitor-1, inhibitor-2, dopamine- and cyclic AMP-regulated phosphoprotein-32 (DARPP-32), and PP-1 nuclear targeting subunit (PNUTS), which facilitate complex integrations of multiple cellular signaling pathways (Kim et al., 2003; Watanabe et al., 2001). PP-1 was initially identified based on its role in controlling glycogen metabolism and protein synthesis in skeletal muscle (Shenolikar & Nairn, 1991; Strålfors, Hiraga, & Cohen, 1985), but multiple functions for PP-1 have since been discovered in neurons including roles in neurite outgrowth (Oliver et al., 2002), synapse formation (Malchiodi-Albedi, Petrucci, Picconi, Iosi, & Falchi, 1997), ion channel function (Surmeier, Bargas, Hemmings, Nairn, & Greengard, 1995; Wang, Orser, Brautigan, & MacDonald, 1994) and neurotransmission (Colbran, 2004; Yan et al., 1999). Identification of PP-1 in dendritic spines highlighted its role in higher-order functions such as synaptic plasticity (Morishita et al., 2001; Mulkey, Endo, Shenolikar, & Malenka, 1994), learning and memory, and behavior (Genoux et al., 2002; Yu, Huang, Chang, & Gean, 2016). This review focuses on the roles of PP-1 in dendritic spines including the roles of its binding proteins neurabin and spinophilin in modulating both normal and pathological functions.

2. Expression and targeting of PP-1 in dendritic spines

In mammals, PP-1c is encoded by three genes giving rise to four isoforms: PP-1α, PP-1β, PP-1γ1, PP-1γ2, with the latter two originating by differential splicing of the same gene (Sasaki et al., 1990). The catalytic subunits for all four isoforms are ~80% identical in amino acid sequence and possess distinct tissue distributions and subcellular localizations (Cohen, 2002). Brain immunoreactivity for isoforms PP-1α and PP-1γ1 is heterogeneously distributed, with intense labeling in the prefrontal cortex, striatum, and hippocampal formation (Muly, Greengard, & Goldman-Rakic, 2001; Ouimet, da Cruz e Silva, & Greengard, 1995). Relatively more widespread brain distribution is found for PP-1β (Strack, Kini, Ebner, Wadzinski, & Colbran, 1999), with PP-1γ2 showing greater expression in non-neuronal cells (Shima et al., 1993) compared to neurons. Evidence from immunofluorescence and immuno-electron microscopy also reveals differential subcellular localization of brain PP-1 isoforms. PP-1β is found in discrete areas of the soma and dendrites co-localized with microtubules, while PP-1α and PP-1γ1 are highly enriched in presynaptic terminals and dendritic spines where they largely associate with the actin cytoskeleton (Fig. 1; Muly et al., 2001; Ouimet et al., 1995; Strack et al., 1999). Dendritic spines are actin-rich, postsynaptic structures that compartmentalize biochemical and cell biological processes critical for excitatory synaptic transmission and plasticity. These dynamic structures concentrate second messenger pathways, signaling enzymes, cytoskeletal elements, and transmembrane and scaffolding molecules appropriate for integration of regulated signaling. PP-1 complexes purified from rat cytoskeletal extracts include neurabin and spinophilin as scaffolding proteins that target PP-1α and PP-1γ1 to dendritic spines (Allen, Ouimet, & Greengard, 1997; MacMillan et al., 1999; Terry-Lorenzo et al., 2002). This facilitates efficient regulation of synaptic phosphoproteins involved in spine formation, signaling, and synaptic plasticity.

Neurabin and spinophilin, also known as neurabin 2, are structurally similar proteins containing shared regions with 43–86% homology (Fig. 2; Satoh et al., 1998): N-terminal actin-binding domains, PP-1 binding domains, PDZ domains (transmembrane receptor binding), and C-terminal coiled-coil domains (GTPase regulatory protein binding) (Kelker et al., 2007; Ryan et al., 2005). In addition, neurabin, but not spinophilin, contains a sterile α motif (SAM) domain in its C-terminus that may mediate

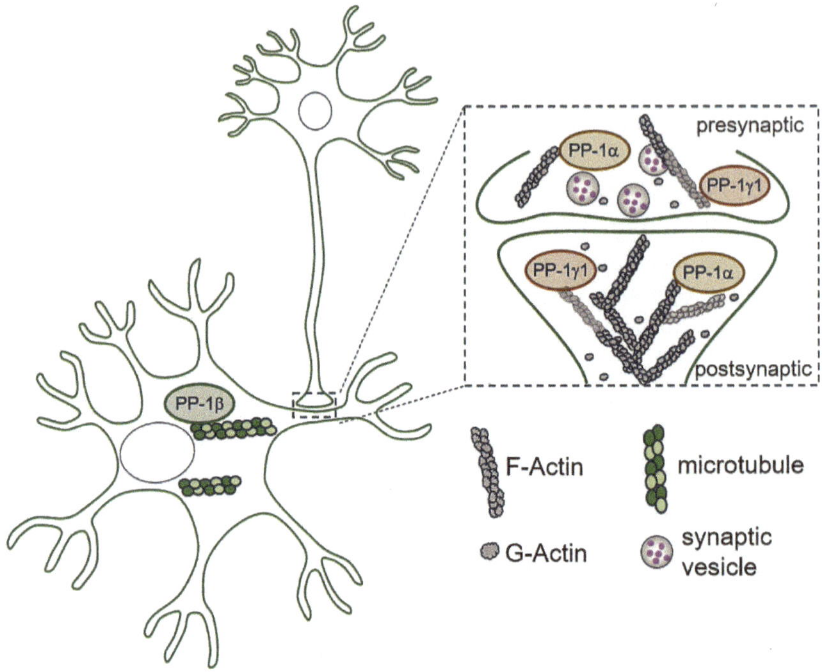

Fig. 1 Schematic diagram showing subcellular localizations of protein phosphatase-1 isoforms. PP-1β is found in the soma and dendrites co-localized with microtubules (left). PP-1α and PP-1γ1 are enriched in presynaptic terminals and postsynaptic dendritic spines associated with the actin cytoskeleton (inset).

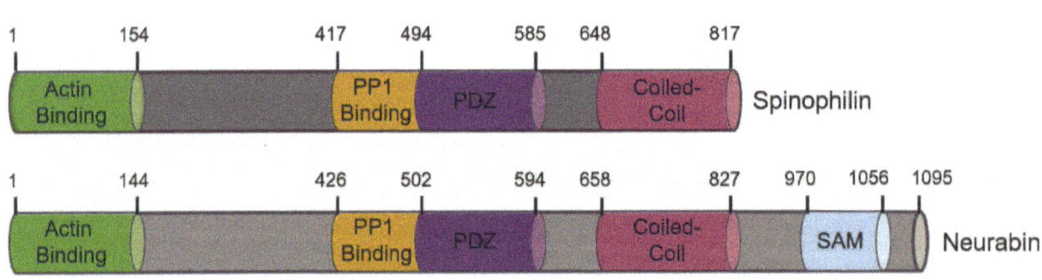

Fig. 2 Schematic diagram showing domain structures of spinophilin (top) and neurabin-1 (bottom) with corresponding amino acid residue numbers (Kelker et al., 2007).

additional protein interactions (Ju, Ragusa, Hudak, Nairn, & Peti, 2007). Both proteins are highly concentrated in the postsynaptic density [PSD] (Muly et al., 2004) and promote F-actin crosslinking in a phosphorylation-dependent manner (Grossman et al., 2004; Hsieh-Wilson, Allen, Watanabe, Nairn, & Greengard, 1999), and thereby play an important role in the formation and function of dendritic spines (Nakanishi et al., 1997). Deletion and genetic knockout studies reveal a role for neurabin in regulating F-actin polymerization involved in spine morphogenesis and glutamatergic synapse formation (Terry-Lorenzo et al., 2005; Zito, Knott, Shepherd, Shenolikar, & Svoboda, 2004), while spinophilin modulates spine morphology and density, and glutamatergic transmission (Evans, Robinson, Shi, & Webb, 2015; Feng et al., 2000).

3. Regulation of protein phosphatase-1 by neurabin and spinophilin

PP-1 interactions with neurabin, spinophilin, and the actin cytoskeleton within dendritic spines are ideally positioned to regulate dephosphorylation of substrates such as NMDA and AMPA glutamate receptors (Snyder, Fienberg, Huganir, & Greengard, 1998; Yan et al., 1999), calcium and potassium ion channels (Endo, Critz, Byrne, & Shenolikar, 1995; Surmeier et al., 1995), and calmodulin-dependent protein kinase II (CaMKII) and protein kinase A (PKA) signaling (Allen, 2004; Blitzer et al., 1998). Interestingly, neurabin, spinophilin, and many of their interacting partners are regulated by reversible phosphorylation, further modulating assembly and/or activity (McAvoy et al., 1999; Sarrouilhe, di Tommaso, Métayé, & Ladeveze, 2006). These multi-protein complexes regulate rapid signaling cascades involved in PP-1-mediated synaptic transmission and plasticity.

3.1 Activity

Neurabin is a F-actin binding protein that copurifies with PP-1α and PP-1γ from rodent brain extracts, interacts with PP-1α in a yeast two-hybrid screen, and potently inhibits the catalytic activity of PP-1α (McAvoy et al., 1999). Neurabin migrates at ~180 kDa on SDS-PAGE, but based on its amino acid composition is ~123 kDa (Nakanishi et al., 1997). At least two domains in neurabin have been identified to bind and target PP-1 isoforms to F-actin *in vitro* and in intact cells. The canonical PP-1 binding motif, particularly Phe-460, can interact with both PP-1α and PP-1γ1 isoforms, but auxiliary residues (473–479) C-terminal to the PP-1 binding domain further stabilize targeting of PP-1γ1 (Carmody, Baucum, Bass, & Colbran, 2008). Regulation of neurabin interactions with PP-1 is further modulated by phosphorylation. For example, phosphorylation of Ser-461 in neurabin by PKA, a site located C-terminal to the PP-1 binding domain, attenuates PP-1c interactions with neurabin, reducing its inhibition of PP-1c activity and revealing a novel mechanism whereby neuromodulators of the PKA pathway can regulate downstream activity of PP-1 (McAvoy et al., 1999; Oliver et al., 2002).

Spinophilin, named for its enrichment in dendritic spines, also has a lower molecular weight (89 kDa) compared to its apparent mass (134 kDa) estimated by SDS-PAGE (Allen et al., 1997). It has similar structural interactions with PP-1α and PP-1γ1 to those of neurabin, including the RVxF PP-1c-binding motif as well as residues outside this domain (478–494) that determine binding of PP-1c and inhibition of its activity, respectively (Hsieh-Wilson et al., 1999). Mutation of Phe-451 or deletion of the conserved motif abolishes binding of PP-1 as observed by co-precipitation and competition binding assays (Hsieh-Wilson et al., 1999). Phosphorylation of residues in the actin-binding domain by PKA reduces the affinity of spinophilin for F-actin and shifts its subcellular localization away from the PSD, with no major effect on its PP-1c binding affinity (Hsieh-Wilson et al., 2003). These phosphorylation sites (Ser-94 and Ser-177) are not conserved in neurabin, and suggest further differential regulation through phosphorylation. In addition to PKA, spinophilin interaction with F-actin is regulated through phosphorylation by CaMKII, cyclin-dependent kinase 5 (cdk5), extracellular signal-regulated kinase (ERK), and protein kinase C (PKC) (Futter et al., 2005; Grossman et al., 2004).

3.2 Spine formation and maturation

Spine density and morphology are dynamic during development as well as in the adult brain, which demands active remodeling of the cytoskeleton (Harris & Kater, 1994; Rochefort & Konnerth, 2012) and suggests key roles for neurabin, spinophilin, and PP-1 in spine modulation. Early studies using heterologous expression in non-neuronal cells identified a role for neurabin in neurite outgrowth (Nakanishi et al., 1997) and for PP-1-dependent regulation of cell morphology (Oliver et al., 2002). Subsequent studies in cultured hippocampal neurons showed that the isolated N-terminal actin-binding domains of both neurabin and spinophilin can induce filopodia extension, delaying spine formation and maturation (Terry-Lorenzo et al., 2005; Zito et al., 2004). This effect is antagonized not only by mutation of the actin-binding domains, but also by association of neurabin with PP-1. The neurabin/PP1 complex remodels F-actin to transform filopodia into spines, increases surface expression of GluA1 AMPA receptor subunits, and enhances AMPA receptor currents underlying functional maturation of excitatory synapses (Terry-Lorenzo et al., 2005; Zito et al., 2004). Potential postsynaptic substrates that may be dephosphorylated by neurabin/PP-1 to regulate the spine actin cytoskeleton include actin-depolymerizing factor (ADF)/cofilin (Meberg, Ono, Minamide, Takahashi, & Bamburg, 1998), and CaMKII (Lisman & Zhabotinsky, 2001).

In addition to actin remodeling, PP-1 modulates the function of various ion channels through dephosphorylation, including glutamate receptors (Greengard, Allen, & Nairn, 1999; Wang, Salter, & MacDonald, 1991) involved in spine formation and function (McKinney, Capogna, Dürr, Gähwiler, & Thompson, 1999; Moser, Trommald, & Andersen, 1994). Spinophilin regulates excitatory synaptic transmission by targeting PP-1 to AMPA and NMDA glutamate receptors *via* the PDZ domain (Kelker et al., 2007) and promotes channel down-regulation through dephosphorylation of GluA1 at Ser-845 (Snyder et al., 2000) and NR1 NMDA receptor subunits at Ser-890 and Ser-897 (Snyder et al., 1998; Yan et al., 1999). Deletion of the spinophilin gene reduces this ability of PP-1 to regulate glutamatergic synaptic transmission by uncoupling PP-1 from glutamate receptor channels and producing persistent AMPA currents and reducing long-term depression (LTD; Feng et al., 2000). Moreover, mice lacking neurabin or spinophilin have reduced PP-1 expression in striatum and hippocampus, further affecting phosphatase activity (Allen et al., 2006; Salek, Edler, McBride, & Baucum II, 2019).

Structural spine changes from alterations in synaptic transmission depend on the brain region: in the caudatoputamen, spinophilin knockout increases or has no effect on spine density depending on age (Feng et al., 2000). Alternatively, in hippocampal neurons, removal of spinophilin decreases dendritic spine density (Evans et al., 2015). As multifunctional scaffolding proteins, association of neurabin or spinophilin with different binding partners may also influence phenotypic differences in spine modulation. Neurabin and spinophilin are localized to spines *via* a conserved N terminal F-actin binding domain (Grossman, Hsieh-Wilson, Allen, Nairn, & Greengard, 2002) and also share a PP-1 binding domain to target PP-1 to dendritic spines (Allen et al., 1997; Hsieh-Wilson et al., 1999). In addition to F-actin and PP-1 binding domains, both neurabin and spinophilin contain a PDZ and C-terminal coiled coil domains that have been implicated in regulating dendritic spine morphology. An interaction between neurabin and the Rho guanine nucleotide exchange factor (GEF) Lfc was identified in a yeast two-hybrid analysis showing a novel mechanism for F-actin reorganization, and in turn, regulation of spine morphology (Ryan et al., 2005). Upon neuronal stimulation, Lfc accumulates in spines through neurabin/spinophilin interaction, locally activating Rho to stabilize F-actin and cause spine shrinkage (Ryan et al., 2005). In contrast, Asef2, another GTPase activating GEF, is recruited to synaptic sites by spinophilin, promoting formation of dendritic spines and synapses in hippocampal neurons by a Rac-dependent mechanism (Evans et al., 2015).

3.3 Synaptic plasticity

3.3.1 Hippocampal-dependent plasticity

Synaptic plasticity is the strengthening or weakening of synapses in response to activity patterns; it involves complex modulation by distinct signaling proteins that alter cellular activity. The two main types of synaptic plasticity are either a persistent decrease [LTD] or increase [long-term potentiation (LTP)] in synaptic efficiency (Citri & Malenka, 2008), involving in part endocytosis or increased surface expression of synaptic AMPA receptors, respectively (Carroll, Lissin, von Zastrow, Nicholl, & Malenka, 1999; Luscher et al., 1999; Man, Ju, Ahmadian, & Wang, 2000). LTD, like LTP, is predominantly mediated by activation of synaptic NMDA receptors (NMDAR-LTD; Mulkey & Malenka, 1992) or by mGluRs (mGluR-LTD; Bellone, Lüscher, & Mameli, 2008; Oliet, Malenka, & Nicoll, 1997) at hippocampal synapses.

In addition to synaptic stimulation, pharmacological agents can induce NMDAR- or mGluR-LTD. The low-frequency pattern of synaptic activity necessary to induce NMDAR-LTD is ineffective in activating specific protein kinases, but does activate PP-1 *via* dephosphorylation of I-1 by calcineurin (Mulkey, Herron, & Malenka, 1993). Induction of LTD *via* NMDARs recruits PP-1 to the activated synapses (Fig. 3; Morishita et al., 2001), where internalized AMPARs are stabilized through dephosphorylation of Ser-845 in GluA1 (Fig. 3; Ehlers, 2000) or Ser-880 in GluA2 (Matsuda, Mikawa, & Hirai, 1999), with additional involvement of protein tyrosine phosphatases (Collingridge, Isaac, & Wang, 2004). AMPAR endocytosis is further permitted by dephosphorylation of Ser-295 of PSD-95 by PP-1, causing dispersal of PSD-95 from synaptic sites and subsequent internalization of AMPAR (Kim et al., 2007). Initially presumed to involve phosphatases, various kinases have also been implicated in NMDAR-LTD, including PP-1 activation of GSK-3β by dephosphorylation of GSK3β itself and its upstream inhibitor, Akt (Szatmari et al., 2005). Targeting of PP-1 to its substrates necessary for LTD requires the scaffolding

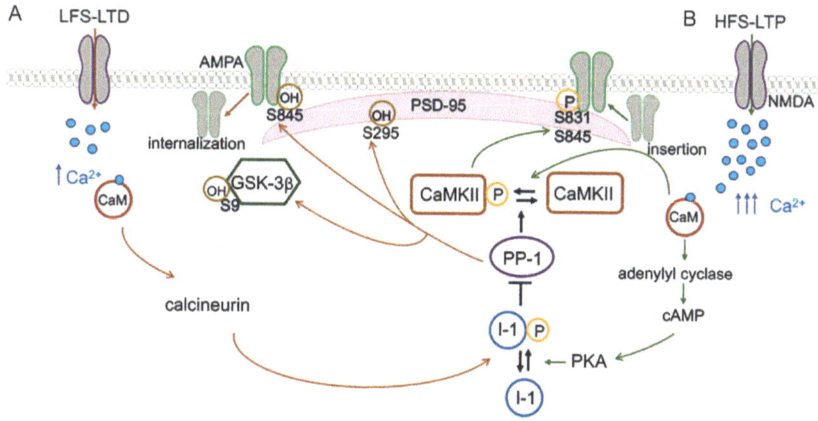

Fig. 3 Role of PP-1 activity in the bidirectional control of hippocampal NMDA-mediated synaptic plasticity. (A) Low frequency stimulation-long-term depression (LFS-LTD, orange lines): LFS activates a calcineurin cascade that leads to inhibitor-1 (I-1) dephosphorylation and disinhibition of PP-1 activity. PP-1 then dephosphorylates Ser-845 on GluA1 leading to internalization of dephosphorylated AMPA receptors. Additional dephosphorylation of Ser-295 on PSD-95 and activation of GSK-3β (dephosphorylation of Ser-9) further permits AMPAR endocytosis and expression of LTD. (B) High frequency stimulation-long-term potentiation (HFS-LTP, green lines): HFS leads to phosphorylation of I-1 by PKA and subsequent inhibition of PP-1. Activation of PKA and of CaMKII leads to GluA1 phosphorylation at Ser-831 and Ser-845, leading to increased conductance, membrane insertion of AMPA receptors and expression of LTP. CaM, calmodulin; CaMKII, calcium/calmodulin-dependent protein kinase II; cAMP, cyclic adenosine monophosphate; GSK-3β, glycogen synthase kinase-3β; I-1, inhibitor-1; PKA, protein kinase A; PP-1, protein phosphatase-1; PSD-95, post-synaptic density-95.

protein spinophilin, as peptides that prevent the PP-1-spinophilin interaction and examination of glutamatergic responses in spinophilin knockout mice reveal potentiation of glutamate receptor responses (Yan et al., 1999) and a failure to elicit NMDAR-LTD (Allen et al., 2006; Morishita et al., 2001).

Spinophilin also interacts with Group I mGluRs in the hippocampus to regulate receptor trafficking and signaling involved in mGluR-mediated synaptic plasticity. Binding of spinophilin to the C-terminal PDZ domain of mGluRs and subsequent prevention of endocytosis is necessary for mGluR activity, as chemically (DHPG)-induced LTD mediated by mGluR5 (Palmer, Irving, Seabrook, Jane, & Collingridge, 1997) is impaired in spinophilin knock-out mice (di Sebastiano et al., 2016). However, acute peptide disruption of PP-1 interaction with spinophilin did not inhibit mGluR-LTD (Morishita et al., 2001). Tyrosine dephosphorylation of

GluA2 also plays a role in internalization of AMPARs during DHPG-LTD (Collingridge, Peineau, Howland, & Wang, 2010; Gladding et al., 2009). The specific roles of various regulatory subunits of PP-1 in synaptic plasticity thus require further study.

Unlike LTD, inhibition of PP-1 activity occurs in NMDAR-LTP (Fig. 3; Mulkey et al., 1993, 1994). Large depolarizations lead to activation of kinases such as CaMKII following influx of Ca^{2+} (Pettit, Perlman, & Malinow, 1994). However, CaMKII also activates enzymes such as adenylyl cyclase and calcineurin with opposing actions that determine the phosphorylation state of inhibitor-1(I-1), a potent inhibitor of PP-1 activity and of LTP. Calcineurin, by dephosphorylating and inactivating I-1, allows PP-1 to disrupt CaMKII signaling and thus LTP (Mulkey et al., 1994). Alternatively, adenylyl cyclase antagonizes effects of calcineurin by producing cAMP and activating PKA, which inhibits PP-1 by phosphorylating I-1 (Blitzer, Wong, Nouranifar, Iyengar, & Landau, 1995). Thus, regulation of these opposing enzyme activities (Blitzer et al., 1995, 1998) is necessary for persistent strengthening of synapses underlying learning and memory (Bliss & Collingridge, 1993).

In addition to spinophilin, the neurabin-PP-1 complex also modulates synaptic transmission in the hippocampus, further solidifying the role of PP-1 in synaptic plasticity. For example, in rat CA1 pyramidal neurons, mutant neurabins that are unable to bind to either PP-1 or F-actin enhance LTP and inhibit LTD (Hu, Huang, Roadcap, Shenolikar, & Xia, 2006), while wild-type neurabin inhibits LTP and elicits more robust LTD (Hu et al., 2006). However, genetic deletion of neurabin reduces LTP and hippocampus-dependent fear memory suggesting that developmental modulation by neurabin of synaptic plasticity may differ from acute knockdown (Wu et al., 2008).

3.3.2 Striatal-dependent plasticity

Principal activity in the striatum is largely controlled by glutamatergic synapses onto medium spiny neurons (Calabresi, Pisani, Mercuri, & Bernardi, 1996). High-frequency stimulation (HFS) or negative spike timing of this pathway leads to LTD of excitatory synaptic transmission (Calabresi, Maj, Pisani, Mercuri, & Bernardi, 1992; Lovinger, Tyler, & Merrit, 1993). Unlike plasticity mechanisms in the hippocampus, striatal LTD does not require glutamate receptor trafficking and is functionally expressed as a reduction in the probability of glutamate release (Choi & Lovinger, 1997) mediated by retrograde endocannabinoid (eCB) signaling (Gerdeman,

Ronesi, & Lovinger, 2002). Postsynaptic activation of mGluRs and L-type calcium channels lead to production and release of endocannabinoids that cross the synaptic cleft and activate presynaptic CB1 receptors (Adermark & Lovinger, 2007; Sung, Choi, & Lovinger, 2001).

Dopamine plays a prominent neuromodulatory role in regulating fast synaptic transmission in the striatum associated with motor control and psychological function. Successful induction of eCB-LTD requires activation of dopamine D1 or D2 receptors, depending on striatal pathway (Calabresi, Maj, et al., 1992; Calabresi, Pisani, Mercuri, & Bernardi, 1992; Shen, Flajolet, Greengard, & Surmeier, 2008). D1 and D2 receptors exhibit opposing effects on adenylyl cyclase to regulate intracellular levels of cAMP and in turn, PKA activity (Stoof & Kebabian, 1981). Phosphorylation by PKA in response to D1 receptor stimulation converts DARPP-32 into a potent inhibitor of PP-1, removing antagonism of downstream PKA signaling involved in ion channel activity, neurotransmitter release, and locomotor activity (Feng et al., 2000; Fienberg et al., 1998). LTD and LTP are absent in DARPP-32 knock-out mice and are restored by pharmacological inhibition of PP-1, suggesting a critical involvement of the DARPP-2/PP-1 cascade in corticostriatal synaptic plasticity (Calabresi et al., 2000). PP-1 mediated regulation in neuromodulatory signal transduction is further revealed in mice lacking spinophilin; genetic deletion of spinophilin reduces striatal PP-1 levels and prevents LTD in a dopamine-dependent manner (Allen et al., 2006). Spinophilin serves to promote PP-1 activity toward substrates critical for synaptic depression, but specific targets are unclear. Although AMPAR trafficking is not associated with eCB-LTD, regulation of glutamate receptors by phosphorylation may still play a role as AMPAR-mediated membrane depolarization is needed to open voltage-gated calcium channels crucial for LTD induction (Wang et al., 2006).

In contrast, striatal LTP does require NMDA receptor activation (Calabresi, Pisani, et al., 1992), and dopaminergic neurotransmission regulates a variety of substrates in a DARPP-32/PP-1-dependent manner (Calabresi et al., 2000) including NMDA receptor function (Calabresi, Maj, et al., 1992; Calabresi, Pisani, et al., 1992; Flores-Hernandez et al., 2002). The absence of LTP in mice lacking DARPP-32 or D1 receptors suggests inhibition of dephosphorylation by the D1/cAMP/PKA/DARPP-32/PP-1 pathway along with activation of kinases leading to increased phosphorylation and enhancement of NMDA currents (Calabresi et al., 2000; Centonze et al., 2003; Flores-Hernandez et al., 2002). Collectively, these findings confirm the role of dopamine transmission in both forms of striatal plasticity, but demonstrate involvement of distinct signaling cascades. Moreover, despite similar PP-1 interactions, spinophilin and neurabin are required for distinct, but converging aspects of dopaminergic neurotransmission. Deletion of spinophilin or neurabin results specifically in loss of LTD or LTP induction, respectively, but are both rescued by exogenous application of dopamine receptor agonists (Allen et al., 2006).

3.4 Behavior

3.4.1 Learning and memory

Potentiation of LTD by PP-1 emphasizes its physiological importance as a suppressor of learning and memory, as well as a key factor in age-related cognitive decline. Repetition and practice in learning are required for formation of accurate and long-lasting memories. PP-1 activation limits acquisition and favors memory decline. Genetic deletion of PP-1 in mutant mice expressing a constitutively active form of inhibitor-1 decreases the time and number of training episodes for optimal performance during a spatial memory task (Genoux et al., 2002). Biochemically, this effect correlates with increased phosphorylation of both CaMKII (Thr-286) and GluA1 (Ser-845), two known PP-1 targets (Genoux et al., 2002). Furthermore, inhibition of PP-1 prolongs memory when induced after learning, suggesting that PP-1 also promotes forgetting, particularly in aging animals (Genoux et al., 2002).

3.4.2 Drug addiction

Synaptic plasticity mechanisms, such as LTP, are physiological correlates of learning and memory. Memory consolidation is a dynamic process, and consolidated memory can become destabilized under various conditions or treatments (Nader, 2003; Nader, Schafe, & Le Doux, 2000). The NMDA receptor subunits GluN2B and GluN2A have been reported to be necessary for memory destabilization and re-stabilization, respectively (Milton et al., 2013). Other studies have identified roles for AMPA receptor subunit GluA2 and PP-1 in memory stabilization (Yu et al., 2016). Drug addiction is a process of strengthened learning, and re-instatement of drug motivation is reinforced when encountered with drug-related environmental cues (Tang & Dani, 2009; Thanos, Bermeo, Wang, & Volkow, 2009). Destabilization of drug memory is mechanistically consistent with a form of LTD; memory retrieval induces activation of GluN2B-containing NMDA receptors resulting in Ca^{2+} influx and activation of PP-1, leading to dephosphorylation of GluA1 and subsequent endocytosis of synaptic AMPA receptors (Yu et al., 2016). In contrast, cellular adaptations that accompany drug sensitization and addiction include up-regulation of AMPA receptor surface expression in the nucleus accumbens (Berke & Hyman, 2000; Boudreau & Wolf, 2005). Corticostriatal LTP is a correlate of reward-related learning (Reynolds, Hyland, & Wickens, 2001), and enhancement of the rewarding effects of cocaine seen in spinophilin knock-out mice may be related to preferential expression of LTP over LTD at cortico-striatal synapses (Allen et al., 2006). Progressive increases in locomotor activity is a hallmark effect of consecutive drug administrations associated with increased dopaminergic neurotransmission (Henry & White, 1991; Kalivas & Duffy, 1990) and LTP induction (Borgland, Malenka, & Bonci, 2004). These drug-induced changes in behavioral sensitization paradigms are also influenced by scaffolding proteins. Standard immunocytochemistry and cell-type specific proteomic screening show increased striatal levels of spinophilin following psychostimulant administration (Boikess & Marshall, 2008; Watkins, True, Mosley, & Baucum II, 2018), enhancing its interactions with various proteins involved in synaptic signaling (Watkins et al., 2018) and concomitantly leading to more dendritic spines (Lee et al., 2006; Li, Kolb, & Robinson, 2003). These alterations indicate greater targeting of PP-1 to its many substrates and greater regulation of its activity. Behaviorally, deletion of spinophilin has no effect on the acute locomotor responses to cocaine, but attenuates cocaine-induced locomotor sensitization compared to wild type controls (Areal, Hamilton, Martins-Silva, Pires, & Ferguson, 2019). Similar findings were also reported in spinophilin-deficient mice administered amphetamine (Morris, Watkins, Salek, Edler, & Baucum 2nd, 2018). Importantly, these results may be protocol-dependent as a shorter observation time and higher cocaine dosage in mice lacking spinophilin or neurabin did lead to acute hyperactivity with preserved locomotor sensitization (Allen et al., 2006).

4. Protein phosphatase-1 and neurodegenerative disorders

Disorders such as Alzheimer's Disease (AD), Parkinson's Disease (PD), and schizophrenia are correlated to dysfunction in learning and memory, and are characterized by functional and structural changes in dendritic spines. This implicates dysregulation of PP-1 as a candidate mechanism in the pathophysiology of various neurodegenerative and psychiatric disorders.

Although few human diseases are reported to be caused by defects in PP-1 *per se*, neurodegenerative diseases are correlated with dysregulation of protein phosphorylation and/or decreased availability and function of PP-1 regulatory/targeting subunits.

Alzheimer's disease is a progressive, degenerative disorder characterized by the presence of extracellular amyloid-beta (Aβ) plaques and intracellular neurofibrillary tangles (NFT; Braak & Braak, 1991; Terry, Gonatas, & Weiss, 1964). Alterations in spine number and size, caused by oligomeric forms of the Aβ peptide, precede these hallmark changes and are directly associated with early memory loss (Masliah, Terry, DeTeresa, & Hansen, 1989; Selkoe, 2002) and severity of disease (Terry et al., 1991). Aβ is proteolytically cleaved from the amyloid precursor protein (APP), a process regulated by PKC (Rebelo et al., 2007) and PP-1 (da Cruz e Silva, da Cruz e Silva, Zaia, & Greengard, 1995). The activity of different isoforms of PP-1 is specifically and potently inhibited by Aβ, an effect that is further potentiated by Aβ aggregation (Vintém, Henriques, da Cruz e Silva, & da Cruz e Silva, 2009). Thus, concomitant activation of PKC and inhibition of PP-1 may contribute to hyperphosphorylation of key proteins associated with AD pathology such as APP and tau (Bennecib, Gong, Grundke-Iqbal, & Iqbal, 2000). Moreover, LTP impairment induced by Aβ oligomers can be reversed by PP-1 inhibition *in vitro* (Knobloch, Farinelli, Konietzko, Nitsch, & Mansuy, 2007). Taken together, increased Aβ production can lead to abnormal PP-1 activity and contribute to AD pathology by mediating reduced synaptic contacts, LTD (Morishita et al., 2001) and age-related memory defects (Genoux et al., 2002).

PP-1 regulatory proteins are also affected by AD. Human AD patients show a marked reduction in spinophilin-labeled hippocampal dendritic spines, which correlates directly with cognitive dysfunction as assessed by both a global neuropsychological measure (MMSE) and a dementia severity scale (CDR; Akram et al., 2008). Moreover, lower spinophilin-reactive dendritic spine numbers also correlate with greater Aβ plaque burden (Mi et al., 2017).

In both human and animal models of PD, there is a specific loss of dopamine neurons that project from the substantia nigra to the striatum leading to progressive motor deficits (Calabresi, Mercuri, Sancesario, & Bernardi, 1993; Stephens et al., 2005). These neurons synapse with dendritic spines in the striatal medium spiny neurons (MSNs) predominantly onto the necks of spines (Freund, Powell, & Smith, 1984) whereas excitatory synaptic input from the cortex and thalamus synapse primarily onto spine heads (Bolam,

Hanley, Booth, & Bevan, 2000). Loss of dopamine signaling leads to a significant reduction in MSN spine density (Ingman, Hood, van Maldegem, Weenink, & Arbuthnott, 1993; Villalba, Lee, & Smith, 2009), glutamatergic synapses (Day et al., 2006) and synaptic plasticity, particularly LTD (Calabresi, Maj, et al., 1992; Calabresi, Pisani, et al., 1992; Calabresi et al., 1993). Dysregulation of kinase and phosphatase activities are observed in animal models of PD including reduction of PP-1γ1 activity in striatal MSNs (Brown, Baucum, Bass, & Colbran, 2008). Decreased activity of PP-1 occurs concurrently with increased association between PP-1 and spinophilin (Brown et al., 2008), consistent with spinophilin's ability to inhibit PP-1 activity toward specific substrates (Ragusa et al., 2010), which influences spine density (Feng et al., 2000) and synaptic plasticity (Allen et al., 2006). Moreover, proteomics-based assays of dopamine depletion in a PD mouse model observed overall reduction in spinophilin association with various substrates including synaptic signaling, cytoskeletal, and scaffolding proteins (Hiday et al., 2017). Decreased spinophilin association with possible PP-1 targets may further lead to reduced PP-1 activity. Attenuated PP-1 activity leads to less dephosphorylation and unopposed kinase activity, and hyperphosphorylation of glutamate subunits (GluN2A and GluN2B) by CaMKII induces motor disability and maladaptive striatal plasticity in a PD mouse model (Brown, Deutch, & Colbran, 2005; Picconi et al., 2004). Spinophilin-dependent PP-1 targeting and activity may underlie these motor effects as spinophilin-deficient mice have deficits in motor behaviors and motor learning (Edler et al., 2018).

5. Protein phosphatase-1 and neuropsychiatric disorders

Neuropsychiatric conditions such as schizophrenia, obsessive compulsive disorder (OCD), and mental retardation alter synaptic and dendritic spine function, making PP-1 a likely factor in their pathophysiology. Schizophrenia is a neurodevelopmental disorder described by impairments in perception, affect, and cognition, reflecting altered connectivity within and between multiple brain regions. Structural imaging studies have shown smaller whole brain volumes (Levitt, Bobrow, Lucia, & Srinivasan, 2010) and reductions in gray matter underlying smaller cortical and hippocampal volumes (Glahn et al., 2008). Electron microscopy of postmortem brain shows synapse- and region-specific effects on spine density; consistent with the imaging studies, spine density was reduced in multiple neocortical areas

(Garey et al., 1998), while hippocampal (Kolomeets, Orlovskaya, Rachmanova, & Uranova, 2005; Rosoklija et al., 2000) and striatal (Roberts, Conley, Kung, Peretti, & Chute, 1996; Roberts, Roche, & Conley, 2005) spines show variable effects based on sub-regions or type of synapses. Changes in spinophilin expression may contribute to these differences as genetic deletion of spinophilin increases the number of spines in the caudatoputamen of young mice, while its acute knockdown reduces spine number in hippocampal cultures (Evans et al., 2015).

Additional evidence that disparate spinophilin regulation in schizophrenia may be brain region-specific is observed at the transcript level. Measurements of spinophilin mRNA show increased or unchanged levels in dorsolateral prefrontal cortex (Baracskay, Haroutunian, & Meador-Woodruff, 2006; Weickert et al., 2004), whereas spinophilin transcript levels are increased in several sub-regions of the hippocampus (Law, Weickert, Hyde, Kleinman, & Harrison, 2004). PP-1 and spinophilin are also implicated in OCD, a disease that is characterized by persistent intrusive thoughts, repetitive actions, and excessive anxiety. Loss of the scaffolding protein SAP90/PSD95-associated protein 3 (SAPAP3) in rodent models leads to OCD-like behaviors such as excessive grooming due to increased AMPAR internalization *via* mGluR5 signaling (Chen et al., 2011; Wan, Feng, & Calakos, 2011; Welch et al., 2007). Spinophilin is associated with both SAPAP3 and mGluR5 in mouse brain (Morris et al., 2018). Association of spinophilin with mGluR5 is enhanced by SAPAP3, while mGluR5 increases association of spinophilin and SAPAP3 (Morris et al., 2018). Normally, spinophilin and SAPAP3 regulate anchoring and trafficking of mGluR5 leading to silencing or potentiation of AMPA signaling, respectively (di Sebastiano et al., 2016; Wan et al., 2011). However, aberrant regulation of the spinophilin/mGluR5/SAPAP3 complex may underlie OCD pathology as loss of spinophilin enhances mGluR endocytosis (di Sebastiano et al., 2016), decreases reduction of AMPA signaling (Allen et al., 2006), and attenuates behaviors associated with OCD (Morris et al., 2018). Moreover, a role for spinophilin/PP-1 interaction is implicated in OCD as overexpression of the catalytic subunit of PP-1α abolishes the association of spinophilin with SAPAP3 and mGluR5 (Morris et al., 2018).

Several mental retardation disorders are caused by mutations in the gene encoding ATRX, a chromatin remodeling protein. A milder form of this disorder has been recapitulated in ATRX$^{\Delta E2}$ mice, mimicking an exon 2 mutation seen in patients that causes learning and memory dysfunction. Mental retardation is associated with changes in dendrite arborization and dendrite spine morphology (Kaufmann & Moser, 2000). ATRX$^{\Delta E2}$ mice have longer and thinner spines in the medial prefrontal cortex compared to wild-type mice, which is mediated by abnormal elevation of CaMKII activity due to reduced expression and activity of PP-1 (Shioda et al., 2011). CaMKII localized in the rat forebrain PSD fraction is predominantly dephosphorylated by PP-1 (Strack, Barban, Wadzinski, & Colbran, 1997), and inhibition of PP-1 in cultured hippocampal or cortical neurons enhances autophosphorylation of CaMKII and spine elongation (Jourdain, Fukunaga, & Muller, 2003) by spinophilin targeting. Disrupting the spinophilin/PP-1 complex *in vitro* enhances spine elongation and filopodia in cultured HEK293 cells (Oliver et al., 2002) and dissociated rat hippocampal neurons (Terry-Lorenzo et al., 2005). Similarly, decreased PP-1 activity correlates with increased phosphorylation of hippocampal CaMKII in the PSD with disruption of synaptic plasticity, learning, and memory in a mouse model of Angelman syndrome (Weeber et al., 2003).

Synaptic dysfunction is implicated in affective disorders such as anxiety and depression, and both neurabin and spinophilin play distinct age-dependent roles in their regulation. Loss of neurabin by genetic deletion is anxiolytic in young adult mice compared to wild-type controls (Kim et al., 2011; Wu et al., 2017). In contrast, there is reduced anxiety-like behavior in middle-aged spinophilin knock-out mice, whereas the anxiolytic effect of neurabin loss is absent in older animals. However, attenuation of anxiety-related behaviors in neurabin or spinophilin knock-out mice was not consistent across different types of behavioral testing, suggesting selective sensitivity to particular anxiogenic conditions (Kim et al., 2011; Wu et al., 2017). Opposing age-dependent regulation of depression-like behavior were also seen in both knock-out strains as loss of spinophilin increased behaviors of depression in young adult mice (Wu et al., 2017), while conflicting findings were reported in mice lacking neurabin (Kim et al., 2011; Wu et al., 2017). In contrast, loss of spinophilin provided protection from depression-like behavior in aged mice (Wu et al., 2017). These distinct phenotypes are of interest as overall protein expression levels did not change in these knock-out mouse models (Wu et al., 2017), suggesting an interplay of region-specific protein expression, age, and differences in synaptic plasticity. Selective inhibition of neurabin in the anterior cingulate cortex using siRNA reproduced anxiety-like behavior without affecting depression-like behavior (Kim et al., 2011); similar studies will be necessary to exclude developmental abnormalities or compensation.

Together these data describe mechanisms modulating the interactions between PP-1 and its regulatory proteins involved in neuropsychiatric disease pathology. Understanding how PP-1 regulates the phosphorylation status of these substrates *in vivo* and in specific cell types promises to provide insights into disease mechanisms, therapeutic treatments, and prevention.

6. Conclusion

Aberrant PP-1 regulation has been linked to several pathological states, making pharmacological manipulation of phosphatase activity or levels an attractive therapeutic strategy. Drugs that target specific phosphatase complexes may provide useful approaches with target specificity. For example, deletion of the C terminus of the PP-1 catalytic subunit prevents PP-1 inhibition by endogenous inhibitors (Conner, Kleeman, Barik, Honkanen, & Shenolikar, 1999), identifying this region as an appealing target for the design of novel, selective inhibitors that prevent substrate access. Disorders that are treated by protein kinase inhibitors may also be responsive to phosphatase activators. Synthetic small molecule peptides can activate PP-1 in the absence or presence of endogenous inhibitors, indicating that binding of these peptides to the regulatory domain of PP-1 can directly influence phosphatase activity as well as its interaction with regulatory proteins (Tappan & Chamberlin, 2008).

The ability to target a specific phosphatase complex directly as opposed to overall PP-1 activity is an appealing approach to prevent unwanted toxic side effects of broad catalytic subunit inhibitors. Methods to accomplish this include disruption of interactions between the phosphatase (catalytic or regulatory subunit) and its substrates and disruption of interactions between catalytic and regulatory subunits (McConnell & Wadzinski, 2009). There are several examples of molecules that affect multiprotein complexes (Vassilev et al., 2004), including phosphatase complexes (McConnell & Wadzinski, 2009), to impair phosphatase-substrate interaction. Targeted dissociation of the catalytic subunit from the associated regulatory subunit can also influence the function of PP-1 holoenzymes. For example, introduction of synthetic peptides that disrupt PP-1 complexes has been shown to influence synaptic transmission (Morishita et al., 2001; Yan et al., 1999), apoptosis (Boyce et al., 2005), and cancer progression (Chen, Weng, Tseng, Lin, & Chen, 2005). Thus, synthetic or natural compounds that regulate PP-1 activity have a broad range of potential therapeutic uses.

Acknowledgments

The authors acknowledge their long and productive collaborations with Paul Greengard and his outstanding collaborators and trainees. Much of the work described in this chapter originated or was inspired by his many fundamental discoveries in cell signaling.

Conflict of interest statement

The authors declare that they have no conflicts of interest.

References

Adermark, L., & Lovinger, D. M. (2007). Retrograde endocannabinoid signaling at striatal synapses requires a regulated postsynaptic release step. *Proceedings of the National Academy of Sciences of the United States of America*, *104*, 20564–20569.

Akram, A., Christoffel, D., Rocher, A. B., Bouras, C., Kövari, E., Perl, D. P., et al. (2008). Stereological estimates of total spinophilin-immunoreactive spine number in area 9 and the CA1 field: Relationship with the progression of Alzheimer's disease. *Neurobiology of Aging*, *29*, 1296–1307.

Allen, P. B. (2004). Functional plasticity in the organization of signaling complexes in the striatum. *Parkinsonism & Related Disorders*, *10*, 287–292.

Allen, P. B., Ouimet, C. C., & Greengard, P. (1997). Spinophilin, a novel protein phosphatase 1 binding protein localized to dendritic spines. *Proceedings of the National Academy of Sciences of the United States of America*, *94*, 9956–9961.

Allen, P. B., Zachariou, V., Svenningsson, P., Lepore, A. C., Centonze, D., Costa, C., et al. (2006). Distinct roles for spinophilin and neurabin in dopamine-mediated plasticity. *Neuroscience*, *140*, 897–911.

Areal, L. B., Hamiltion, A., Martins-Silva, C., Pires, R. G. W., & Ferguson, S. S. G. (2019). Neuronal scaffolding protein spinophilin is integral for cocaine-induced behavioral sensitization and ERK1/2 activation. *Molecular Brain*, *12*, 15.

Baracskay, K. L., Haroutunian, V., & Meador-Woodruff, J. H. (2006). Dopamine receptor signaling molecules are altered in elderly schizophrenic cortex. *Synapse*, *60*, 271–279.

Bellone, C., Lüscher, C., & Mameli, M. (2008). Mechanisms of synaptic depression triggered by metabotropic glutamate receptors. *Cellular and Molecular Life Sciences*, *65*, 2913–2923.

Bennecib, M., Gong, C. X., Grundke-Iqbal, I., & Iqbal, K. (2000). Role of protein phosphatase-2A and −1 in the regulation of GSK-3, cdk5 and cdc2 and the phosphorylation of tau in rat forebrain. *FEBS Letters*, *485*, 87–93.

Berke, J. D., & Hyman, S. E. (2000). Addiction, dopamine, and the molecular mechanisms of memory. *Neuron*, *25*, 515–532.

Bliss, T. V., & Collingridge, G. L. (1993). A synaptic model of memory: Long-term potentiation in the hippocampus. *Nature*, *361*, 31–39.

Blitzer, R. D., Connor, J. H., Brown, G. P., Wong, T., Shenolikar, S., Iyenagar, R., et al. (1998). Gating of CaMKII by cAMP-regulated protein phosphatase activity during LTP. *Science*, *280*, 1940–1942.

Blitzer, R. D., Wong, T., Nouranifar, R., Iyengar, R., & Landau, E. M. (1995). Postsynaptic cAMP pathway gates early LTP in hippocampal CA1 region. *Neuron*, *15*, 1403–1414.

Boikess, S. R., & Marshall, J. F. (2008). A sensitizing d-amphetamine regimen induces long-lasting spinophilin protein upregulation in the rat striatum and limbic forebrain. *European Journal of Neuroscience*, *28*, 2099–2107.

Bolam, J. P., Hanley, J. J., Booth, P. A., & Bevan, M. D. (2000). Synaptic organization of the basal ganglia. *Journal of Anatomy*, *196*, 527–542.

Borgland, S. L., Malenka, R. C., & Bonci, A. (2004). Acute and chronic cocaine-induced potentiation of synaptic strength in the ventral tegmental area: Electrophysiological and behavioral correlates in individual rats. *Journal of Neuroscience*, *24*, 7482–7490.

Boudreau, A. C., & Wolf, M. E. (2005). Behavioral sensitization to cocaine is associated with increased AMPA receptor surface expression in the nucleus accumbens. *Journal of Neuroscience*, *25*, 9144–9151.

Boyce, M., Bryant, K. F., Jousee, C., Long, K., Harding, H. P., Scheuner, D., et al. (2005). A selective inhibitor of eIF2alpha dephosphorylation protects cells from ER stress. *Science*, *307*, 935–939.

Braak, H., & Braak, E. (1991). Neuropathological stageing of Alzheimer-related changes. *Acta Neuropathologica*, *82*, 239–259.

Brown, A. M., Baucum, A. J., Bass, M. A., & Colbran, R. J. (2008). Association of protein phosphatase 1 gamma 1 with spinophilin suppresses phosphatase activity in a Parkinson disease model. *Journal of Biological Chemistry*, *283*, 14286–14294.

Brown, A. M., Deutch, A. Y., & Colbran, R. J. (2005). Dopamine depletion alters phosphorylation of striatal proteins in a model of Parkinsonism. *European Journal of Neuroscience*, *22*, 247–256.

Calabresi, P., Gubellini, P., Centonze, D., Picconi, B., Bernardi, G., Chergui, K., et al. (2000). Dopamine and cAMP-regulated phosphoprotein 32 kDa controls both striatal long-term depression and long-term potentiation, opposing forms of synaptic plasticity. *Journal of Neuroscience*, *20*, 8443–8451.

Calabresi, P., Maj, R., Pisani, A., Mercuri, N. B., & Bernardi, G. (1992). Long-term synaptic depression in the striatum: Physiological and pharmacological characterization. *Journal of Neuroscience*, *12*, 4224–4233.

Calabresi, P., Mercuri, N. B., Sancesario, G., & Bernardi, G. (1993). Electrophysiology of dopamine-denervated striatal neurons. Implications for Parkinson's disease. *Brain*, *116*, 433–452.

Calabresi, P., Pisani, A., Mercuri, N. B., & Bernardi, G. (1992). Long-term potentiation in the striatum is unmasked by removing the voltage-dependent magnesium block of NMDA receptor channels. *European Journal of Neuroscience*, *4*, 929–935.

Calabresi, P., Pisani, A., Mercuri, N. B., & Bernardi, G. (1996). The corticostriatal projection: From synaptic plasticity to dysfunctions of the basal ganglia. *Trends in Neurosciences*, *19*, 19–24.

Carmody, L. C., Baucum, A. J., 2nd, Bass, M. A., & Colbran, R. J. (2008). Selective targeting of the gamma1 isoform of protein phosphatase-1 to F-actin in intact cells requires multiple domains in spinophilin and neurabin. *The FASEB Journal*, *22*, 1660–1671.

Carroll, R. C., Lissin, D. V., von Zastrow, M., Nicholl, R. A., & Malenka, R. C. (1999). Rapid distribution of glutamate receptors contributes to long-term depression in hippocampal cultures. *Nature Neuroscience*, *2*, 454–460.

Centonze, D., Grande, C., Saulle, E., Martin, A. B., Gubellini, P., Pavon, N., et al. (2003). Distinct roles of D1 and D5 dopamine receptors in motor activity and striatal synaptic plasticity. *Journal of Neuroscience*, *23*, 8506–8512.

Chen, M., Wan, Y., Ade, K., Ting, J., Feng, G., & Calakos, N. (2011). Sapap3 deletion anomalously activates short-term endocannabinoid-mediated synaptic plasticity. *Journal of Neuroscience*, *31*, 9563–9573.

Chen, C., Weng, S., Tseng, P., Lin, H. L., & Chen, C. (2005). Histone acetylation-independent effect of histone deacetylase inhibitors on Akt through the reshuffling of protein phosphatase 1 complexes. *Journal of Biological Chemistry*, *280*, 38879–38887.

Choi, S., & Lovinger, D. M. (1997). Decreased probability of neurotransmitter release underlies striatal long-term depression and postnatal developmefvnt of corticostriatal synapses. *Proceedings of the National Academy of Sciences of the United States of America*, *94*, 2665–2670.

Citri, A., & Malenka, R. C. (2008). Synaptic plasticity: Multiple forms, functions, and mechanisms. *Neurospychopharmacology, 33*, 18–41.

Cohen, P. T. W. (2002). Protein phosphatase 1- targeted in many directions. *Journal of Cell Science, 115*, 241–256.

Colbran, R. J. (2004). Protein phosphatases and calcium/calmodulin-dedendent protein kinase II-dependent synaptic plasticity. *Journal of Neuroscience, 24*, 8404–8409.

Collingridge, G. L., Isaac, J. T. R., & Wang, Y. T. (2004). Receptor trafficking and synaptic plasticity. *Nature Reviews Neuroscience, 5*, 952–962.

Collingridge, G. L., Peineau, S., Howland, J. G., & Wang, Y. T. (2010). Long-term depression in the CNS. *Nature Reviews Neuroscience, 11*, 459–473.

Conner, J. H., Kleeman, T., Barik, S., Honkanen, R. E., & Shenolikar, S. (1999). Importance of the b12-b13 loop in protein phosphatase-1 catalytic subunit for inhibition by toxins and mammalian protein inhibitors. *Journal of Biological Chemistry, 274*, 22366–22372.

da Cruz e Silva, E. F., da Cruz e Silva, O. A., Zaia, C. T., & Greengard, P. (1995). Inhibition of protein phosphatase 1 stimulates secretion of Alzheimer amyloid precursor protein. *Molecular Medicine, 1*, 535–541.

Day, M., Wang, Z., Ding, J., An, X., Ingham, C. A., Shering, A. F., et al. (2006). Selective elimination of glutamatergic synapses on striatopallidal neurons in Parkinson disease models. *Nature Neuroscience, 9*, 251–259.

di Sebastiano, E. R., Fahim, S., Dunn, H. A., Walther, C., Ribeiro, F. M., Cregan, S. P., et al. (2016). Role of spinophilin in Group I metabotropic glutamate receptor endocytosis, signaling, and synaptic plasticity. *Journal of Biological Chemistry, 291*, 17602–17615.

Edler, M. C., Salek, A. B., Watkins, D. S., Kaur, H., Morris, C. W., Yamamoto, B. K., et al. (2018). Mechanisms regulating the association of protein phosphatase-1 with spinophilin and neurabin. *Pharmacology and Toxicology, 9*, 2701–2712.

Ehlers, M. D. (2000). Reinsertion or degradation of AMPA receptors determined by activity-dependent endocytic sorting. *Neuron, 28*, 511–525.

Endo, S., Critz, S. D., Byrne, J. H., & Shenolikar, S. (1995). Protein phosphatase-1 regulates outward K+ currents in sensory neurons of *Aplysia californica. Journal of Neurochemistry, 64*, 1833–1840.

Evans, J. C., Robinson, C. M., Shi, M., & Webb, D. J. (2015). The guanine nucleotide exchange factor (GEF) Asef2 promotes dendritic spine formation via Rac activation and spinophilin-dependent targeting. *Journal of Biological Chemistry, 290*, 10295–10308.

Feng, J., Yan, Z., Ferreira, A., Tomizawa, K., Liauw, J. A., Zhuo, M., et al. (2000). Spinophilin regulates the formation and function of dendritic spines. *Proceedings of the National Academy of Sciences of the United States of America, 97*, 9287–9292.

Fienberg, A. A., Hiroi, N., Mermelstein, P. G., Song, W., Snyder, G. L., Nishi, A., et al. (1998). DARPP-32: Regulator of the efficacy of dopaminergic neurotransmission. *Science, 281*, 838–842.

Flores-Hernandez, J., Cepeda, C., Hernandez-Echeagaray, E., Calvert, C. R., Jokel, E. S., Fienberg, A. A., et al. (2002). Dopamine enhancement of NMDA currents in dissociated medium-sized striatal neurons; role of D1 receptors and DARPP-32. *Journal of Neurophysiology, 88*, 3010–3020.

Freund, T. F., Powell, J. F., & Smith, A. D. (1984). Tyrosine hydroxylase-immunoreactive boutons in synaptic contact with identified striatonigral neurons, with particular reference to dendritic spines. *Neuroscience, 13*, 1189–1215.

Futter, M., Uematsu, K., Bullock, S. A., Kim, Y., Hemmings, H. C., Jr., Nishi, A., et al. (2005). Phosphorylation of spinophilin by ERK and cyclin-dependent PK 5 (Cdk5). *Proceedings of the National Academy of Sciences of the United States of America, 102*, 3489–3494.

Garey, L. J., Ong, W. Y., Patel, T. S., Kanani, M., Davis, A., Mortimer, A. M., et al. (1998). Reduced dendritic spine density on cerebral cortical pyramidal neurons in schizophrenia. *Journal of Neurology, Neurosurgery and Psychiatry, 65*, 446–453.

Genoux, D., Haditsch, U., Knobloch, M., Michalon, A., Storm, D., & Mansuy, I. M. (2002). Protein phosphatase 1 is a molecular constraint on learning and memory. *Nature, 418*, 970–975.

Gerdeman, G. L., Ronesi, J., & Lovinger, D. M. (2002). Postsynaptic endocannabinoid release is critical to long-term depression in the striatum. *Nature Neuroscience, 5*, 446–451.

Gladding, C. M., Collett, V. J., Jia, Z., Bashir, Z. I., Collingridge, G. L., & Molnar, E. (2009). Tyrosine dephosphorylation regulates AMPAR internalisation in mGluR-LTD. *Molecular and Cellular Neuroscience, 40*, 267–279.

Glahn, D. C., Laird, A. R., Ellison-Wright, I., Thelen, S. M., Robinson, J. L., Lancaster, J. L., et al. (2008). Meta-analysis of gray matter anomalies in schizophrenia: Application of anatomic likelihood estimation and network analysis. *Biological Psychiatry, 64*, 774–781.

Greengard, P., Allen, P. B., & Nairn, A. C. (1999). Beyond the dopamine receptor: The DARPP-32/protein phosphatase-1 cascade. *Neuron, 23*, 435–447.

Grossman, S. D., Futter, M., Snyder, G. L., Allen, P. B., Nairn, A. C., Greengard, P., et al. (2004). Spinophilin is phosphorylated by $Ca^{2+/}$calmodulin-dependent protein kinase II resulting in regulation of its binding to F-actin. *Journal of Neurochemistry, 90*, 317–324.

Grossman, S. D., Hsieh-Wilson, L. C., Allen, P. B., Nairn, A. C., & Greengard, P. (2002). The actin-binding domain of spinophilin is necessary and sufficient for targeting to dendritic spines. *NeuroMolecular Medicine, 2*, 61–69.

Harris, K. M., & Kater, S. B. (1994). Dendritic spines: Cellular specializations imparting both stability and flexibility to synaptic function. *Annual Review of Neuroscience, 17*, 341–371.

Henry, D. J., & White, F. J. (1991). Repeated cocaine administration causes persistent enhancement of D1 dopamine receptor sensitivity within the rat nucleus accumbens. *Journal of Pharmacology and Experimental Therapeutics, 258*, 882–890.

Hiday, A. C., Edler, M. C., Salek, S. B., Morris, C. W., Thang, M., Rentz, T. J., et al. (2017). Mechanisms and consequences of dopamine depletion-induced attenuation of the spinophilin/neurofilament medium interaction. *Neural Plasticity, 2017*, 1–16.

Hsieh-Wilson, L. C., Allen, P. B., Watanabe, T., Nairn, A. C., & Greengard, P. (1999). Characterization of the neuronal targeting protein spinophilin and its interactions with protein phosphatase-1. *Biochemistry, 38*, 4365–4373.

Hsieh-Wilson, L. C., Benfenati, F., Snyder, G. L., Allen, P. B., Nairn, A. C., & Greengard, P. (2003). Phosphorylation of spinophilin modulates its interaction with actin filaments. *The Journal of Biological Chemistry, 278*, 1186–1194.

Hu, X. D., Huang, Q., Roadcap, D. W., Shenolikar, S. S., & Xia, H. (2006). Actin-associated neurabin-protein phosphatase-1 complex regulates hippocampal plasticity. *Journal of Neurochemistry, 98*, 1841–1851.

Ingman, C. A., Hood, S. H., van Maldegem, B., Weenink, A., & Arbuthnott, G. W. (1993). Morphological changes in the rat neostriatum after unilateral 6 hydroxydopamine injections into the nigrostriatal pathway. *Experimental Brain Research, 93*, 17–27.

Jourdain, P., Fukunaga, K., & Muller, D. (2003). Calcium/calmodulin-dependent protein kinase II contributes o activity-dependent filopodia growth and spine formation. *Journal of Neuroscience, 23*, 10645–10649.

Ju, T., Ragusa, M. J., Hudak, J., Nairn, A. C., & Peti, W. (2007). Structural characterization of the neurabin sterile alpha motif domain. *Proteins, 69*, 192–198.

Kalivas, P. W., & Duffy, P. (1990). Effect of acute and daily cocaine treatment on extracellular dopamine in the nucleus accumbens. *Synapse, 5*, 48–58.

Kaufmann, W. E., & Moser, H. W. (2000). Dendritic anomalies in disorders associated with mental retardation. *Cerebral Cortex, 10*, 981–991.

Kelker, M. S., Dancheck, B., Ju, T., Kessler, R. P., Hudak, J., Nairn, A. C., et al. (2007). Structural basis for spinophilin-neurabin receptor interaction. *Biochemistry, 46*, 2333–2344.

Kim, M. J., Futai, K., Jo, J., Hayashi, Y., Cho, K., & Sheng, M. (2007). Synaptic accumulation of PSD-95 and synaptic function regulated by phosphorylated of serine-295 of PSD-95. *Neurology, 56*, 488–502.

Kim, S. S., Wang, H., Li, X.-Y., Chen, T., Mercaldo, V., Descalzi, G., et al. (2011). Neurabin in the anterior cingulate cortex regulates anxiety-like behavior in adult mice. *Molecular Brain, 4*, 6.

Kim, Y., Watanabe, T., Allen, P. B., Kim, Y., Lee, S., Greengard, P., et al. (2003). PNUTS, a protein phosphatase 1 (PP1) nuclear targeting subunit. Characterization of its PP1- and RNA-binding domains and regulation by phosphorylation. *Journal of Biological Chemistry, 278*, 13819–13828.

Knobloch, M., Farinelli, M., Konietzko, U., Nitsch, R. M., & Mansuy, I. M. (2007). Abeta oligomer-mediated long-term potentiation impairment involves protein phosphatase 1-dependent mechanisms. *Journal of Neuroscience, 27*, 7648–7653.

Kolomeets, N. S., Orlovskaya, D. D., Rachmanova, V. I., & Uranova, N. A. (2005). Ultrastructural alterations in hippocampal mossy fiber synapses in schizophrenia: A postmortem morphometric study. *Synapse, 57*, 47–55.

Law, A. J., Weickert, C. S., Hyde, T. M., Kleinman, J. E., & Harrison, P. J. (2004). Reduced spinophilin but not microtubule-associated protein 2 expression in the hippocampal formation in schizophrenia and mood disorders: Molecular evidence for a pathology of dendritic spines. *American Journal of Psychiatry, 161*, 1848–1855.

Lee, K. W., Kim, Y., Kim, A. M., Helmin, K., Nairn, A. C., & Greengard, P. (2006). Cocaine-induced dendritic spine formation in D1 and D2 dopamine receptor-containing medium spiny neurons in nucleus accumbens. *Proceedings of the National Academy of Sciences of the United States of America, 103*, 3399–3404.

Levitt, J. J., Bobrow, L., Lucia, D., & Srinivasan, P. (2010). A selective review of volumetric and morphometric imaging in schizophrenia. *Current Topics in Behavioral Neurosciences, 4*, 243–281.

Li, Y., Kolb, B., & Robinson, T. E. (2003). The location of persistent amphetamine-induced changes in the density of dendritic spines on medium spiny neurosn in the nucleus accumbens and caudate-putamen. *Neuropsychopharmacology, 28*, 1082–1085.

Lisman, J. E., & Zhabotinsky, A. M. (2001). A model of synaptic memory: A CaMKII/PP1 switch that potentiates transmission by organizing an AMPA receptor anchoring assembly. *Neuron, 31*, 191–201.

Lovinger, D. M., Tyler, E. C., & Merrit, A. (1993). Short-and long-term synaptic depression in rat neostriatum. *Journal of Neurophysiology, 70*, 1937–1949.

Luscher, C., Xia, H., Beattie, E. C., Carroll, R. C., von Zastrow, M., Malenka, R. C., et al. (1999). Role of AMPA receptor cycling in synaptic transmission and plasticity. *Neuron, 24*, 649–658.

MacMillan, L. B., Bass, M. A., Cheng, N., Howard, E. F., Tamura, M., Strack, S., et al. (1999). Brain actin-associated protein phosphatase 1 holoenzymes containing spinophilin, neurabin, and selected catalytic subunit isoforms. *Journal of Biological Chemistry, 274*, 35845–35854.

Malchiodi-Albedi, F., Petrucci, T. C., Picconi, B., Iosi, F., & Falchi, M. (1997). Protein phosphatase inhibitors induce modification of synapse structure and tau hyperphosphorylation in cultured rat hippocampal neurons. *Journal of Neuroscience Research, 48*, 425–438.

Man, H. Y., Ju, W., Ahmadian, G., & Wang, Y. T. (2000). Intracellular trafficking of AMPA receptors in synaptic plasticity. *Cellular and Molecular Life Sciences, 57*, 1526–1534.

Masliah, E., Terry, R. D., DeTeresa, R. M., & Hansen, L. A. (1989). Immunohistochemical quantification of the synapse-related protein synaptophysin in Alzheimer disease. *Neuroscience Letters*, *103*, 234–239.

Matsuda, S., Mikawa, S., & Hirai, H. (1999). Phosphorylation of serine-880 in GluR2 by protein kinase C prevents its C terminus from binding with glutamate receptor-interacting protein. *Journal of Neurochemistry*, *73*, 1765–1768.

McAvoy, T., Allen, P. B., Obaishi, H., Nakanishi, H., Takai, Y., Greengard, P., et al. (1999). Regulation of neurabin I interaction with protein phosphatase 1 by phosphorylation. *Biochemistry*, *38*, 12943–12949.

McConnell, J. L., & Wadzinski, B. E. (2009). Targeting protein serine/threonine phosphatases for drug development. *Molecular Pharmacology*, *75*, 1249–1261.

McKinney, R. A., Capogna, M., Dürr, R., Gähwiler, B. H., & Thompson, S. M. (1999). Miniature synaptic events maintain dendritic spines via AMPA receptor activation. *Nature Neuroscience*, *2*, 44–49.

Meberg, P. J., Ono, S., Minamide, L. S., Takahashi, M., & Bamburg, J. R. (1998). Actin depolymerizing factor and cofilin phosphorylation dynamics: Response to signals that regulate neurite extension. *Cell Motility and the Cytoskeleton*, *39*, 172–190.

Mi, Z., Abrahamson, E. E., Ryu, A. Y., Fish, K. N., Sweet, R. A., Mufson, E. J., et al. (2017). Loss of precuneus dendritic spines immopositive for spinophilin is related to cognitive impairment in early Alzheimer's disease. *Neurobiology of Aging*, *55*, 159–166.

Milton, A. L., Merlo, E., Ratano, P., Gregory, B. L., Dumbreck, J. K., & Everitt, B. J. (2013). Double dissociation of the requirement for GluN2B- and GluN2A-containing NMDA receptors in the destabilization and restabilization of reconsolidating memory. *Journal of Neuroscience*, *33*, 1109–1115.

Morishita, W., Connor, J. H., Xia, H., Quinlan, E. M., Shenolikar, S., & Malenka, R. C. (2001). Regulation of synaptic strength by protein phosphatase 1. *Neuron*, *32*, 1133–1148.

Morris, C. W., Watkins, D. S., Salek, A. B., Edler, M. C., & Baucum, A. J., 2nd. (2018). The association of spinophilin with disks large-associated protein 3 (SAPAP3) is regulated by metabotropic glutamate receptor (mGluR) 5. *Molecular and Cellular Neuroscience*, *90*, 60–69.

Moser, M. B., Trommald, M., & Andersen, P. (1994). An increase in dendritic spine density on hippocampal CA1 pyramidal cells following spatial learning in adult rats suggests the formation of new synapses. *Proceedings of the National Academy of Sciences of the United States of America*, *91*, 12673–12675.

Mulkey, R. M., Endo, S., Shenolikar, S., & Malenka, R. C. (1994). Involvement of a calcineurin/inhibitor-1 phosphatase cascade in hippocampal long-term depression. *Nature*, *369*, 486–488.

Mulkey, R. M., Herron, C. E., & Malenka, R. C. (1993). An essential role for protein phosphatases in hippocampal long-term depression. *Science*, *261*, 1051–1055.

Mulkey, R. M., & Malenka, R. C. (1992). Mechanisms underlying induction of homosynaptic long-term depression in area CA1 of the hippocampus. *Neuron*, *9*, 967–975.

Muly, E. C., Allen, P., Mazloom, M., Aranbayeva, A., Greenfield, A. T., & Greengard, P. (2004). Subcellular distribution of neurabin immunolabeling in primate prefrontal cortex: Comparison with spinophilin. *Cerebral Cortex*, *14*, 1398–1407.

Muly, E. C., Greengard, P., & Goldman-Rakic, P. S. (2001). Distribution of protein phosphatases-1 alpha and −1 gamma 1 and the D (1) dopamine receptor in primate prefrontal cortex: Evidence for discrete populations of spines. *Journal of Comparative Neurology*, *440*, 261–270.

Nader, K. (2003). Memory traces unbound. *Trends in Neurosciences*, *26*, 65–72.

Nader, K., Schafe, G. E., & Le Doux, J. E. (2000). Fear memories require protein synthesis in the amygdala for reconsolidation after retrieval. *Nature*, *406*, 722–726.

Nakanishi, H., Obaishi, H., Satoh, A., Wada, M., Mandai, K., Satoh, K., et al. (1997). Neurabin: A novel neural tissue-specific actin filament-binding protein involved in neurite formation. *Journal of Cell Biology*, *139*, 951–961.

Oliet, S. H., Malenka, R. C., & Nicoll, R. A. (1997). Two distinct forms of long-term depression coexist in CA1 hippocampal pyramidal cells. *Neuron*, *18*, 969–982.

Oliver, C. J., Terry-Lorenzo, R. T., Elliott, E., Bloomer, W. A. C., Li, L., Brautigan, D. L., et al. (2002). Targeting protein phosphatase 1 (PP1) to the actin cytoskeleton: The neurabin I/PP1 complex regulates cell morphology. *Molecular and Cellular Biology*, *22*, 4690–4701.

Ouimet, C. C., da Cruz e Silva, E. F., & Greengard, P. (1995). The alpha and gamma 1 isoforms of protein phosphatase 1 are highly and specifically concentrated in dendritic spines. *Proceedings of the National Academy of Sciences of the United States of America*, *92*, 3396–3400.

Palmer, M. J., Irving, A. J., Seabrook, G. R., Jane, D. E., & Collingridge, G. L. (1997). The group I mGlu receptor agonist DHPG induces a novel form of LTD in the CA1 region of the hippocampus. *Neuropharmacology*, *36*, 1517–1532.

Pettit, D. L., Perlman, S., & Malinow, R. (1994). Potentiated transmission and prevention of further LTP by increased CaMKII activity in postsynaptic hippocampal slice neurons. *Science*, *266*, 1881–1885.

Picconi, B., Gardoni, F., Centonze, D., Mauceri, D., Cenci, M. A., Bernardi, G., et al. (2004). Abnormal Ca2+−calmodulin-dependent protein kinase II function mediates synaptic and motor deficits in experimental parkinsonism. *Journal of Neuroscience*, *24*, 5283–5291.

Ragusa, M. J., Dancheck, B., Critton, D. A., Nairn, A. C., Page, R., & Peti, W. (2010). Spinophilin directs protein phosphatase 1 specificity by blocking substrate binding sites. *Nature Structural and Molecular Biology*, *17*, 459–464.

Rebelo, S., Vieira, S. I., Esselmann, H., Wiltfang, J., da Cruz e Silva, E. F., & da Cruz e Silva, O. A. B. (2007). Tyrosine 687 phosphorylated Alzheimer's amyloid precursor protin is retained intracellularly and exhibits a decreased turnover rate. *Neurodegenerative Diseases*, *4*, 78–87.

Reynolds, J. N., Hyland, B. I., & Wickens, J. R. (2001). A cellular mechanism of reward-related learning. *Nature*, *413*, 67–70.

Roberts, R. C., Conley, R., Kung, L., Peretti, F. J., & Chute, D. J. (1996). Reduced striatal spine size in schizophrenia: A postmortem ultrastructural study. *Neuroreport*, *7*, 1214–1218.

Roberts, R. C., Roche, J. K., & Conley, R. R. (2005). Synaptic differences in the postmortem striatum of subjects with schizophrenia: A stereological ultrastructural analysis. *Synapse*, *56*, 185–197.

Rochefort, N. L., & Konnerth, A. (2012). Dendritic spines: From structure to in vivo function. *EMBO Reports*, *13*, 699–708.

Rosoklija, G., Toomayan, G., Ellis, S. P., Keilp, J., Mann, J. J., Latov, N., et al. (2000). Structural abnormalities of subicular dendrites in subjects in schizophrenia and mood disorders: Preliminary findings. *Archives of General Psychiatry*, *57*, 349–356.

Ryan, X. P., Alldritt, J., Svenningsson, P., Allen, P. B., Wu, G., Nairn, A. C., et al. (2005). The Rho-specific GEF Lfc interacts with neurabin and spinophilin to regulate dendritic spine morphology. *Neuron*, *47*, 85–100.

Salek, A. B., Edler, M. C., McBride, J. P., & Baucum, A. J., II. (2019). Spinophilin regulates phosphorylation and interactions of the GluN2B subunit of the *N*-methyl-*d*-aspartate receptor. *Journal of Neurochemistry*, *151*, 185–203.

Sarrouilhe, D., di Tommaso, A., Métayé, T., & Ladeveze, V. (2006). Spinophilin: From partners to functions. *Biochimie*, *88*, 1099–1113.
Sasaki, K., Shima, H., Kitagawa, Y., Irino, S., Sugimura, T., & Nagao, M. (1990). Identification of members of the protein phosphatase 1 gene family in the rat and enhanced expression of protein phosphatase 1 alpha gene in rat hepatocellular carcinomas. *Japanese Journal of Cancer Research*, *81*, 1271–1280.
Satoh, S., Nakanishi, H., Obaishi, H., Wada, M., Takahashi, K., Satoh, K., et al. (1998). Neurabin-II/spinophilin: An actin-filament-binding protein with one PDZ domain localized at cadherin-based cell-cell adhesion sites. *Journal of Biological Chemistry*, *273*, 3470–3475.
Selkoe, D. J. (2002). Alzheimer's disease is a synaptic failure. *Science*, *298*, 789–791.
Shen, W., Flajolet, M., Greengard, P., & Surmeier, D. J. (2008). Dichotomous dopaminergic control of striatal synaptic plasticity. *Science*, *321*, 848–851.
Shenolikar, S., & Nairn, A. C. (1991). Protein phosphatases: Recent progress. *Advances in Second Messenger and Phosphoprotein Research*, *23*, 1–121.
Shima, H., Haneji, T., Hatano, Y., Kasugai, I., Sugimura, T., & Nagao, M. (1993). Protein phosphatase 1 gamma 2 is associated with nuclei of meiotic cells in rat testis. *Biochemical and Biophysical Research Communications*, *194*, 930–937.
Shioda, N., Beppu, H., Fukuda, T., Li, E., Kitajima, I., & Fukunaga, K. (2011). Aberrant calcium/calmodulin-dependent protein kinase II (CaMKII) activity is associated with abnormal dendritic spine morphology in the ATRX mutant mouse brain. *Journal of Neuroscience*, *31*, 346–358.
Snyder, G. L., Allen, P. B., Fienberg, A. A., Valle, C. G., Huganir, R. L., Nairn, A. C., et al. (2000). Regulation of phosphorylation of the GluR1 AMPA receptor in the neostriatum by dopamine and psychostimulants in vivo. *Journal of Neuroscience*, *20*, 4480–4488.
Snyder, G. L., Fienberg, A. A., Huganir, R. L., & Greengard, P. (1998). A dopamine/D1 receptor/protein kinase A/dopamine-and cAMP-regulated phosphoprotein (Mr 32 kDa)/protein phosphatase-1 pathway regulates dephosphorylation of the NMDA receptor. *Journal of Neuroscience*, *18*, 10297–102303.
Stephens, B., Mueller, A. J., Shering, A. F., Hood, S. H., Taggart, P., Arbuthnott, G. W., et al. (2005). Evidence of a breakdown of corticostriatal connections in Parkinson's disease. *Neuroscience*, *132*, 741–754.
Stoof, J. C., & Kebabian, J. W. (1981). Opposing roles for D-1 and D-2 dopamine receptors in efflux of cyclic AMP from rat neostriatum. *Nature*, *294*, 366–368.
Strack, S., Barban, M. A., Wadzinski, B. E., & Colbran, R. J. (1997). Differential inactivation of postsynaptic density-associated and soluble Ca2+/calmodulin-dependent protein kinase II by protein phosphatases 1 and 2A. *Journal of Neurochemistry*, *68*, 2119–2128.
Strack, S., Kini, S., Ebner, F. F., Wadzinski, B. E., & Colbran, R. J. (1999). Differential cellular and subcellular localization of protein phosphatase 1 isoforms in brain. *Journal of Comparative Neurology*, *413*, 373–384.
Strålfors, P., Hiraga, A., & Cohen, P. (1985). The protein phosphatases involved in cellular regulation. Purification and characterization of the glycogen-bound form of protein phosphatase-1 from rabbit skeletal muscle. *European Journal of Biochemistry*, *149*, 295–303.
Sung, K. W., Choi, S., & Lovinger, D. M. (2001). Activation of group I mGluRs is necessary for induction of long-term depression at striatal synapses. *Journal of Neurophysiology*, *86*, 2405–2412.
Surmeier, D. J., Bargas, J., Hemmings, H. C., Jr., Nairn, A. C., & Greengard, P. (1995). Modulation of calcium currents by a D1 dopaminergic protein kinase/phosphatase cascade in rat neostriatal neurons. *Neuron*, *14*, 385–397.
Szatmari, E., Habas, A., Yang, P., Zheng, J., Hagg, T., & Hetman, M. (2005). A positive feedback loop between glycogen synthase kinase 3b and protein phosphatase 1 after

stimulation of NR2B NMDA receptors in forebrain neurons. *Journal of Biological Chemistry, 280*, 37526–37535.

Tang, J., & Dani, J. A. (2009). Dopamine enables in vivo synaptic plasticity associated with the addictive drug nicotine. *Neuron, 63*, 673–682.

Tappan, E., & Chamberlin, A. R. (2008). Activation of protein phosphatase 1 by a small molecule designed to bind to the enzyme's regulatory site. *Chemistry and Biology, 15*, 167–174.

Terry, R. D., Gonatas, N. K., & Weiss, M. (1964). The ultrastructure of the cerebral cortex in Alzheimer's disease. *Transactions of the American Neurological Association, 89*, 12.

Terry, R. D., Masliah, E., Salmon, D. P., Butters, N., DeTeresa, R., Hill, R., et al. (1991). Physical basis of cognitive alterations in Alzheimer's disease: Synapse loss is the major correlate of cognitive impairment. *Annals of Neurology, 30*, 572–580.

Terry-Lorenzo, R. T., Carmody, L. C., Voltz, J. W., Connor, J. H., Li, S., Smith, F. D., et al. (2002). The neuronal actin-binding proteins, neurabin I and neurabin II, recruit specific isoforms of protein phosphatase-1 catalytic subunits. *Journal of Biological Chemistry, 277*, 27716–27724.

Terry-Lorenzo, R. T., Roadcap, D. W., Otsuka, T., Blanpied, T. A., Zamorano, P. L., Garner, C. C., et al. (2005). Neurabin/protein phosphatase-1 complex regulates dendritic spine morphogenesis and maturation. *Molecular Biology of the Cell, 16*, 2349–2362.

Thanos, P. K., Bermeo, C., Wang, G., & Volkow, N. D. (2009). D-cycloserine accelerates the extinction of cocaine-induced conditioned place preference in C57bL/c mice. *Behavioral Brain Research, 199*, 345–349.

Vassilev, L. T., Vu, B. T., Graves, B., Carvajal, D., Podlaski, F., Filipovic, Z., et al. (2004). In vivo activation of the p53 pathway by small molecule antagonists of MDM2. *Science, 303*, 844–848.

Villalba, R. M., Lee, H., & Smith, Y. (2009). Dopaminergic denervation and spine loss in the striatum of MPTP-treated monkeys. *Experimental Neurology, 215*, 220–227.

Vintém, A. P. B., Henriques, A. G., da Cruz E Silva, O. A. B., & da Cruz E Silva, E. F. (2009). PP1 inhibition by Abeta peptide as a potential pathological mechanism in Alzhemer's disease. *Neurotoxicology and Teratology, 31*, 85–88.

Wan, Y., Feng, G., & Calakos, N. (2011). Sapap3 deletion causes mGluR5-dependent silencing of AMPAR synapses. *Journal of Neuroscience, 31*, 16685–16691.

Wang, Z., Kai, L., Day, M., Ronesi, J., Yin, H. H., Ding, J., et al. (2006). Dopaminergic control of corticostriatal long-term synaptic depression in medium spiny neurons is mediated by cholinergic interneurons. *Neuron, 50*, 443–452.

Wang, L. Y., Orser, B. A., Brautigan, D. L., & MacDonald, J. F. (1994). Regulation of NMDA receptors in cultured hippocampal neurons by protein phosphatases 1 and 2A. *Nature, 369*, 230–323.

Wang, L. Y., Salter, M. W., & MacDonald, J. F. (1991). Regulation of kainate receptors by cAMP-dependent protein kinase and phosphatases. *Science, 253*, 1132–1135.

Watanabe, T., Huang, H. B., Horiuchi, A., da Cruze Silva, E. F., Hsieh-Wilson, L., Allen, P. B., et al. (2001). Protein phosphatase 1 regulation by inhibitors and targeting subunits. *Proceedings of the National Academy of Sciences of the United States of America, 98*, 3080–3085.

Watkins, D. S., True, J. D., Mosley, A. L., & Baucum, A. J., II. (2018). Proteomic analysis of the spinophilin interactome in rodent striatum following psychostimulant sensitization. *Proteomics, 6*, 53.

Weeber, E. J., Jiang, Y., Elgersma, Y., Varga, A. W., Carrasquillo, Y., Brown, S. E., et al. (2003). Derangements of hippocampal calcium/calmodulin-dependent protein kinase II in a mouse model for Angelman mental retardation syndrome. *Journal of Neuroscience, 23*, 2634–2644.

Weickert, C. S., Straub, R. E., McClintock, B. W., Matsumoto, M., Hashimoto, R., Hyde, T. M., et al. (2004). Human dysbindin (DTNBP1) gene expression in normal brain and in schizophrenia prefrontal cortex and midbrain. *Archives of General Psychiatry*, *61*, 544–555.

Welch, J. M., Lu, J., Rodriguiz, R. M., Trotta, N. C., Peca, J., Ding, J., et al. (2007). Cortico-striatal synaptic defects and OCD-like behaviours in *Sapap3*-mutant mice. *Nature*, *448*, 894–900.

Wu, H., Cottingham, C., Chen, L., Wang, H., Che, P., Liu, K., et al. (2017). Age-dependent differential regulation of anxiety-and depression-related behaviors by neurabin and spinophilin. *PLoS One*, *12*, e0180638.

Wu, L., Ren, M., Wang, H., Kim, S. S., Cao, X., & Zhuo, M. (2008). Neurabin contributes to hippocampal long-term potentiation and contextual fear memory. *PLoS One*, *3*, e1407.

Yan, Z., Hsieh-Wilson, L., Feng, J., Tomizawa, K., Allen, P. B., Fienberg, A. A., et al. (1999). Protein phosphatase 1 modulation of neostriatal AMPA channels: Regulation by DARPP-32 and spinophilin. *Nature Neuroscience*, *2*, 13–17.

Yu, Y., Huang, C., Chang, C., & Gean, P. (2016). Involvement of protein phosphatases in the destabilization of methamphetamine-associated contextual memory. *Learning and Memory*, *23*, 486–493.

Zito, K., Knott, G., Shepherd, G. M. G., Shenolikar, S., & Svoboda, K. (2004). Induction of spine growth and synapse formation by regulation of the spine actin cytoskeleton. *Neuron*, *44*, 321–334.

CHAPTER SEVEN

Deciphering cell-type specific signal transduction in the brain: Challenges and promises

Jean-Pierre Roussarie[a,*] and Patricia Rodriguez-Rodriguez[a,b]
[a]Laboratory of Molecular and Cellular Neuroscience, The Rockefeller University, New York, NY, United States
[b]Department of Neurobiology, Care Sciences and Society, Division of Neurogeriatrics, Karolinska Institutet, Solna, Sweden
[*]Corresponding author: e-mail address: jroussarie@rockefeller.edu

Contents

Abstract

Signal transduction designates the set of molecular events that take place within a cell upon extracellular stimulation to mediate a functional outcome. Decades after the discovery that dopamine triggers opposing signaling pathways in D1- and D2-expressing medium spiny neurons, it is now clear that there are as many different flavors of signaling pathways in the brain as there are neuron types. One of the biggest challenges in molecular neuroscience is to elucidate cell-type specific signaling, in order to understand neurological diseases with regional vulnerability, but also to identify targets for precision drugs devoid of off-target effects. Here, we make a case for the importance of the study of neuron-type specific molecular characteristics. We then review the technologies that exist to study neurons in their full diversity and highlight their disease-relevant idiosyncrasies.

Advances in Pharmacology, Volume 90
ISSN 1054-3589
https://doi.org/10.1016/bs.apha.2020.09.009

List of abbreviations

AD	Alzheimer's disease
ARACNe	algorithm for the reconstruction of accurate cellular networks
bacTRAP	bacterial artificial chromosome—translating ribosome affinity purification
BioID	proximity-dependent biotin identification
ECII	layer II of the entorhinal cortex
FACS	fluorescence activated cell sorting
FUNCAT	fluorescent non-canonical amino acid tagging
GWAS	genome-wide association study
HD	Huntington's disease
MARINA	master regulator inference algorithm
MDD	major depressive disorder
MS	mass spectrometry
MSN	medium spiny neuron
NetWAS	network-wide association study
PD	Parkinson's disease
RNAseq	RNA sequencing
SLIC	synthetic lethal in the central nervous system
SNpc	substantia nigra pars compacta
SORT	stochastic orthogonal recoding of translation

1. Introduction

1.1 Early steps of neuronal signaling pathway dissection

At the beginning of the 1970s, Paul Greengard made his first series of groundbreaking observations that would pave the way for much of modern molecular neuroscience: he discovered the existence of slow synaptic transmission modes, where neurotransmitters like dopamine trigger a series of biochemical changes within a neuron, modulating its function (reviewed in Girault & Greengard, 2004). He first noted that exposure to dopamine triggers biochemical events within dopaminoceptive neurons, specifically an increase of the second messenger cyclic AMP (Kebabian & Greengard, 1971). This laid the groundwork for the exploration of signal transduction in neurons, i.e., the biochemical cascades that, upon receipt of an extracellular signal, and through the successive activation of kinases and phosphorylation of their substrates eventually change neuronal morphology, excitability, plasticity, and can also potentially trigger the onset of neurodegenerative processes. Among many molecular outcomes, signal transduction pathways would later be shown to modify, within a neuron, the presence of ion channels at the plasma membrane, its responsiveness to neurotransmitters, the outgrowth of neuronal processes, the genesis and consolidation of synapses and the regulation of transcription and translation (Girault & Greengard, 1999, 2004; Kuo & Greengard, 1969).

The discovery that there are two types of dopamine receptors, D1 and D2, expressed on two different sets of striatal medium spiny neurons (MSNs) (Girault & Greengard, 2004), the activation of which had opposite effects on cAMP levels, demonstrated for the first time that the same stimulus could trigger different transduction pathways in different cell types (Kebabian & Caine, 1979). These opposite effects, due to different biochemical properties of D1 and D2 receptors but also to the differential expression of signaling intermediates in the two types of MSNs eventually led to two very different functional outcomes for these cells (Girault & Greengard, 2004). For Paul Greengard, this created the impulse to precisely describe transduction pathways in a cell-type specific manner, to understand the molecular mechanisms by which different cells, when subjected to the same stimulus, would exhibit different responses. This principle, at the basis of neuron specialization across and within different regions of the brain (Doyle et al., 2008; Fishell & Heintz, 2013), relentlessly occupied Paul Greengard from his initial dopamine discoveries. Of the many methods that became available with time to probe the activity of signal transduction pathways, very few offered the possibility to assess one cell at a time. What electrophysiologist routinely do when they patch a specific cell is a rare luxury for biochemists. Paul Greengard had to develop a number of transformative technologies to dissect signal transduction pathways in individual cell types (Bateup et al., 2008; Brichta et al., 2015; Heiman et al., 2008; Jordi, 2013; Oh et al., 2013; Roussarie et al., 2020), some of which we will outline in this review. The striatum, the ultimate Greengardian brain region, with its two intermingled MSN types that are very similar to one another, but yet differ molecularly by hundreds of differentially expressed genes (Heiman et al., 2008), is a paradigm of choice for the study of cell-type specific processes that he and many others would go back to, time and again.

Our goal here is to review the status of cell-type specific signaling research, and in particular its importance for the study of brain diseases. We will first make the case that most psychiatric and neurodegenerative diseases affect specific cell types, and therefore can only be understood by taking into account this cellular tropism and cell-type specific particularities. After establishing a benchmark of the proteomics, epigenomics and genomics techniques that exist in order to tackle this question, we will review in greater details a few systems-level approaches that could bring new light on cell-type specific signal transduction. Lastly, we will show the immense promises of a cell type specific description of disease pathogenesis, with cell-type specific drugs potentially allowing greater efficacy with minimal side effects. Paul Greengard's intuition during his entire life was that defects in signal transduction underlie the pathogenesis of most brain diseases. As a consequence, the understanding of cell-type specific transduction cascades can yield therapeutic targets for cell-type specific diseases.

2. Psychiatric and neurodegenerative diseases: A cell-specific perspective

Psychiatric and neurodegenerative disorders have in common that the dysfunction of the nervous system is chronic, either progressive or prone to relapse, having a profound impact on families and society. The most prevalent psychiatric disorders are autism spectrum disorders, major depressive disorder (MDD), schizophrenia and bipolar disorder. Some of them frequently co-occur in the same patients, complicating both the diagnosis and the optimization of drug therapies. The available medication is inefficient for a significant subset of patients and is often associated with a wide range of side effects that contribute to disability and noncompliance. Alzheimer's (AD), Parkinson's (PD) and Huntington's disease (HD) are among the most common neurodegenerative disorders and are characterized by the progressive degeneration of specific neuronal subpopulations. They ultimately lead to death and there is no available cure.

One possible explanation for the difficulties to develop successful therapies to treat neurodegenerative disorders like AD or to find efficient treatments that lead to remission of psychiatric disorders with minimal side effects is that the study of these diseases rarely takes into account the cell type or brain region most affected by them.

The necessity to study disease mechanisms from a cell-type specific perspective is relatively obvious in the case of neurodegenerative disorders like AD, PD or HD, where specific sets of neurons are actually degenerating early on in the disease (Fu, Hardy, & Duff, 2018). For each of these diseases, the vulnerable neuron populations have long been described by pathologists, but the reasons behind the selective susceptibility of specific neuronal subpopulations remains to be understood. In the past few years, the complexity of the mechanisms and contribution of different cell types to these diseases is becoming more and more evident. In HD, a ubiquitous autosomal dominant inherited mutation in the gene that codes for Huntington is causative for the disease and leads to the specific loss of MSNs in the striatum by making them more vulnerable to oxidative stress and excitotoxicity (Valencia et al., 2013) and by activating neuronal innate immune response (Wertz et al., 2020). Vulnerability is even more specific since D2-expressing MSNs are more vulnerable than their D1-expressing counterpart (Reiner et al., 1988). There is also a strong contribution of astrocytes to this regional susceptibility, making them potential targets for therapeutic intervention (Ehrnhoefer et al., 2018; Polyzos et al., 2019). PD, the most common neurodegenerative disorder after AD, is associated with the degeneration of dopaminergic neurons in the midbrain, specifically those in the substantia nigra pars compacta (SNpc) (Poewe et al., 2017). It is characterized by the presence of intraneuronal accumulations of the alpha-synuclein protein called Lewy bodies. Despite heritable cases of the disease being triggered by mutations in *SNCA, LRRK2, PINK1, PARKIN* and *DJ-1* genes, the majority of cases are sporadic. The reasons behind the vulnerability of dopaminergic neurons in the SNpc is unknown but thought to be associated with the intrinsic higher sensitivity of these cells to mitochondrial dysfunction and oxidative stress (Surmeier, Obeso, & Halliday, 2017). In the past years increasing evidence suggests a contribution of microglia and astrocytes in the development and progression of the disease by triggering pathological inflammation (Liddelow et al., 2017; Yun et al., 2018). AD is the most common neurodegenerative disorder and the leading cause of dementia. It is characterized by the appearance of amyloid plaques (deposits of amyloid beta, the cleavage product of amyloid precursor protein) and intracellular accumulation of hyperphosphorylated tau protein (neurofibrillary tangles, NFT). The first neurons to degenerate in AD are the excitatory pyramidal neurons of the layer II of the entorhinal cortex (ECII), where NFT appear at prodromal stages of the disease (Braak & Braak, 1996), and the presence of amyloid pathology seems to be necessary for the progression of tau pathology from the EC to the neocortex (Pontecorvo et al., 2019). The familial cases of early-onset AD are associated with mutations in either the gene that codes for amyloid precursor protein (APP) or for APP-processing proteins. However, 95% of the AD cases show a late onset and while old age, *APOE* and *TREM2* mutations are the most significant genetic risk factors, their association with the appearance of the amyloid plaques and NFTs that characterize AD are not understood. In the past few years, a wide range of cell-specific studies have confirmed a strong implication of non-neuronal cells to the disease, including microglia (Ledo, Liebmann, et al., 2020; Ledo, Zhang, et al., 2020; Nott et al., 2019; Sala Frigerio et al., 2019; Shi et al., 2019), where *TREM2* is expressed, modulating their function, astrocytes (Habib et al., 2020; Liddelow et al., 2017), oligodendrocytes (Mathys et al., 2019; Tse, Cheng, Ma, & Herrup, 2018) and even pericytes, that are especially sensitive to injury in APOE4 carriers, leading to breakdown of the blood brain barrier (Montagne et al., 2020). How all these cell types and their crosstalk contribute to the development of the disease, and the cascade of events that lead to the early degeneration of ECII neurons remains unknown.

Perhaps less trivially than for neurodegenerative diseases, psychiatric diseases also do not affect all cells equally, and would greatly benefit from a closer investigation of cell-type specific disease mechanisms. Of course, the impairment in serotonergic and noradrenergic transmission that has traditionally been a major axis of MDD research has warranted investigation of neurons producing these neurotransmitters. But in the past decade, a very large body of work from the Greengard laboratory and collaborators complexified this view of the disease. Different studies revealed that cell-type specific alterations in signal transduction pathways in various glutamatergic, GABAergic, and cholinergic cells could cause a depressed state and affect the responsiveness to selective serotonin reuptake inhibitor treatments, via, for instance, deficits in neurotransmitter receptor or ion channel shuttling to the plasma membrane, or responsiveness to growth factors (Arango-Lievano et al., 2016; Castello et al., 2018; Cheng, Umschweif, Leung, Sagi, & Greengard, 2019; Chottekalapanda et al., 2020; Jin et al., 2020; Lee et al., 2015; Medrihan et al., 2020; Milosevic et al., 2017; Nasca et al., 2017; Sagi et al., 2020; Sargin et al., 2020; Schmidt et al., 2012; Shuto et al., 2020; Virk et al., 2016; Wang et al., 2015; Warner-Schmidt et al., 2012). Schizophrenia, bipolar disorder and autism have also all been associated to modifications in the excitatory-inhibitory balance (Marín, 2012; Yizhar et al., 2011). The interneuron subtypes and the precise mechanisms of neuron-type specific dysfunctions implicated in each of these disorders are far from being understood (Marín, 2012). Common genetic risk variants for schizophrenia map to specific inhibitory neuron subpopulations such as *Drd2/Drd1*-expressing medium spiny neurons and parvalbumin (PV) interneurons in the striatum or *Reln*-expressing interneurons in cortex layer I (Skene et al., 2018). Knocking down the *Erbb4* gene or decreasing NMDA receptor signaling exclusively in PV-interneurons in mice leads to schizophrenia-like behavior (Carlén et al., 2012; Wen et al., 2010).

Moreover, there is a very abundant literature on region-specific variations in brain volume or activity in each of these psychiatric disorders, suggesting differences in synapse or cell density, or connectivity between brain areas, but the precise underlying molecular bases remain to be established (Amaral, Schumann, & Nordahl, 2008; Baumann & Bogerts, 2001; Hercher, Turecki, & Mechawar, 2009; Meyer-Lindenberg et al., 2005). Beyond neurons, glial cells could also play a role in psychiatric disease pathogenesis. Studies in patients with schizophrenia or bipolar disorders have reported a contribution of astrocytes, as they are essential for the maintenance of neuronal and synaptic homeostasis, and they have been shown to be direct targets of lithium (Rivera & Butt, 2019). In MDD, there is a decrease in astrocyte numbers and astrocyte-derived ATP has been shown to modulate depressive-like behavior (Cao et al., 2013; Oh, Son, Hwang, & Kim, 2012; Toker, Mancarci, Tripathy, & Pavlidis, 2018). Also, single-nucleus RNA-seq in MDD patients compared to controls found some of the most significant gene expression differences in immature oligodendrocyte precursor cells. These changes could suggest impairment in oligodendrocyte lineage differentiation (Nagy et al., 2020).

Together, this evidence supports the notion that we will only be able to develop efficient therapies against psychiatric and neurodegenerative diseases by studying disease mechanisms from a cell-type specific perspective, identifying how genetic variation associated with disease modifies cell-type specific pathways (Hekselman & Yeger-Lotem, 2020), and also how the interplay between different brain cells contributes to disease progression.

3. Cell-type specific identification of pathological pathways: Current advances and remaining challenges

To probe a signaling pathway in a cell-type specific way, one would ideally separate physically the cell type before using it for biochemical assays. Yet among all organs, the brain poses a unique challenge. Its cellular heterogeneity is extremely complex and neurons and glial cells are all intermingled. Dissociation of the brain might thus damage cells, first and foremost neurons, since their processes are longer and more complex than the ones from all the other cell types. In spite of this caveat, brain dissociation and cell sorting has been successfully used in multiple studies, and we will discuss some of these studies, as well as available alternatives.

The second challenge is to conduct, on the cell-type specific isolate, an assay that will yield insight into a signal transduction pathway. Activity of a pathway involves the complex regulation of protein function and activity, including synthesis, degradation, posttranslational modifications (phosphorylation, truncation, glycosylation, acetylation, etc.) and transport to specific cellular compartments (Hirokawa & Takemura, 2005; Liu, Beyer, & Aebersold, 2016). It is thus crucial to study all of these levels of regulation in order to evaluate cell-type specific transduction. Unfortunately, even though mass spectrometry (MS) techniques are improving in sensitivity, cell-type specific proteomics are still methodologically challenging. One lingering problem in the field is that proteins cannot be amplified like mRNAs, and after isolation from sparse cells are often below the current detection limits. For this reason, the availability of cell-type specific proteomic data is still very limited. Brain dissociation (with the caveats highlighted above), followed by fluorescence-activated cell sorting (FACS) or magnetic activated cell sorting, and MS allows for cell-type specific proteomics, and has been used to characterize the proteome of specific cell types in AD mouse models (Rayaprolu et al., 2020). Dissociated cells can also be analyzed by single-cell mass cytometry (CyTOF), where different proteins can be analyzed at the single cell level in multiplex. However, it relies on the use of a battery of antibodies, so it does not allow for unbiased proteomics analysis, and the number of proteins that can be measured is limited (Bendall et al., 2011).

An alternative to brain dissociation, which is still at its early stages, is to label the proteome *in vivo* in a cell-type specific manner. This relies on the incorporation of a non-canonical amino acid into the proteome and requires the overexpression of a modified tRNA synthetase in a cell type of interest either by generation of a transgenic mouse model like for FUNCAT (Fluorescent non-canonical amino acid tagging) (Alvarez-Castelao et al., 2017) or by the injection, in the region of interest, of an adeno-associated virus (AAV) with a cell-type specific promoter like for SORT (Stochastic orthogonal recoding of translation) (Krogager et al., 2018). Only cells that express the modified tRNA synthetase incorporate the non-canonical amino acid into their proteome. This non-canonical amino acid can then be immunoprecipitated and all labeled proteins can be analyzed by MS. Alternatively, in a technique called BioID (for proximity-dependent biotin identification), enzyme catalyzed proximity labeling consists of using engineered biotin ligases fused to a protein of interest to tag neighboring proteins in a radius of approximately 10 nm from the ligase (Roux, Kim, Raida, & Burke, 2012).

Biotinylated proteins are then immunoprecipitated with neutravidin and identified by MS. By expressing the ligase under a cell-type specific promoter, this technique allows for cell-type specific proteomics analysis with subcellular resolution (Uezu et al., 2016). These techniques have a huge potential although some challenges remain, namely the amount of mice required to have enough cell-type specific proteins for MS, and specificity issues requiring to always compare two carefully controlled conditions, in order to rule out the isolation of any protein coming from unwanted cell types.

On the other end of the throughput spectrum, cell-type specific genetic tools can also be used elegantly to study particular signal transduction pathways. Bateup and colleagues from the Greengard lab generated mouse lines expressing a tagged DARPP-32—a central signaling protein of the striatum (Greengard & Fienberg, 1998)—in D1- or D2-MSNs. Isolation of cell-type specific DARPP-32 by immunoprecipitation allowed the study of DARPP-32 phosphorylation specifically in each type of MSN and yielded unprecedented insight into D1- vs. D2-MSN posttranslational modification of this major signaling intermediate (Bateup et al., 2008). Opposite effects of a number of psychostimulant and antipsychotic drugs on both types of MSNs were thus shown for the first time.

In the case of human brain samples, collected *postmortem* and often frozen, the impossibility to perform any of the aforementioned protein tagging techniques makes the generation of cell-type specific proteomics data more challenging. For this reason, the only available neuron-type specific data has been obtained by laser capture microdissection (Drummond, Nayak, Ueberheide, & Wisniewski, 2015). However, it is time consuming and relies on proper identification of the cell type of interest using antibodies. To date, most of the proteomics data from patients with psychiatric and neurodegenerative diseases is obtained from bulk tissue from specific brain regions (Bereczki et al., 2018; Mendonça et al., 2019; Xu et al., 2018), including a recent study of the proteome and phosphoproteome in AD (Bai et al., 2020) and would benefit of being integrated with single-cell genomics and transcriptomics data (Canchi et al., 2019).

While the dissociation of the brain into individual cells can be challenging for reasons outlined above, breaking all plasma membranes to isolate nuclei allows the isolation of easily FACS-sortable nucleus suspensions from all brain cells. This makes the study of chromatin and nuclear proteins or mRNA easier than the study of cytoplasmic material and opens up the possibility to easily study cell-type specific chromatin regulation.

Interestingly, Genome-wide association studies (GWASs), that help identify genetic polymorphisms associated with a disease, have found that in psychiatric and neurodegenerative disorders many of the loci are located in non-coding regions of the genome (Zhou et al., 2019). This suggests that mechanisms that regulate gene expression may play an essential role in the development of these diseases (Jakovcevski & Akbarian, 2012). Indeed, histone deacetylases inhibitors have been proposed as potential therapies to treat a wide range of diseases affecting the central nervous system, including HD (Jia, Kast, Steffan, & Thomas, 2012; Kazantsev & Thompson, 2008). Differences in histone acetylation were also found in patients with autism spectrum disorder (Sun et al., 2016). Furthermore, changes in DNA methylation during development and neurodifferentiation have been found to be enriched in genomic regions associated with risk for schizophrenia by GWAS (Jaffe et al., 2015). GWAS for psychiatric disorders have also identified histone methylation as some of the top pathways associated with schizophrenia and bipolar disorder (Hannon et al., 2015; O'dushlaine et al., 2015). Epigenetic modifications also play an important role in aging, and have been shown to be associated with tau pathology and AD (De Jager et al., 2014; Gjoneska et al., 2015; Klein et al., 2019; Smith et al., 2018). Since epigenetic modifications can greatly differ between different cell subtypes, it is important to study epigenomics in a cell-type specific manner (Kozlenkov et al., 2014; Mendizabal et al., 2019). To gain insight into cell-type specific epigenetic modifications FACS-sorted nuclei can be subjected to either whole-genome bisulfite sequencing, to identify DNA methylation patterns (Mendizabal et al., 2019), or ChIP-seq to identify DNA-protein interactions or histone modifications (Girdhar et al., 2018). However, the limitation of nucleus sorting is that it relies on antibody- or genetic tagging-based labeling, limiting the cell subtypes that can be studied. The molecular characterization of cell types from an increasing number of brain regions will likely generalize the availability of nuclear markers to identify nuclei from specific sets of neurons, in the mouse as well as in humans (Xu et al., 2018). The use of bacterial artificial chromosome translational ribosome affinity purification mice (bacTRAP), where nucleoli of specific neuron populations are labeled by an eGFP-L10a fusion protein permits the isolation of nuclei of restricted cell types, for chromatin studies (Kriaucionis & Heintz, 2009). For instance, Mellen and colleagues used this technique to study genome-wide deposition of methylated and hydroxymethylated DNA marks in different cell types of the cerebellum (Mellén, Ayata, Dewell, Kriaucionis, & Heintz, 2012). Very elegant studies in the striatum have also yielded more targeted insight into cell type specific chromatin regulation in MSNs (Jordi, 2013; Schaefer et al., 2009). Jordi and colleagues from the Greengard lab demonstrated that cocaine has differential effects on various histone posttranslational modifications in D1- and D2-expressing MSNs, using D1- and D2-bacTRAP mice. These different approaches could be used in neurodegenerative disease and psychiatric disease models, in order to study the cell-type specific epigenetic dysregulation in these pathological contexts.

Alleviating the need for cell-type specific tagging, the assay for transposase-accessible chromatin sequencing (ATAC-seq), that identifies genome-wide open chromatin regions, was recently made possible at the single-cell resolution (Buenrostro et al., 2015; Cusanovich et al., 2015), and chromatin accessibility can thus be studied in all the cell types of a given brain region.

While the study of cell-type specific proteome and chromatin conformation has long remained elusive, earlier progress was made with the isolation of cell-type specific mRNA. A real breakthrough came when Paul Greengard and Nathaniel Heintz developed the first mammalian *in vivo* ribosomal profiling technique (Doyle et al., 2008; Heiman et al., 2008). It relies on the construction of bacTRAP mice that overexpress an eGFP-tagged ribosomal protein L10a exclusively in a cell type of interest. In these cells, polysomes are bound by eGFP-tagged L10a, which can then be immunoprecipitated for subsequent profiling using RNA sequencing (RNAseq). For a number of cell types and bacTRAP mice, only one mouse is enough to isolate enough RNA for RNAseq (Roussarie et al., 2020). This then allows to correlate gene expression with behavioral traits or with disease endophenotypes, by using disease mouse models (Heiman et al., 2008; Heiman, Kulicke, Fenster, Greengard, & Heintz, 2014). It is a real *ex vivo* mRNA profiling technique where RNA is isolated, unaltered, within minutes after sacrificing the animal. Long before the advent of single-cell RNAseq, this method allowed cell-type specific isolation of mRNA, opening the door to a comprehensive understanding of the unique molecular characteristics of different cells (Roussarie et al., 2020).

More recently though, single-cell and -nucleus RNAseq emerged for the comprehensive characterization of all cells within a given brain region. These methods are either sorting cells and placing them in individual tubes where they will be used for the generation of a single-cell cDNA library or they trap single cells within microdroplets along with barcodes, generating cDNA libraries where material from each individual cell or nucleus is barcoded (Islam et al., 2012; Macosko et al., 2015). As discussed above, single-nucleus sequencing alleviates the need of a dissociated cell suspension, and RNA content will probably more faithfully reflect physiological RNA content (Habib et al., 2017). The main limitations of these techniques are their high price, and that they only allow a relatively shallow sequencing of each cell or nucleus.

While the bacTRAP technology can be tedious to develop because it requires the construction of a transgenic mouse with cell-type restricted expression of eGFP-L10a, it is still the preferred technique to test the effect of a genetic mutation or a drug treatment. Since only mRNA bound to ribosomes are immunoprecipitated, the cell-type specific profile obtained is a reflection of the translatome, rather than the transcriptome, and thus slightly closer to the protein content of the cells (Heiman et al., 2008). Also, the profiling of a cell type is much deeper than what is possible with single-cell RNAseq. For instance *Nmur2*, is one of the genes most significantly enriched in ECII neurons in our bacTRAP data (Roussarie et al., 2020), but it is too sparsely detected in our EC single-nucleus sequencing data to show as enriched (unpublished data). Furthermore bacTRAP mRNA is also amenable to the study of differential exon usage (Furlanis, Traunmüller, Fucile, & Scheiffele, 2019). Lastly, it is much cheaper than single-cell RNAseq, and thus makes it possible to run as many replicates as needed to achieve desired power for differential expression analysis. Altogether, bacTRAP is a very powerful technique to catalog, with a large dynamic range, the mRNA isoforms actively translated in a specific cell type, and how they are modulated by genetic or pharmacological intervention.

4. Gaining functional understanding of the cell from systems-level approaches

Profiling specific cell types in normal conditions or in a disease context is only a first necessary step. The ongoing challenge for cell-type specific signaling research has been to transform profiling data into a readout of the functional status of the cells. One technique to derive functional knowledge from RNA studies is to study the coexpression between genes. Genes within a common pathway are likely regulated together. The activation of a specific functional program it is not triggered by one gene in isolation, but rather by, for instance, all the targets of a transcription factor or a microRNA that are activated in a coordinated manner. Modules of genes that are coregulated will thus yield insight into functionally coherent groups of genes, and signaling pathways (Eisen, Spellman, Brown, & Botstein, 1998). A widely used technique is weighted-gene coexpression analysis (WGCNA) (Langfelder & Horvath, 2008) which identifies modules of coexpressed genes, and can correlate these modules with disease traits. Very often, coexpression modules are enriched in cell-type specific markers. However, they generally represent entire sets of cell-type specific genes, or groups of massively coexpressed genes like inflammatory genes rather than more subtle functional modules within neurons, for instance, and will yield only little insight into specific neuronal regulatory modules.

In the past years, we and others set out to design analysis frameworks that integrate cell-type specific expression data along with other data to gain functional insight into specific cell types in the context of neurodegenerative diseases. We will review a few cases where bacTRAP was used to profile a vulnerable neuron type, and where functional insight came from a systems-level use of publicly available data or simply from the screening of many candidate genes. While these techniques are ambitious endeavors at early stages of cell-type specific modeling, they represent a promising direction of what can be achieved by modeling cells *in silico* and testing cells *in vivo* for the study of cell-type specific processes.

Gene expression patterns do not reveal function when taken in isolation. They represent a cross-section of a cell at a given time and in a given context. Analyzed in conjunction with large data compendia that include many of these cross-sections for a particular organan, as well as additional functional genomics data, the transcriptome (or even better the translatome) can eventually reveal functional signal. This was exemplified with the MPTP model of PD (Brichta et al., 2015). Brichta and colleagues used bacTRAP to profile dopaminergic neurons right before they degenerate as a result of treatment with the neurotoxin MPTP in the mouse. This yielded a list of differentially expressed transcripts. However, it was difficult to disentangle active drivers of degeneration from secondary changes with no functional consequence for the cells. The solution to this issue was the generation of networks to predict upstream regulators of gene expression. Brichta et al. used the combination of two algorithms named ARACNe (Algorithm for the Reconstruction of Accurate Cellular Networks) and MARINA (MAster Regulator INference Algorithm). ARACNe first mapped all the relationships between transcription factors and potential target genes using a large compendium of publicly available mouse whole brain expression data. This brain-specific model of all interactions between genes, was then leveraged by MARINA along with the gene signature of MPTP-treated dopaminergic neurons to predict the upstream regulatory changes that led to neurodegeneration. MARINA returned a ranked list of transcription factors inferred to direct gene expression changes in dopaminergic neurons subjected to MPTP. While ARACNe's mappings are not cell-type specific, MARINA returned cell-type specific transcription factor predictions because cell-type specific gene signatures were used as an input. One of the most striking results of this analysis was the prediction of MPTP-induced changes in the activity of the transcription factor SATB1, while the expression level of SATB1 is not affected by MPTP. Interestingly SATB1 is expressed at higher levels in the vulnerable SNpc and at much lower levels in the more resistant dopaminergic neurons from the ventral tegmental area. Follow-up analyses further proved that the invalidation of SATB1 triggered senescence in human dopaminergic neurons but not cortical neurons (Riessland et al., 2019). Strikingly, SATB1 was later found to be genetically associated with PD in a large GWAS (Chang et al., 2017). Altogether this proved the ability of MARINA and ARACNe to identify functional changes that go beyond pure gene expression, and to highlight cell-type specific molecular features associated with disease. Much work is needed in order to understand how MPTP triggers a series of molecular events specifically in dopaminergic neurons that culminate with the inhibition of SATB1 and ensuing neurodegeneration, but these results show that SATB1 plays a major part in pathological signaling in dopaminergic neurons.

The identity of all members of a signal transduction pathway is often determined by overexpressing or silencing putative members of the pathway, while probing a functional outcome for the cell. In the field of neurodegeneration, the influence of a gene on the neurodegeneration phenotype can be determined by injecting viral vectors stereotaxically in the region of interest in a mouse model of the disease, while monitoring cell survival. Unfortunately, this approach is difficult to scale up to rapidly screen for dozens of potential gene candidates. It is nonetheless the tour de force proposed by Shema et al., a major advance in the field (Shema et al., 2015). In this approach coined SLIC (for Synthetic Lethal In the Central nervous system), literally an *in vivo* toxic lethality screen, a library of lentiviruses each containing a silencing shRNA against a different gene, as well as a unique barcode was injected into the striatum of HD mouse models or controls. Four weeks after injection, the comparative presence or absence of each barcode in HD or controls was determined by RNAseq. Silencing a gene involved in neuronal survival in the context of HD will be toxic and the corresponding barcode will be lost in HD but not in control mice. On the contrary, if an shRNA is directed against a gene that is not involved in neuronal survival, the cell will survive, and the barcode will remain present. This impressive and unique strategy that Heiman and colleagues achieved, first with a couple hundred genes shortlisted based on previous bacTRAP data (Shema et al., 2015), and then with the entire genome (Wertz et al., 2020) paves the way to identify the transduction pathways at play during HD pathogenesis.

A further example of the use of functional genomics to investigate cell-type specific signal transduction is a study that we recently published, aimed at understanding the reasons for selective neuronal vulnerability in AD (Roussarie et al., 2020). In this study, like in the ones described above, we heavily relied on bacTRAP data in order to guide our systems-level analysis. We compared the profile of the neurons most vulnerable to AD, the ones from ECII, and to some extent CA1 pyramidal neurons, with more resistant neurons, like pyramidal cells from CA2, CA3, from primary visual and somatosensory cortices and granule cells from the dentate gyrus. We used bacTRAP to compare these neurons in wild type mice at three different ages and profiled ECII neurons in a mouse model of amyloid accumulation. We identified dozens of genes enriched in vulnerable neurons, a number of them also modulated by aging and amyloid accumulation. However, like in previous examples, this was not sufficient to gain unequivocal insight into the molecular drivers of cell-type specific vulnerability to AD. To identify functionally meaningful features of vulnerable neurons, we adopted a systems-level strategy: we constructed functional networks, i.e., *in silico* models for each type of vulnerable and resistant neurons studied. For that, we used our neuron type specific profiles as a hook to extract neuron-type specific relationships between genes from a large compendium of functional genomics data. Functional relationships between genes are evaluated based on gene-gene co-expression, but also protein–protein interactions, shared transcription factor binding sites in promoters, shared microRNA binding sites, and shared membership to pathways. Proteins members of a common signal transduction pathway in a given neuron type will likely be significantly connected with one another. The data compendium is composed of an array of data diverse enough to capture relationships relevant to both healthy and disease brain but also to a number of different brain regions. The functional networks are thus a tool to identify functional partners for any gene of the genome, in the context of a specific cell type.

We then analyzed these functional networks in an unbiased data-driven way and identified the pathways that best differentiate vulnerable neurons from resistant ones: a number of microtubule remodeling pathways were the most salient ones in vulnerable compared to resistant neurons.

Very interestingly, members of these pathways were not enriched in vulnerable neurons. Rather the saliency of these pathways was driven by two genes, *MAPT* and *SNCA* (genes encoding tau and alpha-synuclein, respectively), that have much larger connectivity in ECII neurons, without being differentially expressed between vulnerable and resistant neurons. This result was remarkable not only because it identified non-trivial functional patterns in vulnerable neurons, but also because of the nature of the identified pathways: vulnerable neurons develop NFT (aggregates of the microtubule associated protein tau) before any other neuron type, and microtubule dysfunction have been proposed to be at the center of AD pathogenesis.

In order to gain insight into the most relevant mechanisms for AD in vulnerable neurons, we then leveraged the disease-specific signal present in GWAS data for NFT formation using the NetWAS 2.0 algorithm (for Network-wide association study). NetWAS 2.0 is a machine-learning based algorithm which ranks genes based on their predicted functional association with a trait (e.g., NFT formation), by using functional relationships between genes in a cell type relevant for this trait (e.g., the vulnerable ECII neurons) and GWAS for this trait (e.g., data from Beecham et al., 2014 for Braak stage, a pathological staging for NFT formation). Very strikingly, this completely unbiased data-driven approach ranked tau number 1, showing, perhaps expectedly, that tau is occupying a central role in the AD process. More informatively it also showed that a module of genes involved in axon plasticity underlies vulnerability to tau pathology in AD. Not all genes in this module will represent therapeutic targets or central drivers in the pathogenesis. But further analysis can help identify "hub" genes, very connected to many other genes, or to find genes that are very close functional partners of MAPT. One such example is the purely data-driven identification of the splice factor PTBP1 as a very close functional partner of MAPT in ECII neurons. We were able to demonstrate experimentally that PTBP1 is a modulator of tau exon 10 splicing, an exon that is very relevant for neurodegeneration in tauopathies (Liu & Gong, 2008). These findings show the ability of our networks to capture functional interactions between genes beyond mere coexpression.

While the approach does not provide direct knowledge of signal transduction pathways within vulnerable neurons, it sheds light on the genes and pathways that are likely to be at play during incipient AD in these neurons, genes and pathways that should be targeted in priority to halt pathological processes in these cells. The next challenge will be to understand how different types of cells are communicating with one another, and how signal transduction cascades are communicating intercellularly through extracellular ligand-receptor interactions. This is particularly relevant for the study of diseases where different cell types are involved, i.e., for most neurological diseases.

5. Cell-specific and network approaches in drug development and repurposing

Network analysis of molecular pathways can be a transformative tool to find common pathological mechanisms between different diseases and to predict the potential side effects of a drug, facilitating drug repositioning. Considering that the development of a new drug can take up to 20 years and is risky and expensive, there is a great interest in this kind of approach by the pharmaceutical industry (Ashburn & Thor, 2004). By integrating information about known targets and side effects of approved drugs with drug-drug interaction datasets and protein-protein interactions into a network, von Eichborn and colleagues developed PROMISCUOUS (von Eichborn et al., 2011). It allows to search for an approved drug, for example the AD drug memantine, that is an antagonist of a specific type of glutamate receptor and causes nausea as a side effect. The network identifies drugs that share the same target and that have side effects with known molecular mechanisms, such as amantadine, that besides the glutamate receptor, targets D2 dopamine receptor. D2 dopamine receptors antagonists are known drugs used as antiemetic (to prevent nausea and vomiting), so it is likely that memantine side effect is mediated by an off-target activation of D2 dopamine receptor. Furthermore, higher doses of D2 receptors antagonists, such as haloperidol, are the most widely used antipsychotics, for schizophrenia and bipolar disorder. On the other hand, dopamine receptors agonists, such as bromocriptine, are used to treat PD, and show nausea, vomiting and hallucinations as side effects. This simple example gives an outlook on how these networks can be built and shows the potential of this kind of approach for drug development.

The current availability of cell-type specific transcriptomics, epigenomics and proteomics data, provides a unique opportunity not only to identify the molecular mechanisms behind diseases, but also to predict the impact and the differential effects that a certain therapeutic drug or combination of drugs might have in different cell types. The next step will be to further take into consideration the highly cell-type specific expression of certain receptors, and the differential effect that the activation of a receptor can have in different cell types (as Paul Greengard first described for dopamine receptors and their response in different striatal MSNs). This was shown for p38a protein kinase inhibitors used to treat immune-mediated disorders, that can show a therapeutic or adverse effect depending on the cell type (Ritprajak, Hayakawa, Sano, Otsu, & Park, 2012). In the neuroscience field, cell-type specific data has been used to develop CVN424, a new drug to treat PD that is in clinical trial: L-dopa, traditionally used to treat PD, produces dyskinesia (uncontrollable movements) as a side effect, due to the generalized increase in dopamine in the brain, that leads to non-specific dopamine signaling activation. CVN424 targets a protein exclusively expressed in MSNs in the striatum, showing the same benefits as L-dopa without the side effects. The same company (Cerevance) has developed CVN417 to treat L-dopa induced dyskinesia by inhibiting a receptor exclusively expressed by dopaminergic neurons in the midbrain and noradrenergic neurons in the locus coeruleus.

6. Future outlook

In this review, we gave a historical perspective of the cell-type specific signal transduction field and showed how incremental technological developments have made it possible to investigate the activity of a pathway in a distinct set of cells rather than in the entire tissue. Unfortunately, the technique that arguably evaluates signal transduction most accurately—proteomics—because it allows the measurement of post-translational protein modifications is the one that is most challenging to implement at the cell-type specific level. But the proteomics field is now at a transformative moment similar to the transcriptomics field a decade ago: as we discussed above, the technologies now exist to go beyond bulk tissue proteomics, and the next years will probably see the emergence of a number of tools, and the establishment of numerous cell-type specific proteomes in healthy and diseased states. A real game-changer will certainly be the development of single-cell proteomics for high-throughput analysis of hundreds of cell types across the brain in many different conditions, without the need for exogenous cell-type specific expression of a labeling protein (Slavov, 2020).

But since the functional status of a cell is a complex composite not only of its protein content but also of its RNA profile, its chromatin conformation, and many other aspects not discussed here, like its lipid or metabolite composition, profiling along a single functional modality will not yield comprehensive characterization of cell-type specific transduction pathways.

Both cutting-edge technological developments and novel computational methods will propel signal transduction in the multi-omics era: on the one hand, *in silico* integration of multiple omics levels to achieve more precise *in silico* cell models will refine our understanding of cell-type specific processes. Some network strategies highlighted above were already built with both protein–protein interaction and transcriptomic data (Roussarie et al., 2020). RNA and protein expression data can also be integrated to get insight into cell function: a recent study drew from bulk and cell-type specific transcriptomics, proteomics and phosphoproteomics to uncover drivers of dendritic cell differentiation (Du et al., 2018). On the other hand, there are already first examples of simultaneous measurements within single cells (previewed in Zhu, Preissl, & Ren, 2020). For instance, simultaneous analysis of transcriptome and surface expression of immune checkpoint proteins on single cells allowed for the identification of transcriptional networks at play for the regulation of PD-L1 surface levels on tumor cells (Papalexi et al., 2020). Such an approach could be applied to the brain *in vivo*, to understand the pathways that regulate, for instance, serotonin receptor levels, or surface expression of neuronal regulators of microglial phagocytosis. Altogether we think that the complexity of the regulatory processes that make the identity of neuron types and determines their vulnerability to disease can only be approached with the complex frameworks that modern computational and multi-omics experimental biology are starting to build together.

7. Conclusion

Fifty years after Paul Greengard co-founded the field of signal transduction in neurons, tremendous progress has been made in the understanding of how different types of neurons react to their environment. But we still need low- and high throughput analyses of the different genes and pathways at play in physiological and pathological processes in specific sets of neurons. The perspective of fully understanding signaling pathways in a cell-type specific manner holds great promise for finding new therapies because we might be able to design precision drugs acting on targets that regulate a pathway exclusively in a specific cell type. In the case of psychiatric diseases, where the available therapies are associated to extensive side effects and disability, it will help to develop more efficient therapies while improving the patient's quality of life. The example of the PD drugs highlighted above show the sophistication that can be achieved once we gain knowledge of cell-type specific characteristics, and cell-type specific pathological mechanisms. In the case of neurodegenerative diseases, it is precisely the cell-type specific signaling mechanisms that dictate selective neuronal vulnerability, and disease-modifying drugs will most likely hit these vulnerability pathways. In this review, we made the case for the complexity of cell-type specific regulatory mechanisms, and the challenges of the identification of functionally relevant processes. We also showed an array of technological frameworks, many of them pioneered by Paul Greengard, that are now available to reveal cell-type specific targets for treatment of neurological disorders, making us hopeful that we will soon be able to target specific process in specific sets of neurons with next-generation designer drugs.

Acknowledgments

J.-P.R. and P.R.-R. are supported by the Fisher Center for Alzheimer's Disease Research. J.-P.R is supported by Cure Alzheimer's Fund, and the National Institute on Aging of the NIH award RF1AG054564. P.R.-R. is supported in part by the European Union Horizon 2020 Research and Innovation Program under Marie Sklodowska-Curie grant agreement 799638. Opinions, interpretations, conclusions, and recommendations are those of the author and are not necessarily endorsed by the sponsors.

Conflict of interest

The authors have no conflict of interest to declare.

References

Alvarez-Castelao, B., Schanzenbächer, C. T., Hanus, C., Glock, C., Dieck, S.t., Dörrbaum, A. R., et al. (2017). Cell-type-specific metabolic labeling of nascent proteomes in vivo. *Nature Biotechnology*, *35*, 1196–1201.

Amaral, D. G., Schumann, C. M., & Nordahl, C. W. (2008). Neuroanatomy of autism. *Trends in Neurosciences*, *31*(3), 137–145.

Ashburn, T. T., & Thor, K. B. (2004). Drug repositioning: Identifying and developing new uses for existing drugs. *Nature Reviews Drug Discovery*, *3*(8), 673–683.

Bai, B., Wang, X., Li, Y., Chen, P. C., Yu, K., Dey, K. K., et al. (2020). Deep multilayer brain proteomics identifies molecular networks in Alzheimer's disease progression. *Neuron*, *105*, 975–991.e7.

Bateup, H. S., Svenningsson, P., Kuroiwa, M., Gong, S., Nishi, A., Heintz, N., et al. (2008). Cell type-specific regulation of DARPP-32 phosphorylation by psychostimulant and antipsychotic drugs. *Nature Neuroscience*, *11*(8), 932–939.

Baumann, B., & Bogerts, B. (2001). Neuroanatomical studies on bipolar disorder. *British Journal of Psychiatry*, *178*, S142–S147.

Beecham, G. W., Hamilton, K., Naj, A. C., Martin, E. R., Huentelman, M., Myers, A. J., et al. (2014). Genome-wide association meta-analysis of neuropathologic features of Alzheimer's disease and related dementias. edited by G. Gibson *PLoS Genetics*, *10*(9), e1004606.

Bendall, S. C., Simonds, E. F., Qiu, P., Amir, E.-a. D., Krutzik, P. O., Finck, R., et al. (2011). Single-cell mass cytometry of differential immune and drug responses across a human hematopoietic continuum. *Science, 332*, 687–696.

Bereczki, E., Branca, R. M., Francis, P. T., Pereira, J. B., Baek, J. H., Hortobágyi, T., et al. (2018). Synaptic markers of cognitive decline in neurodegenerative diseases: A proteomic approach. *Brain, 141*(2), 582–595.

Braak, H., & Braak, E. (1996). Evolution of the neuropathology of Alzheimer's disease. *Acta Neurologica Scandinavica, 165*, 3–12.

Brichta, L., Shin, W., Jackson-Lewis, V., Blesa, J., Yap, E. L., Walker, Z., et al. (2015). Identification of neurodegenerative factors using translatome-regulatory network analysis. *Nature Neuroscience, 18*(9), 1325–1333.

Buenrostro, J. D., Wu, B., Litzenburger, U. M., Ruff, D., Gonzales, M. L., Snyder, M. P., et al. (2015). Single-cell chromatin accessibility reveals principles of regulatory variation. *Nature, 523*, 486–490.

Canchi, S., Raao, B., Masliah, D., Rosenthal, S. B., Sasik, R., Fisch, K. M., et al. (2019). Integrating gene and protein expression reveals perturbed functional networks in Alzheimer's disease. *Cell Reports, 28*, 1103–1116.e4.

Cao, X., Li, L. P., Wang, Q., Wu, Q., Hu, H. H., Zhang, M., et al. (2013). Astrocyte-derived ATP modulates depressive-like behaviors. *Nature Medicine, 19*, 773–777.

Carlén, M., Meletis, K., Siegle, J. H., Cardin, J. A., Futai, K., Vierling-Claassen, D., et al. (2012). A critical role for NMDA receptors in parvalbumin interneurons for gamma rhythm induction and behavior. *Molecular Psychiatry, 17*, 537–548.

Castello, J., Lefrancois, B., Flajolet, M., Greengard, P., Friedman, E., & Rebholz, H. (2018). CK2 regulates 5-HT4 receptor signaling and modulates depressive-like behavior. *Molecular Psychiatry, 23*(4), 872–882.

Chang, D., Nalls, M. A., Hallgrímsdóttir, I. B., Hunkapiller, J., van der Brug, M., Cai, F., et al. (2017). A meta-analysis of genome-wide association studies identifies 17 new Parkinson's disease risk loci. *Nature Genetics, 49*, 1511–1516.

Cheng, J., Umschweif, G., Leung, J., Sagi, Y., & Greengard, P. (2019). HCN2 channels in cholinergic interneurons of nucleus accumbens shell regulate depressive behaviors. *Neuron, 101*(4), 662–672.e5.

Chottekalapanda, R. U., Kalik, S., Gresack, J., Ayala, A., Gao, M., Wang, W., et al. (2020). AP-1 controls the P11-dependent antidepressant response. *Molecular Psychiatry, 25*, 1364–1381.

Cusanovich, D. A., Daza, R., Adey, A., Pliner, H. A., Christiansen, L., Gunderson, K. L., et al. (2015). Multiplex single-cell profiling of chromatin accessibility by combinatorial cellular indexing. *Science, 348*, 910–914.

De Jager, P. L., Srivastava, G., Lunnon, K., Burgess, J., Schalkwyk, L. C., Yu, L., et al. (2014). Alzheimer's disease pathology is associated with early alterations in brain DNA methylation at ANK1, BIN1, RHBDF2 and other loci HHS public access author manuscript. *Nature Neuroscience, 17*(9), 1156–1163.

Doyle, J. P., Dougherty, J. D., Heiman, M., Schmidt, E. F., Stevens, T. R., Ma, G., et al. (2008). Application of a translational profiling approach for the comparative analysis of CNS cell types. *Cell, 135*(4), 749–762.

Drummond, E. S., Nayak, S., Ueberheide, B., & Wisniewski, T. (2015). Proteomic analysis of neurons microdissected from formalin-fixed, paraffin-embedded Alzheimer's disease brain tissue. *Scientific Reports, 5*(15456).

Du, X., Wen, J., Wang, Y., Karmaus, P. W. F., Khatamian, A., Tan, H., et al. (2018) Hippo/Mst signalling couples metabolic state and immune function of CD8α + dendritic cells. *Nature, 558*(7708), 141–145.

Ehrnhoefer, D. E., Southwell, A. L., Sivasubramanian, M., Qiu, X., Villanueva, E. B., Xie, Y., et al. (2018). HACE1 is essential for astrocyte mitochondrial function and influences Huntington disease phenotypes in vivo. *Human Molecular Genetics, 27*(2), 239–253.

Eisen, M. B., Spellman, P. T., Brown, P. O., & Botstein, D. (1998). Cluster analysis and display of genome-wide expression patterns. *Proceedings of the National Academy of Sciences of the United States of America, 95*(25), 14863–14868.

Fishell, G., & Heintz, N. (2013). The neuron identity problem: Form meets function. *Neuron, 80*(3), 602–612.

Fu, H., Hardy, J., & Duff, K. E. (2018). Selective vulnerability in neurodegenerative diseases. *Nature Neuroscience, 21*(10), 1350–1358.

Furlanis, E., Traunmüller, L., Fucile, G., & Scheiffele, P. (2019). Landscape of ribosome-engaged transcript isoforms reveals extensive neuronal-cell-class-specific alternative splicing programs. *Nature Neuroscience, 22*(10), 1709–1717.

Girault, J.-A., & Greengard, P. (1999). Principles of signal transduction. In *Neurobiology of mental illness*.

Girault, J.-A., & Greengard, P. (2004). The neurobiology of dopamine signaling. *Archieves of Neurology, 61*(5), 641–644.

Girdhar, K., Hoffman, G. E., Jiang, Y., Brown, L., Kundakovic, M., Hauberg, M. E., et al. (2018). Cell-specific histone modification maps in the human frontal lobe link schizophrenia risk to the neuronal epigenome. *Nature Neuroscience, 21*(8), 1126–1136.

Gjoneska, E., Pfenning, A. R., Mathys, H., Quon, G., Kundaje, A., Tsai, L. H., et al. (2015). Conserved epigenomic signals in mice and humans reveal immune basis of Alzheimer's disease. *Nature, 518*(7539), 365–369.

Greengard, P., & Fienberg, A. (1998). 261. DARPP-32: Regulator of the efficacy of dopaminergic neurotransmission. *Biological Psychiatry, 281*(5378), 838–842.

Habib, N., Avraham-Davidi, I., Basu, A., Burks, T., Shekhar, K., Hofree, M., et al. (2017). Massively parallel single-nucleus RNA-Seq with DroNc-Seq. *Nature Methods, 14*(10), 955–958.

Habib, N., McCabe, C., Medina, S., Varshavsky, M., Kitsberg, D., Dvir-Szternfeld, R., et al. (2020). Disease-associated astrocytes in Alzheimer's disease and aging. *Nature Neuroscience, 23*(6), 701–706.

Hannon, E., Spiers, H., Viana, J., Pidsley, R., Burrage, J., Murphy, T. M., et al. (2015). Methylation QTLs in the developing brain and their enrichment in schizophrenia risk loci. *Nature Neuroscience, 19*(1), 48–54.

Heiman, M., Kulicke, R., Fenster, R. J., Greengard, P., & Heintz, N. (2014). Cell type-specific MRNA purification by translating ribosome affinity purification (TRAP). *Nature Protocols, 9*(6), 1282–1291.

Heiman, M., Schaefer, A., Gong, S., Peterson, J. D., Day, M., Ramsey, K. E., et al. (2008). A translational profiling approach for the molecular characterization of CNS cell types. *Cell, 135*(4), 738–748.

Hekselman, I., & Yeger-Lotem, E. (2020). Mechanisms of tissue and cell-type specificity in heritable traits and diseases. *Nature Reviews Genetics, 21*(3), 137–150.

Hercher, C., Turecki, G., & Mechawar, N. (2009). Through the looking glass: Examining neuroanatomical evidence for cellular alterations in major depression. *Journal of Psychiatric Research, 43*(11), 947–961.

Hirokawa, N., & Takemura, R. (2005). Molecular motors and mechanisms of directional transport in neurons. *Nature Reviews Neuroscience, 6*(3), 201–214.

Islam, S., Kjällquist, U., Moliner, A., Zajac, P., Fan, J. B., Lönnerberg, P., et al. (2012). Highly multiplexed and strand-specific single-cell RNA 5′ end sequencing. *Nature Protocols, 7*(5), 813–828.

Jaffe, A. E., Gao, Y., Deep-Soboslay, A., Tao, R., Hyde, T. M., Weinberger, D. R., et al. (2015). Mapping DNA methylation across development, genotype and schizophrenia in the human frontal cortex. *Nature Neuroscience, 19*(1), 40–47.

Jakovcevski, M., & Akbarian, S. (2012). Epigenetic mechanisms in neurological disease. *Nature Medicine, 18*(8), 1194–1204.

Jia, H., Kast, R. J., Steffan, J. S., & Thomas, E. A. (2012). Selective histone deacetylase (HDAC) inhibition imparts beneficial effects in Huntington's disease mice: Implications for the ubiquitin-proteasomal and autophagy systems. *Human Molecular Genetics*, *21*(24), 5280–5293.

Jin, J., Bhatti, D. L., Lee, K. W., Medrihan, L., Cheng, J., Wei, J., et al. (2020). Ahnak scaffolds P11/Anxa2 complex and L-type voltage-gated calcium channel and modulates depressive behavior. *Molecular Psychiatry*, *25*(5), 1035–1049.

Jordi, E. (2013). Histone post-translational modifications in the nuclei of striatal D1 and D2 neurons: Development of a novel method of study and effects of cocaine. *Proceedings of the National Academy of Sciences of the United States of America*, *110*(23), 9511–9516.

Kazantsev, A. G., & Thompson, L. M. (2008). Therapeutic application of histone deacetylase inhibitors for central nervous system disorders. *Nature Reviews Drug Discovery*, 7(10), 854–868.

Kebabian, J. W., & Caine, D. B. (1979). *Review article multiple receptors for dopamine. Vol. 277.*

Kebabian, J. W., & Greengard, P. (1971). Dopamine-sensitive adenyl cyclase: Possible role in synaptic transmission. *Science*, *174*(4016), 1346–1349.

Klein, H. U., McCabe, C., Gjoneska, E., Sullivan, S. E., Kaskow, B. J., Tang, A., et al. (2019). Epigenome-wide study uncovers large-scale changes in histone acetylation driven by tau pathology in aging and Alzheimer's human brains. *Nature Neuroscience*, *22*(1), 37–46.

Kozlenkov, A., Roussos, P., Timashpolsky, A., Barbu, M., Rudchenko, S., Bibikova, M., et al. (2014). Differences in DNA methylation between human neuronal and glial cells are concentrated in enhancers and non-CpG sites. *Nucleic Acids Research*, *42*(1), 109–127.

Kriaucionis, S., & Heintz, N. (2009). The nuclear DNA base 5-hydroxymethylcytosine is present in purkinje neurons and the brain. *Science*, *324*(5929), 929–930.

Krogager, T. P., Ernst, R. J., Elliott, T. S., Calo, L, Beránek, V, Ciabatti, E, et al. (2018). Labeling and identifying cell-specific proteomes in the mouse brain. *Nature Biotechnology*, *36*(2), 156–159.

Kuo, J. F., & Greengard, P. (1969). *Cyclic nucleotide-dependent protein kinases III. Purification and properties of adenosine 3′,5′-monophosphate-dependent protein kinase from bovine brain. Vol. 244.*

Langfelder, P., & Horvath, S. (2008). WGCNA: An R package for weighted correlation network analysis. *BMC Bioinformatics*, *9*(1), 1–13.

Ledo, J. H., Liebmann, T., Zhang, R., Chang, J. C., Azevedo, E. P., Wong, E., et al. (2020). Presenilin 1 phosphorylation regulates amyloid-β degradation by microglia. *Molecular Psychiatry*.

Ledo, J. H., Zhang, R., Mesin, L., Mourão-Sá, D., Azevedo, E. P., Troyanskaya, O. G., et al. (2020). Lack of a site-specific phosphorylation of presenilin 1 disrupts microglial gene networks and progenitors during development. *PLoS One*, *15*(8), e0237773.

Lee, K. W., Westin, L., Kim, J., Chang, J. C., Oh, Y. S., Amreen, B., et al. (2015). Alteration by P11 of MGluR5 localization regulates depression-like behaviors. *Molecular Psychiatry*, *20*(12), 1546–1556.

Liddelow, S. A., Guttenplan, K. A., Clarke, L. E., Bennett, F. C., Bohlen, C. J., Schirmer, L., et al. (2017). Neurotoxic reactive astrocytes are induced by activated microglia. *Nature*, *541*(7638), 481–487.

Liu, Y., Beyer, A., & Aebersold, R. (2016). On the dependency of cellular protein levels on MRNA abundance. *Cell*, *165*(3), 535–550.

Liu, F., & Gong, C.-X. (2008). Tau exon 10 alternative splicing and tauopathies. *Molecular Neurodegeneration*, *3*(1), 8.

Macosko, E. Z., Basu, A., Satija, R., Nemesh, J., Shekhar, K., Goldman, M., et al. (2015). Highly parallel genome-wide expression profiling of individual cells using nanoliter droplets. *Cell*, *161*(5), 1202–1214.

Marín, O. (2012). Interneuron dysfunction in psychiatric disorders. *Nature Reviews Neuroscience*, *13*(2), 107–120.

Marongiu, R., Arango-Lievano, M., Francardo, V., Morgenstern, P., Zhang, X., Angela Cenci, M., et al. (2016). Gene therapy blockade of dorsal striatal P11 improves motor function and dyskinesia in parkinsonian mice. *Proceedings of the National Academy of Sciences of the United States of America*, *113*(5), 1423–1428.

Mathys, H., Davila-Velderrain, J., Peng, Z., Gao, F., Mohammadi, S., Young, J. Z., et al. (2019). Single-cell transcriptomic analysis of Alzheimer's disease. *Nature*, *570*(7761), 332–337.

Medrihan, L., Umschweif, G., Sinha, A., Reed, S., Lee, J., Gindinova, K., et al. (2020). Reduced Kv3.1 activity in dentate gyrus parvalbumin cells induces vulnerability to depression. *Biological Psychiatry*, *88*, 405–414.

Mellén, M., Ayata, P., Dewell, S., Kriaucionis, S., & Heintz, N. (2012). MeCP2 binds to 5hmC enriched within active genes and accessible chromatin in the nervous system. *Cell*, *151*(7), 1417–1430.

Mendizabal, I., Berto, S., Usui, N., Toriumi, K., Chatterjee, P., Douglas, C., et al. (2019). Cell type-specific epigenetic links to schizophrenia risk in the Brain. *Genome Biology*, *20*(1), 1–21.

Mendonça, C. F., Kuras, M, Nogueira, F, Plá, I, Hortobágyi, T, Csiba, L, et al. (2019). Proteomic signatures of brain regions affected by tau pathology in early and late stages of Alzheimer's disease. *Neurobiology of Disease*, *130*(104509).

Meyer-Lindenberg, A. S., Olsen, R. K., Kohn, P. D., Brown, T., Egan, M. F., Weinberger, D. R., et al. (2005). Regionally specific disturbance of dorsolateral prefrontal–hippocampal functional connectivity in schizophrenia. *Archives of General Psychiatry*, *62*(4), 379–386.

Milosevic, A., Liebmann, T., Knudsen, M., Schintu, N., Svenningsson, P., & Greengard, P. (2017). Cell- and region-specific expression of depression-related protein P11 (S100a10) in the brain. *Journal of Comparative Neurology*, *525*(4), 955–975.

Montagne, A., Nation, D. A., Sagare, A. P., Barisano, G., Sweeney, M. D., Chakhoyan, A., et al. (2020). APOE4 leads to blood–brain barrier dysfunction predicting cognitive decline. *Nature*, *581*(7806), 71–76.

Nagy, C., Maitra, M., Tanti, A., Suderman, M., Théroux, J. F., Davoli, M. A., et al. (2020). Single-nucleus transcriptomics of the prefrontal cortex in major depressive disorder implicates oligodendrocyte precursor cells and excitatory neurons. *Nature Neuroscience*, *23*(6), 771–781.

Nasca, C., Bigio, B., Zelli, D., de Angelis, P., Lau, T., Okamoto, M., et al. (2017). Role of the astroglial glutamate exchanger XCT in ventral hippocampus in resilience to stress. *Neuron*, *96*(2), 402–413.e5.

Nott, A., Holtman, I. R., Coufal, N. G., Schlachetzki, J. C. M., Miao, Y., Rong, H., et al. (2019). Brain cell type–specific enhancer–promoter interactome maps and disease-risk association. *Science*, *366*(6469), 1134–1139.

O'dushlaine, C., Rossin, L., Lee, P. H., Duncan, L., Parikshak, N. N., Newhouse, S., et al. (2015). Psychiatric genome-wide association study analyses implicate neuronal, immune and histone pathways. *Nature Neuroscience*, *18*, 199–209.

Oh, Y. S., Gao, P., Lee, K. W., Ceglia, I., Seo, J. S., Zhang, X., et al. (2013). SMARCA3, a chromatin-remodeling factor, is required for P11-dependent antidepressant action. *Cell*, *152*(4), 831–843.

Oh, D. H., Son, H., Hwang, S., & Kim, S. H. (2012). Neuropathological abnormalities of astrocytes, GABAergic neurons, and pyramidal neurons in the dorsolateral prefrontal cortices of patients with major depressive disorder. *European Neuropsychopharmacology*, *22*, 330–338.

Papalexi, E., Mimitou, E., Butler, A. W., Foster, S., Bracken, B., Mauck, W. M., et al. (2020). Characterizing the molecular regulation of inhibitory immune checkpoints with multi-modal single-cell screens. *BioRxiv*. 2020.06.28.175596.

Poewe, W., Seppi, K., Tanner, C. M., Halliday, G. M., Brundin, P., Volkmann, J., et al. (2017). Parkinson disease. *Nature Reviews Disease Primers*, *3*(17013).

Polyzos, A. A., Lee, D. Y., Datta, R., Hauser, M., Budworth, H., Holt, A., et al. (2019). Metabolic reprogramming in astrocytes distinguishes region-specific neuronal susceptibility in Huntington mice. *Cell Metabolism*, *29*(6), 1258–1273.

Pontecorvo, M. J., Devous, M. D., Kennedy, I., Navitsky, M., Ming, L., Galante, N., et al. (2019). A multicentre longitudinal study of Flortaucipir (18F) in normal ageing, mild cognitive impairment and Alzheimer's disease dementia. *Brain: A Journal of Neurology*, *142*(6), 1723–1735.

Rayaprolu, S, Gao, T, Xiao, H, Ramesha, S, Weinstock, L. D., Shah, J, et al. (2020). Flow-cytometric microglial sorting coupled with quantitative proteomics identifies moesin as a highly-abundant microglial protein with relevance to Alzheimer's disease. *Molecular Neurodegeneration*, *15*(1), 28.

Reiner, A., Albin, R. L., Anderson, K. D., D'Amato, C. J., Penney, J. B., & Young, A. B. (1988). Differential loss of striatal projection neurons in Huntington disease. *Proceedings of the National Academy of Sciences of the United States of America*, *85*(15), 5733–5737.

Riessland, M., Kolisnyk, B., Kim, T. W., Cheng, J., Ni, J., Pearson, J. A., et al. (2019). Loss of SATB1 induces P21-dependent cellular senescence in post-mitotic dopaminergic neurons. *Cell Stem Cell*, *25*(4), 514–530.e8.

Ritprajak, P, Hayakawa, M, Sano, Y, Otsu, K, & Park, J. M. (2012). Cell type-specific targeting dissociates the therapeutic from the adverse effects of protein kinase inhibition in allergic skin disease. *Proceedings of the National Academy of Sciences of the United States of America.*, *109*(23), 9089–9094.

Rivera, A. D., & Butt, A. M. (2019). Astrocytes are direct cellular targets of lithium treatment: Novel roles for lysyl oxidase and peroxisome-proliferator activated receptor-γ as astroglial targets of lithium. *Translational Psychiatry*, *9*, 211.

Roussarie, J. P., Yao, V., Rodriguez-Rodriguez, P., Oughtred, R., Rust, J., Plautz, Z., et al. (2020). Selective neuronal vulnerability in alzheimer's disease: A network-based analysis. *Neuron*, *107*(5), 821–835.

Roux, K. J., Kim, D. I., Raida, M, & Burke, B. (2012). A promiscuous biotin ligase fusion protein identifies proximal and interacting proteins in mammalian cells. *Journal of Cell Biology*, *196*(6), 801–810.

Sagi, Y., Medrihan, L., George, K., Barney, M., McCabe, K. A., & Greengard, P. (2020). Emergence of 5-HT5A signaling in parvalbumin neurons mediates delayed antidepressant action. *Molecular Psychiatry*, *25*(6), 1191–1201.

Sala Frigerio, C., Wolfs, L., Fattorelli, N., Thrupp, N., Voytyuk, I., Schmidt, I., et al. (2019). The major risk factors for Alzheimer's disease: Age, sex, and genes modulate the microglia response to Aβ plaques. *Cell Reports*, *27*(4), 1293–1306.

Sargin, D., Chottekalapanda, R. U., Perit, K. E., Yao, V., Chu, D., Sparks, D. W., et al. (2020). Mapping the physiological and molecular markers of stress and SSRI antidepressant treatment in S100a10 corticostriatal neurons. *Molecular Psychiatry*, *25*(5), 1112–1129.

Schaefer, A., Sampath, S. C., Intrator, A., Min, A., Gertler, T. S., James Surmeier, D., et al. (2009). Control of cognition and adaptive behavior by the GLP/G9a epigenetic suppressor complex. *Neuron*, *64*(5), 678–691.

Schmidt, E. F., Warner-Schmidt, J. L., Otopalik, B. G., Pickett, S. B., Greengard, P., & Heintz, N. (2012). Identification of the cortical neurons that mediate antidepressant responses. *Cell*, *149*(5), 1152–1163.

Shema, R., Kulicke, R., Cowley, G. S., Stein, R., Root, D. E., & Heiman, M. (2015). Synthetic lethal screening in the mammalian central nervous system Identifies Gpx6 as a modulator of Huntington's disease. *Proceedings of the National Academy of Sciences of the United States of America, 112*(1), 268–272.

Shi, Y., Manis, M., Long, J., Wang, K., Sullivan, P. M., Remolina Serrano, J., et al. (2019). Microglia drive apoe-dependent neurodegeneration in a tauopathy mouse model. *Journal of Experimental Medicine, 216*, 2546–2561.

Shuto, T., Kuroiwa, M., Sotogaku, N., Kawahara, Y., Oh, Y. S., Jang, J. H., et al. (2020). Obligatory roles of dopamine D1 receptors in the dentate gyrus in antidepressant actions of a selective serotonin reuptake inhibitor, fluoxetine. *Molecular Psychiatry, 25*(6), 1229–1244.

Skene, N. G., Bryois, J., Bakken, T. E., Breen, G., Crowley, J. J., Gaspar, H. A., et al. (2018). Genetic identification of brain cell types underlying schizophrenia. *Nature Genetics, 50*, 825–833.

Slavov, N. (2020). Unpicking the proteome in single cells. *Science, 367*(6477), 512–513.

Smith, R. G., Hannon, E., De Jager, P. L., Chibnik, L., Lott, S. J., Condliffe, D., et al. (2018). Elevated DNA methylation across a 48-Kb region spanning the HOXA gene cluster is associated with Alzheimer's disease neuropathology. *Alzheimer's & Dementia, 14*, 1580–1588.

Sun, W., Poschmann, J., Cruz-Herrera del Rosario, R., Parikshak, N. N., Hajan, H. S., Kumar, V., et al. (2016). Histone acetylome-wide association study of autism spectrum disorder. *Cell, 167*(5), 1385–1397.e11.

Surmeier, D. J., Obeso, J. A., & Halliday, G. M. (2017). Selective neuronal vulnerability in Parkinson disease. *Nature Reviews Neuroscience, 18*, 101–113.

Toker, L., Mancarci, B. O., Tripathy, S., & Pavlidis, P. (2018). Transcriptomic evidence for alterations in astrocytes and parvalbumin interneurons in subjects with bipolar disorder and schizophrenia. *Biological Psychiatry, 84*(11), 787–796.

Tse, K. H., Cheng, A., Ma, F., & Herrup, K. (2018). DNA damage-associated oligodendrocyte degeneration precedes amyloid pathology and contributes to Alzheimer's disease and Dementia. *Alzheimer's & Dementia, 14*(5), 664–679.

Uezu, A, Kanak, D. L., Bradshaw, T. W. A., Soderblom, E. J., Catavero, C. M., Burette, A. C., et al. (2016). Identification of an elaborate complex mediating postsynaptic inhibition. *Science, 353*(6304), 1123–1129.

Valencia, A., Sapp, E., Kimm, J. S., McClory, H., Reeves, P. B., Alexander, J., et al. (2013). Elevated NADPH oxidase activity contributes to oxidative stress and cell death in Huntington's disease. *Human Molecular Genetics, 22*, 1112–1131.

Virk, M. S., Sagi, Y., Medrihan, L., Leung, J., Kaplitt, M. G., & Greengard, P. (2016). Opposing roles for serotonin in cholinergic neurons of the ventral and dorsal striatum. *Proceedings of the National Academy of Sciences of the United States of America, 113*(3), 734–739.

von Eichborn, J, Murgueitio, M. S., Dunkel, M, Koerner, S, Bourne, P. E., & Preissner, R. (2011). PROMISCUOUS: A database for network-based drug-repositioning. *Nucleic Acids Research, 39*(Database issue), D1060–D1066.

Wang, H., Warner-Schmidt, J., Varela, S., Enikolopov, G., Greengard, P., & Flajolet, M. (2015). Norbin ablation results in defective adult hippocampal neurogenesis and depressive-like behavior in mice. *Proceedings of the National Academy of Sciences of the United States of America, 112*(31), 9745–9750.

Warner-Schmidt, J. L., Schmidt, E. F., Marshall, J. J., Rubin, A. J., Arango-Lievano, M., Kaplitt, M. G., et al. (2012). Cholinergic interneurons in the nucleus accumbens regulate depression-like behavior. *Proceedings of the National Academy of Sciences of the United States of America, 109*(28), 11360–11365.

Wen, L., Yi Sheng, L., Zhu, X. H., Li, X. M., Woo, R. S., Chen, Y. J., et al. (2010). Neuregulin 1 regulates pyramidal neuron activity via ErbB4 in parvalbumin-positive interneurons. *Proceedings of the National Academy of Sciences of the United States of America, 107*(3), 1211–1216.

Wertz, M. H., Mitchem, M. R., Pineda, S. S., Hachigian, L. J., Lee, H., Lau, V., et al. (2020). Genome-wide in vivo CNS screening identifies genes that modify CNS neuronal survival and MHTT toxicity. *Neuron, 106*(1), 76–89.

Xu, X., Stoyanova, E. I., Lemiesz, A. E., Xing, J., Mash, D. C., & Heintz, N. (2018). Species and cell-type properties of classically defined human and rodent neurons and glia. *eLife*, 7(e37551).

Yizhar, O., Fenno, L. E., Prigge, M., Schneider, F., Davidson, T. J., Ogshea, D. J., et al. (2011). Neocortical excitation/inhibition balance in information processing and social dysfunction. *Nature, 477*, 171–178.

Yun, S. P., In Kam, T., Panicker, N., Kim, S., Yumin, O., Park, J. S., et al. (2018). Block of A1 astrocyte conversion by microglia is neuroprotective in models of Parkinson's disease. *Nature Medicine, 24*, 931–938.

Zhou, J., Park, C. Y., Theesfeld, C. L., Wong, A. K., Yuan, Y., Scheckel, C., et al. (2019). Whole-genome deep-learning analysis identifies contribution of noncoding mutations to autism risk. *Nature Genetics, 51*, 973–980.

Zhu, C., Preissl, S., & Ren, B. (2020). Single-cell multimodal omics: The power of many. *Nature Methods, 17*, 11–14.

CHAPTER EIGHT

Drug-activated cells: From immediate early genes to neuronal ensembles in addiction

Marine Salery, Arthur Godino, and Eric J. Nestler*
Nash Family Department of Neuroscience and Friedman Brain Institute, Icahn School of Medicine at Mount Sinai, New York, NY, United States
*Corresponding author: e-mail address: eric.nestler@mssm.edu

Contents

Abstract

Beyond their rapid rewarding effects, drugs of abuse can durably alter an individual's response to their environment as illustrated by the compulsive drug seeking and risk of relapse triggered by drug-associated stimuli. The persistence of these associations even long after cessation of drug use demonstrates the enduring mark left by drugs on brain reward circuits. However, within these circuits, neuronal populations are differently affected by drug exposure and growing evidence indicates that relatively small subsets of neurons might be involved in the encoding and expression of drug-mediated associations. The identification of sparse neuronal populations recruited in response to

Advances in Pharmacology, Volume 90
ISSN 1054-3589
https://doi.org/10.1016/bs.apha.2020.09.006

drug exposure has benefited greatly from the study of immediate early genes (IEGs) whose induction is critical in initiating plasticity programs in recently activated neurons. In particular, the development of technologies to manipulate IEG-expressing cells has been fundamental to implicate broadly distributed neuronal ensembles coincidently activated by either drugs or drug-associated stimuli and to then causally establish their involvement in drug responses. In this review, we summarize the literature regarding IEG regulation in different learning paradigms and addiction models to highlight their role as a marker of activity and plasticity. As the exploration of neuronal ensembles in addiction improves our understanding of drug-associated memory encoding, it also raises several questions regarding the cellular and molecular characteristics of these discrete neuronal populations as they become incorporated in drug-associated neuronal ensembles. We review recent efforts towards this goal and discuss how they will offer a more comprehensive understanding of addiction pathophysiology.

Abbreviations

AMPA	α-amino-3-hydroxy-5-methyl-4-isoxazolepropionic acid
Arc	activity regulated cytoskeleton associated protein
ArchT	archaerhodopsin
BAC	bacterial artificial chromosome
CA1	cornus ammonis subfield 1
Cas9	CRISPR associated protein 9
ChR2	channelrhodopsin 2
CPP	conditioned place preference
Cre	Cre recombinase
CREB	cAMP response element-binding protein
$CreER^{T2}$	Cre recombinase fused to a mutant estrogen ligand-binding domain
CRISPR	clustered regularly interspaced short palindromic repeat
DG	dentate gyrus
Dnmt3A	DNA methyltransferase 3 Alpha
Drd1/D1	dopamine receptor D1
D1-MSN	dopamine receptor D1-expressing medium spiny neuron
Drd2/D2	dopamine receptor D2
D2-MSN	dopamine receptor D2-expressing medium spiny neuron
DREADD	designer receptors exclusively activated by designer drugs
Egr1	early growth response 1
Egr2	early growth response 2
Egr3	early growth response 3
Ehmt1	euchromatic histone lysine methyltransferase 1
FACS	fluorescence-activated cell sorting
Fos	FBJ murine osteosarcoma viral oncogene homolog
FosB	FBJ murine osteosarcoma viral oncogene homolog B
GFP	green fluorescent protein
Grin2A	glutamate Ionotropic receptor N-methyl-D-aspartate type subunit 2A
Grin2B	glutamate Ionotropic receptor N-methyl-D-aspartate type subunit 2B
Hdac1	histone deacetylase 1
Hdac3	histone deacetylase 3

Hdac4	histone deacetylase 4
Hdac5	histone deacetylase 5
Homer1A	homer scaffold protein 1A
IEGs	immediate early genes
JunD	JunD proto-oncogene, AP-1 transcription factor subunit
Kdm1a	Lysine demethylase 1A
LA	lateral nucleus of the amygdala
LacZ	bacterial beta-galactosidase gene
mRNA	messenger ribonucleic acid
MSN	medium spiny neuron
NAc	nucleus accumbens
NGFI-A	nerve growth factor-induced protein A
Npas4	neuronal PAS domain-containing protein 4
Nr4a1	nuclear receptor subfamily 4 group A member 1
Nr4a3	nuclear receptor subfamily 4 group A member 3
OFC	orbitofrontal cortex
PFC	prefrontal cortex
TRAP	targeted recombination in active populations
vCA1	ventral cornus ammonis subfield 1
Zif268	zinc finger protein 268

1. Introduction

The integration in the central nervous system of external sensory inputs together with internal information reflecting our physiological state is critical for individuals to produce appropriate behavioral responses and to quickly adapt to a changing environment. This continual adjustment of brain circuits through life experiences paradoxically requires both a highly dynamic remodeling of neuronal networks and the capacity to stabilize these adaptations to support the encoding and storage of relevant information into memory (Kandel, Dudai, & Mayford, 2014). Addiction can be studied through this lens of memory formation, maintenance and updating: the high risk of relapse to drug seeking in abstinent individuals even long after cessation of drug taking is proof of such highly stable alterations (Dong, Taylor, Wolf, & Shaham, 2017; Nestler, 2001; Wolf, 2016). The neuronal networks whose activity is dramatically and durably affected by drug exposure are mostly comprised of the interconnected cortical, striatal and limbic regions of the brain's reward circuitry (Lüscher & Malenka, 2011), which normally integrates midbrain dopamine signals to guide reward-related learning (Hyman, Malenka, & Nestler, 2006; Kelley, 2004).

The persistent imprint of drug exposure onto brain function relies on the ability of neuronal plasticity mechanisms normally engaged in non-pathological processes like reward learning to adjust neuronal physiology in order to modulate the response of brain networks to a given stimulus. The mechanisms that translate rapid and transient electrical and neurochemical changes into persistent cellular adaptations require a coordinated response across neuronal compartments from the synapse to the nucleus (Kandel, 2001; Nestler & Lüscher, 2019). Among the myriad of cellular mechanisms orchestrating neuronal plasticity, changes in gene expression are pivotal in reshaping neuronal networks during learning and memory formation (Alberini & Kandel, 2015). Addiction is similarly associated with complex transcriptional adaptations following drug exposure, which underlie the long-term behavioral alterations observed in this pathology (Nestler, 2013; Robison & Nestler, 2011; Walker et al., 2018).

Gene expression is tightly coupled to synaptic activity with signaling mechanisms transducing and propagating information from the membrane to different cell compartments including the nucleus. Activity-dependent transcription thus links rapid environmental changes to long-term neuronal adaptations via specific transcriptional programs (West & Greenberg, 2011; Yap & Greenberg, 2018). The first wave of these activity-regulated genes are called immediate early genes (IEGs) because of their rapid but transient up-regulation in response to a wide variety of cellular stimuli (Sheng & Greenberg, 1990). Bulk analysis of IEG induction provided the first evidence in favor of a brain region- and task-specific recruitment of activity-regulated transcription (Tischmeyer & Grimm, 1999). Because they are supposedly strictly coupled to synaptic activity, these mechanisms seem likely to be restricted to electrophysiologically activated cells, suggesting that changes detected at the bulk level could be driven by the activity of a discrete subpopulation of neurons specifically recruited in memory encoding (Miyashita, Kubik, Lewandowski, & Guzowski, 2008). This hypothesis was further corroborated by the histological mapping of IEG induction in sparse subsets of neurons during learning and memory retrieval (Guzowski et al., 2005; Miyashita et al., 2008). As a result, activity-dependent transcription progressively emerged as a highly reliable marker of behaviorally relevant activated neuronal populations, later termed neuronal ensembles (Minatohara, Akiyoshi, & Okuno, 2016). Activity-dependent mechanisms, including IEG induction, are similarly recruited by drugs of abuse throughout the brain (Chandra & Lobo, 2017; Manning, Williams,

& Robison, 2017). As the identification and manipulation of these drug-activated cells in multiple addiction models markedly improved our understanding of the biology behind neuronal ensembles, it also provided new insights into the encoding of drug-associated memories at different stages of addiction (Bobadilla et al., 2017; Cruz, Rubio, & Hope, 2015; Whitaker & Hope, 2018).

Here we review the literature published in the last three decades that has supported the concept that drug-related pathological memories are encoded through plasticity changes in discrete neuronal ensembles in key regions of the brain reward circuitry. First, we discuss the up-regulation of IEGs by drugs of abuse in light of their role in general learning and memory processes, and how these markers of transcriptional plasticity can identify drug-activated cells. Second, we examine the various genetic tools that have more recently been developed to track and manipulate activated cells, and how they have been used to causally demonstrate the importance of IEG-expressing neuronal ensembles in mediating memory- and addiction-related learned behaviors. Third, we summarize the emerging and still relatively scarce data describing the circuit, physiological, cellular, and molecular features that specifically characterize the neuronal ensembles recruited by drug exposure. We finally conclude by arguing that the ongoing investigation of the unique signature of drug-activated cells has the potential to greatly deepen our understanding of basic neuronal biology, as well as to yield preclinical data with strong translational potential to better combat drug addiction.

It is very fitting that this review appears in a special issue devoted to the life and career of Paul Greengard, PhD, in whose laboratory one of us (EJN) completed his dissertation research close to 40 years ago. No one better exemplified the ideals of a superb mentor, and provided much of the field's basic understanding of how the molecular constituents and circuit activities of neurons are inter-related, than Paul Greengard (Nestler & Huganir, 2019).

2. Immediate early genes to visualize drug-activated cells: toward neuronal ensembles

2.1 IEG Expression as a proxy for neuronal activity and plasticity

The first evidence that neurons can trigger rapid transcriptional activity in response to environmental changes came from the study of the *Fos* gene, with both the transcript and protein induced within minutes following cell stimulation (Cole, Saffen, Baraban, & Worley, 1989; Greenberg, Ziff, & Greene, 1986; Morgan, Cohen, Hempstead, & Curran, 1987). The idea of a dynamic coupling between extracellular events and transcription was further confirmed through the identification of multiple genes regulated by neuronal activity and referred to as IEGs (Morgan & Curran, 1989; Sheng & Greenberg, 1990). These genes, many of which are expressed at very low levels in basal conditions, are remarkable by their rapid and transient induction in response to a wide range of stimuli. In neurons, IEGs are induced within minutes following synaptic activation and most of them return to their basal levels of expression one to two hours later (Sheng & Greenberg, 1990). Because they encode either transcription factors (e.g., Fos, FosB, JunD, Egr1 [also known as Zif268 or NGFI-A]) or effector proteins involved in activity-dependent plasticity (e.g., Arc, Homer1A) (Lanahan & Worley, 1998; Guzowski, McNaughton, Barnes, & Worley, 1999), these genes were logically proposed to be essential linking blocks that ensure the continuity between the rapid synaptic changes and long-lasting adaptations necessary for neuronal plasticity (Flavell & Greenberg, 2008; Sheng & Greenberg, 1990) that underlie memory formation (Tischmeyer & Grimm, 1999).

The bulk expression of several IEGs such as Fos and Egr-1 is increased within brain regions involved in memory encoding after several behavioral learning tasks (Gallo, Katche, Morici, Medina, & Weisstaub, 2018; Kubik, Miyashita, & Guzowski, 2007). They are induced in the hippocampus following novel environment exploration, spatial memory tasks, object recognition or fear conditioning (Montag-Sallaz, Welzl, Kuhl, Montag, & Schachner, 1999; Guzowski et al., 1999a; Vann, Brown, Erichsen, & Aggleton, 2000; Guzowski, Setlow, Wagner, & McGaugh, 2001; Ramírez-Amaya et al., 2005; Barbosa et al., 2013) and following fear conditioning in the cortex and amygdala as well (Hall, Thomas, & Everitt, 2001; Rosen, Fanselow, Young, Sitcoske, & Maren, 1998). Across these different types of tasks, the spatiotemporal regulation of Fos and Zif268 expression matches the known role and recruitment of specific brain regions during given phases of training and memory encoding (Minatohara et al., 2016). For instance, Zif268 expression is increased in the amygdala after retrieval of both contextual and cued fear associations, and in the hippocampus during contextual fear retrieval only (Hall et al., 2001). Similarly, Arc expression is increased in relevant brain regions during several behavioral tasks, from the exploration of a novel environment to the acquisition of operant behavior (Montag-Sallaz et al., 1999; Guzowski et al., 1999; Kelly & Deadwyler, 2002, 2003). Moreover, the level of Arc expression in the hippocampus positively correlates with novelty (Kelly & Deadwyler, 2002), decreases in trained animals (Kelly & Deadwyler, 2002), and is higher in animals showing higher performance in hippocampus- (Guzowski, McNaughton, Barnes, & Worley, 2001) or striatal- (Daberkow, Riedy, Kesner, & Keefe, 2007) dependent learning paradigms, together suggesting a role in the early phases of learning.

Preliminary evidence showing that patterns of IEG induction reflect the activity of not only given brain regions studied in bulk but also of specific neuronal networks within and across these brain regions came from studies of Arc (Miyashita et al., 2008). Unlike many other IEGs, Arc is localized in the dendritic compartment (Link et al., 1995; Lyford et al., 1995), where it directly regulates synaptic plasticity (Korb & Finkbeiner, 2011). While Arc expression is broadly increased in the brain following the massive and synchronous neuronal activity surge induced by a seizure (Lyford et al., 1995), it also appears to be induced selectively in dendrites exhibiting long-term potentiation (LTP) after electrical stimulation (Moga et al., 2004; Steward, Wallace, Lyford, & Worley, 1998), suggesting that Arc induction could be restricted to recently activated neurons that develop synaptic plasticity. Consistently, more precise histological mapping of IEG-expressing cells demonstrated and confirmed that only subsets of neurons engage these mechanisms in several learning paradigms (Guzowski et al., 2005; Miyashita et al., 2008). In particular, a mRNA labeling method called cellular compartment analysis of temporal activity by fluorescence in situ hybridization (catFISH) has been instrumental in correlating IEG expression with neuronal network activity (Guzowski et al., 1999; Guzowski, McNaughton, et al., 2001). This approach takes advantage of the rapid nuclear induction (within 2 min) and export (within 20 min) of IEG mRNAs such as *Arc*, *Homer1A* and others to distinguish cells activated at two different time points. Using this method, one can backtrack the activity of a given neuron or population of neurons during two different behavioral tasks, such as the exploration of two distinct environments. Exploration of a novel environment increased *Arc* expression in the hippocampus (Guzowski et al., 1999) and cortex (Vazdarjanova, McNaughton, Barnes, Worley, & Guzowski, 2002). In the hippocampus, the sequential exploration of two different environments induced *Arc* mRNA in two separate populations, whereas exploring twice the same environment induced *Arc* expression within the same neuronal population (Guzowski et al., 1999). These studies were fundamental in linking Arc induction with the activation by behavioral experience of precise brain networks and were further used to dissect the activation dynamics of distinct hippocampal subfields (Guzowski, Knierim, & Moser, 2004;

Vazdarjanova & Guzowski, 2004). Together, this seminal data strongly supported the idea that IEGs not only serve as a reliable marker to detect global activation of given brain regions but can also help define discrete neuronal ensembles specifically recruited during learning processes, in which activity-dependent plasticity programs are likely to be engaged (Guzowski et al., 2004; Kubik et al., 2007; Minatohara et al., 2016).

2.2 IEG induction and function in drug-activated neuronal ensembles

Both acute and chronic consumption of drugs of abuse dramatically alter an individual's behavioral, psychological, and cognitive responses in a wide range of situations, and these changes can linger for a very long time after cessation of use (Wolf, 2016). Such enduring effects reflect the development of a pathological form of neuronal and behavioral plasticity likely initiated during the early stages of drug exposure and whose persistence sustains the maladaptations and resulting malfunction of the brain reward circuitry. While decades of work documented the various ways these circuits are altered in addiction (Lüscher & Malenka, 2011), the concept that sparsely activated neuronal populations within those circuits are key in driving drug-induced alterations and network remodeling has emerged more recently and stands as a very promising perspective to refine our understanding of drug-associated memory encoding. IEG expression has been instrumental in identifying these drug-activated cells.

Several IEGs, including *Fos*, *Arc* and *Zif268*, are induced by drugs of abuse in a variety of drug exposure paradigms and across multiple regions of the reward circuitry (Table 1). *Fos* is induced in the nucleus accumbens (NAc), dorsal striatum and prefrontal cortex (PFC) following treatment with cocaine, amphetamine or methamphetamine (Crombag et al., 2002; Graybiel et al., 1990; Hope et al., 1992; Moratalla et al., 1993; Norman et al., 1993; Robertson, Paul, Moratalla, & Graybiel, 1991; Rosen et al., 1994; Torres et al., 2015; Young et al., 1991). Like Fos, Arc expression is increased in the same three brain regions after both acute and chronic cocaine (Fosnaugh et al., 1995; Freeman et al., 2010; Fumagalli et al., 2006; Salery et al., 2017; Tan et al., 2000; Yuferov et al., 2003), methamphetamine (Fujiyama et al., 2003; Kodama et al., 1998) and amphetamine (Tan et al., 2000). Arc expression is also increased in the CA1 region of the hippocampus after chronic treatment with psychostimulants (Fumagalli et al., 2006; Kodama et al., 1998). Similar patterns of induction are observed for *Egr1* in response to psychostimulants (Bhat et al., 1992a,

Table 1 Summary of IEG regulation in rodent brain in response to psychostimulants or opioids.

Arc

Drug	Regimen	Brain region	mRNA	Protein	References
Cocaine	Acute	PFC	↑		Fumagalli et al. (2006)
			↑	↑	Freeman et al. (2010)
		dStri	↑		Fosnaugh, Bhat, Yamagata, Worley, and Baraban (1995)
				↑	Tan, Moratalla, Lyford, Worley, and Graybiel (2000)
			↑	↑	Fumagalli et al. (2006); Salery et al. (2017)
		NAc	↑	↑	Salery et al. (2017)
		HPC	↑		Fumagalli et al. (2006)
	Chronic	PFC	↑		Fumagalli et al. (2006)
		dStri	↑	↑	Fumagalli et al. (2006)
			↑		Yuferov et al. (2003)
Amph/Meth	Acute	PFC, OFC, Cg, PC	↑		Kodama et al. (1998)
		dStri		↑	Tan et al. (2000)
		vStri	↑		Kodama et al. (1998); Tan et al. (2000)
	Chronic	NeoCx	↑		Fujiyama, Kajii, Hiraoka, and Nishikawa (2003)
		PFC, OFC, Cg, PC	↑		Kodama et al. (1998)
		vStri	↑		Kodama et al. (1998)

Continued

Table 1 Summary of IEG regulation in rodent brain in response to psychostimulants or opioids.—cont'd

Arc

Drug	Regimen	Brain region	mRNA	Protein	References
Morphine	Acute	dStri	↑		Ziółkowska, Korostyński, Piechota, Kubik, and Przewłocki (2012)
		NAc		↑	Lv, Xu, Han, and Cui (2011)
	Chronic	PFC	↑		Ammon, Mayer, Riechert, Tischmeyer, and Höllt (2003)
		dStri	↑		Ziółkowska et al. (2012)
					Marie-Claire, Courtin, Roques, and Noble (2004)
	WD	PFC	↑		Ammon et al. (2003)

Egr1

Drug	Regimen	Brain region	mRNA	Protein	References
Cocaine	Acute	NeoCx	↑		Moratalla, Robertson, and Graybiel (1992); Bhat, Cole, and Baraban (1992a, 1992b)
		dStri	↑		Moratalla et al. (1992); Bhat et al. (1992a, 1992b)
		NAc	↑		Moratalla et al. (1992); Bhat et al. (1992a, 1992b); Hope, Kosofsky, Hyman, and Nestler (1992)
	Chronic	Cortex, dStri	↓		Bhat et al. (1992a)
		NAc	=		Hope et al. (1992)
Amph	Acute	NeoCx, dStri, NAC	↑		Moratalla et al. (1992); Bhat et al. (1992b)
Meth	Acute	NAc	↑		Torres et al. (2015)
Morphine	Acute	Striatum	↑		Ziółkowska et al. (2012)
	Chronic	Striatum	↑		

Fos

Drug	Regimen	Brain region	mRNA	Protein	References
Cocaine	Acute	dmLC, vmLC	↑	↑	Graybiel, Moratalla, and Robertson (1990)
		dStri	↑	↑	Graybiel et al. (1990); Rosen, Chuang, and Iadarola (1994)
				↑	Young, Porrino, and Iadarola (1991)
			↑		Moratalla, Vickers, Robertson, Cochran, and Graybiel (1993)
		vStri	↑	↑	Graybiel et al. (1990)
		NAc	↑	↑	Hope et al. (1992)
			↑		Moratalla et al. (1993)
	Chronic	dStri	↓	↓	Rosen et al. (1994)
		NAc	=	=	Hope et al. (1992)
	Chronic (LS)	dStri		↑↑	Crombag, Jedynak, Redmond, Robinson, and Hope (2002)
		NAc		↑↑	
Amph	Acute	dmLC, vmLC	↑		Graybiel et al. (1990)
		dStri	↑		Graybiel et al. (1990)
				↑	Norman, Lu, Klug, and Norgren (1993)
		vStri	↑		Graybiel et al. (1990)
		NAc		↑	Norman et al. (1993)
	Chronic	dStri		↑↑	Norman et al. (1993)
		NAc			

Continued

Table 1 Summary of IEG regulation in rodent brain in response to psychostimulants or opioids.—cont'd

Fos

Drug	Regimen	Brain region	mRNA	Protein	References
	Acute	LC	↓	↓	Hayward, Duman, and Nestler (1990)
		PFC	=		
		dStri	↑		Hayward et al. (1990); Ziółkowska et al. (2012)
		NAc	↑		Hayward et al. (1990)
	Chronic	dStri	↑		Ziółkowska et al. (2012)
		LC	↓	↓	Hayward et al. (1990)
Morphine	WD	LC	↑	↑	Hayward et al. (1990)
		CC, dStri, NAc, VTA	↑		

FosB/ΔFosB

Drug	Regimen	Brain region	mRNA	Protein	References
Cocaine	Acute	Striatum	↑		Chen et al. (1995)
				↑	Hope et al. (1994)
	Chronic	Striatum	↑		Chen et al. (1995)
				↑	Hope et al. (1994); Perrotti et al. (2008); Lobo et al. (2013)
		NAc		↑	Perrotti et al. (2008); Lobo et al. (2013); Lee et al. (2006)
Meth	Acute	NAc	↑		Torres et al. (2015)
Morphine	Chronic	dStri, NAc		↑	Perrotti et al. (2008); Lobo et al. (2013)

Amph, amphetamine; CC, cerebral cortex; Cg, cingulate cortex; dStri, dorsal striatum; dmLC, dorsomedial limbic cortex; vmLC, ventromedial limbic cortex; HPC, Hippocampus; LC, locus coeruleus; LS, locomotor sensitization; Meth, methamphetamine; NAc, nucleus accumbens; NeoCx, neocortex: OFC, orbitofrontal cortex; PFC, prefrontal cortex; PC, parietal cortex; vStri, ventral striatum; WD, withdrawal.

1992b; Hope et al., 1992; Moratalla et al., 1992; Thomas, Arroyo, & Everitt, 2003; Torres et al., 2015). Consistent with their characteristic rapid and transient induction kinetics, IEGs are induced within minutes following psychostimulants exposure and return to their basal level of expression after minutes to hours (Fumagalli et al., 2006; Salery et al., 2017). The expression of these genes is also regulated by acute or chronic exposure to opioids (Ammon et al., 2003; Bisagno & Cadet, 2019; Browne, Godino, Salery, & Nestler, 2020; Hayward et al., 1990; Lv et al., 2011; Marie-Claire et al., 2004; Ziółkowska et al., 2012), albeit, with a slower time-course (Ziółkowska et al., 2012), likely due to different pharmacokinetic properties of the drugs and possibly different signaling mechanisms. In addition to these three well-described IEGs, several others including *FosB* (Alibhai, Green, Potashkin, & Nestler, 2007; Hope et al., 1992), *Homer1A* (Zhang et al., 2007), *Jun* and *JunB* (Hope et al., 1992; Moratalla et al., 1993), *Egr3* (Chandra et al., 2015), *Npas4* (Taniguchi et al., 2017) and *Nr4a1* (Carpenter et al., 2020) are induced in diverse paradigms of drug exposure. However, whether all of these IEGs are induced in the exact same cells has yet to be fully substantiated, even if it seems to be the case at least for *Fos* and *Arc* following acute cocaine (Guez-Barber et al., 2011; Liu et al., 2014; Salery et al., 2017).

In turn, IEG induction in reward-processing circuits contributes to establishing the persistent neuronal and behavioral adaptations characterizing the addicted phenotype in many different ways. Up-regulation of Fos is implicated in downstream changes in gene expression: its selective knock-out in Drd1-containing medium-sized spiny neurons (D1-MSNs) of the NAc alters drug-induced transcriptional programs along with cocaine-induced dendritic remodeling and locomotor sensitization (Xu, 2008; Zhang et al., 2007). The related IEG, *FosB,* has been studied widely in the context of addiction. *FosB* regulation is particularly interesting in the context of chronic drug exposure as a spliced product of the gene called ΔFosB resists degradation and thus accumulates in neurons following chronic treatment with psychostimulants and virtually any other class of abused drug (Hope et al., 1994; Chen et al., 1995; Jingshan Chen, Kelz, Hope, Nakabeppu, & Nestler, 1997; Lee et al., 2006; Robison & Nestler, 2011; Lobo et al., 2013). The long-lasting expression of this transcription factor in multiple brain regions following drug exposure (Perrotti et al., 2008) supports the idea that ΔFosB could act as a key "switch" for the drug-induced maladaptations underlying the transition from acute to compulsive drug taking (Brenhouse & Stellar, 2006; Nestler, 2013; Nestler, Kelz, & Chen, 1999). Consistently, ΔFosB overexpression in D1-MSNs of NAc increases cocaine-induced locomotor sensitization and conditioned place preference (CPP) (Kelz et al., 1999), facilitates acquisition of self-administration at low doses and enhances responses in a progressive ratio schedule of reinforcement (Colby, Whisler, Steffen, Nestler, & Self, 2003). Similar effects are seen with opioids (Zachariou et al., 2006). At the cellular level, ΔFosB overexpression in the NAc affects structural (Robison et al., 2013) and synaptic (Grueter, Robison, Neve, Nestler, & Malenka, 2013) plasticity. ΔFosB also regulates transcriptional programs in the NAc (McClung & Nestler, 2003) and has been mechanistically involved in the epigenetic desensitization of the *Fos* promoter via the recruitment of HDAC1 after chronic amphetamine (Renthal et al., 2008).

The role of Egr1 in drug models appears more subtle than that of Fos family members. Genetic suppression of Egr1 impairs locomotor sensitization but does not affect animals' responses to cocaine CPP (Valjent et al., 2006), advocating for more comprehensive studies of this transcription factor in drug models, which remains surprisingly scarce despite its pivotal role in synaptic plasticity (Duclot & Kabbaj, 2017).

Unlike Fos, FosB/ΔFosB and Egr1, Arc protein does not interact directly with DNA to regulate transcription but rather exerts its function through the interaction with other proteins involved in plasticity. Due to its peculiar dendritic localization, most studies have focused on Arc's canonical role in dendrites, where it regulates – among others – synaptic strength through AMPA glutamate receptor endocytosis (Chowdhury et al., 2006; Shepherd et al., 2006) and long-term neuronal plasticity (Guzowski et al., 2000; Shepherd & Bear, 2011; Waung, Pfeiffer, Nosyreva, Ronesi, & Huber, 2008). Recent evidence demonstrates that a nuclear pool of Arc protein might also contribute to neuronal plasticity in a non-canonical manner via indirect transcriptional regulation (Bloomer, VanDongen, & VanDongen, 2007; Korb, Wilkinson, Delgado, Lovero, & Finkbeiner, 2013; Salery et al., 2017). In drug models, cocaine increases Arc expression in the nucleus, and its suppression is associated with increased RNA-PolII activity and Fos expression (Salery et al., 2017). At the behavioral level, Arc loss of function is associated with increased sensitivity to low doses of cocaine in locomotor sensitization and CPP paradigms (Salery et al., 2017) and the local inhibition of Arc in the dorsal striatum attenuates the extinction of cocaine seeking but not seeking itself (Hearing, Schwendt, & McGinty, 2011). Together, cellular and behavioral studies of Arc in cocaine models argue for a homeostatic role of Arc in drug-induced plasticity, a unique property diametrically opposed to the proposed roles of other IEGs like *Fos*, *FosB* and *Egr1*, which seem to be overall positive regulators of drug-evoked maladaptations.

2.3 Plasticity in IEG expression, a substrate for behavioral plasticity in addiction models

While most IEGs are up-regulated by acute drug treatment independent of their molecular function, their response to prolonged exposure is different. The unique induction of ΔFosB protein after chronic drug exposure was discussed above. Arc too shows different responses to acute vs. chronic drug exposure. Chronic psychostimulant administration is for instance associated with a higher induction of Arc protein levels in animals with a drug history in comparison with those exposed to the drug for the first time (Fumagalli et al., 2006). This sensitization of Arc induction is associated with persistent accumulation of its protein and mRNA over days following the last injection. Arc expression is also chronically up-regulated in the absence of the drug during abstinence from cocaine self-administration (Freeman et al., 2010, 2008). After withdrawal, *Arc* mRNA expression is increased upon re-exposure to a drug-paired context (Hearing et al., 2011) or drug-paired discrete cues (Zavala, Osredkar, Joyce, & Neisewander, 2008), indicating that, through plastic changes, Arc expression tracks not only activation triggered by direct drug exposure but also the retrieval of previously learned drug-related memories.

In an opposite manner, bulk Fos expression is desensitized when cocaine or amphetamine is given in the home cage (Hope et al., 1992, 1994; Rosen et al., 1994), an effect mediated via ΔFosB as noted earlier (Renthal et al., 2008). By contrast, the number of Fos+cells is sensitized when animals are treated in a new environment and exhibit locomotor sensitization (Crombag et al., 2002, Nordquist et al., 2008) and not in the home cage (Mattson et al., 2008). Nonetheless, the absence of Fos sensitization to repeated cocaine or amphetamine when animals are injected in a familiar environment strongly suggests that the Fos+population is involved in the specific encoding of drug-context associations more than in simply tracking drug-evoked neuronal activity in chronically treated animals. Consistent with the persistence of such associations, context-specific Fos sensitization was maintained over 6 months after drug exposure along with locomotor sensitization (Hope, Simmons, Mitchell, Kreuter, & Mattson, 2006). In operant models, Fos expression is chronically up-regulated during abstinence from cocaine self-administration (Freeman et al., 2010, 2008) and can be further induced by re-exposure to contextual or discrete drug-paired cues (Bastle et al., 2012; Bossert et al., 2011; Fanous et al., 2012; Hamlin, Clemens, & McNally, 2008; Kufahl et al., 2009; Neisewander et al., 2000; Rubio et al., 2019; Zavala, Biswas, Harlan, & Neisewander, 2007). Similarly, chronic non-contingent cocaine treatment desensitizes Egr1 expression, with reductions in its basal levels in multiple forebrain areas (Bhat et al., 1992a, 1992b; Daunais & McGinty, 1995; Unal, Beverley, Willuhn, & Steiner, 2009). However, similar to Arc and Fos, in a chronic self-administration model, Egr1 expression was induced by exposure to discrete cues previously associated with cocaine (Thomas et al., 2003). This response was not observed in yoked controls, suggesting that Egr1 may participate in the encoding of stimulus-drug conditioned associations.

Together, these findings argue for complex gene-specific, drug-specific and paradigm-specific patterns of IEG expression and plasticity, which could be explained by numerous factors. First, different signaling cascades might converge onto different epigenetic regulation of a given IEG promoter—which has been described in detail only in the specific case of Fos desensitization after chronic amphetamine (Renthal et al., 2008). Second, the precise pharmacodynamics of different drugs and drug administration regimens can greatly influence IEG induction and sensitization, as for example Arc and Fos induction and locomotor sensitization have all been shown to depend on the rate of intravenous cocaine administration (Samaha, Mallet, Ferguson, Gonon, & Robinson, 2004). Third, given that not all cells are activated by drugs, one cannot exclude drug-induced adaptations in non-activated cells or that the global response might be driven by relatively smaller or larger neuronal ensembles, especially as these methods do not allow the tracking of the initially activated population at subsequent stages of drug-related behaviors. Nevertheless, the one consistent finding is that multiple IEGs are induced following the presentation of previously neutral contextual information now associated with the drug. This could indicate a coordinated transcriptional response within a subset of neurons specifically involved in encoding drug-context associations if it were that those IEGs are induced in the same cells—which has not yet been confirmed. This also strengthens the idea that IEG-expressing cells not only track neuronal activity *per se* but neuronal activity relevant for drug-related learning and plasticity as well. Overall, the fact that the IEG response itself can change over time parallels behavioral plasticity, and that these responses seem to occur in ensembles encoding drug-cue associations reinforces the argument that IEG induction is more than just a good marker of neuronal activity: it can also be used as a proxy for the neuronal plasticity mechanisms engaged in those activated ensembles.

3. Beyond correlation: Causal role of activated cells in controlling behavior

The mapping of endogenous IEG expression across multiple brain regions and learning paradigms has been instrumental in identifying the neuronal populations recruited at different stages of memory formation and expression. We have seen that their activation not only reflects the rapid response of distributed neuronal networks but also contribute to initiate plasticity mechanisms within these neuronal ensembles. While a crucial first step, these early studies remained correlative and did not provide insight into the causal role of IEG-expressing cells in memory processing. The recent advent of optogenetic and chemogenetic approaches has made it possible to assess causality of neuronal ensembles (DeNardo & Luo, 2017; Denny, Lebois, & Ramirez, 2017; Koya, Margetts-Smith, & Hope, 2016; Whitaker & Hope, 2018).

3.1 Genetic tools to tag and manipulate neuronal ensembles

Because of their very transient induction, endogenous IEG expression can only be correlated to performance in recently executed behavioral tasks. Nonetheless, their role in neuronal plasticity suggests that cells where IEGs were initially expressed are likely to be reactivated by further stimulation, and that subsequent and repeated reactivation could be decisive in evoking persistent adaptations in network activity. As a first basis for that argument, the initial peak of Arc expression in the hippocampus after the exploration of a novel environment is followed a few hours later by a second wave of Arc induction in a subset of the originally activated neurons in the absence of any new stimulation (Ramírez-Amaya et al., 2005). Such reactivation—solely driven by network activity—has been proposed to reflect the stabilization of recently activated neuronal networks during memory consolidation, which is corroborated by the fact that Arc is induced by a second exploration of the same environment in the same neurons that were activated during the first exploration (Guzowski et al., 1999a; Vazdarjanova et al., 2002). Yet, studies based on the detection of endogenous IEG expression remain considerably limited in their ability to track the fate of initially activated cells over longer periods of time to decipher their role at later stages of memory encoding and retrieval, which would confirm that they truly represent the neuronal substrates of the corresponding memories. Past and current efforts to establish a causal role for these populations in memory encoding have benefited from the development of research tools allowing for both the permanent labeling (tagging) of activated cells to monitor their reactivation as well as the transient manipulation of their activity during key phases of learning processes (Denny et al., 2017; Garner & Mayford, 2012; Liu, Ramirez, Redondo, & Tonegawa, 2014; Ramirez, Tonegawa, & Liu, 2014).

These transgenic approaches mostly used the promoters of *Arc* or *Fos* to drive the expression of artificial tags, which can be either fluorescent reporters to simply visualize IEG-expressing cells, or optogenetic/chemogenetic constructs to manipulate IEG-expressing cells' activity. The key factor has been to render those tags activity-dependent yet stable, and the persistence of this tagging depends on the system and strategy used. The Arc-GFP knock-in mouse—in which the *Arc* promoter drives the transient expression of a destabilized form of GFP instead of Arc itself—allowed for the visualization of *Arc*-expressing neuronal ensembles in different cortical areas during visual information processing (Gao et al., 2010; Wang et al., 2006) and motor learning (Cao et al., 2015; Gao et al., 2010). While this method is useful for *in vivo* real-time visualization and characterization of *Arc*-inducing cells, the destabilized GFP does not provide a permanent tagging of activated cells. Studying those cells over longer periods of time is feasible using the TetTag mouse line, another genetic model in which the tag expression can last days to weeks (Reijmers & Mayford, 2009; Reijmers, Perkins, Matsuo, & Mayford, 2007). In these mice, the expression of a longer-lasting tag in *Fos*-expressing cells is triggered by doxycycline treatment and can be used to both track and manipulate cells that were Fos+during the time window of doxycycline action, which is usually synchronized with a behavior or experience of interest (Garner et al., 2012; X. Liu et al., 2012; Ramirez et al., 2013, 2015). While this tag persists over days, it fails to offer an indelible labeling of activated neurons over weeks to months. A truly permanent tagging of activated cells was made possible via the development of the *Arc*-Cre/*Arc*-TRAP and *Fos*-Cre/*Fos*-TRAP transgenic mice (Guenthner, Miyamichi, Yang, Heller, & Luo, 2013), as well as the *Arc*-CreER^{T2} bacterial artificial chromosome (BAC) mice (Denny et al., 2014) (Fig. 1). Based on the use of a tamoxifen-inducible CreER^{T2} recombination system, these mouse lines offer improved temporal control over the tagging window to achieve specific and permanent labeling

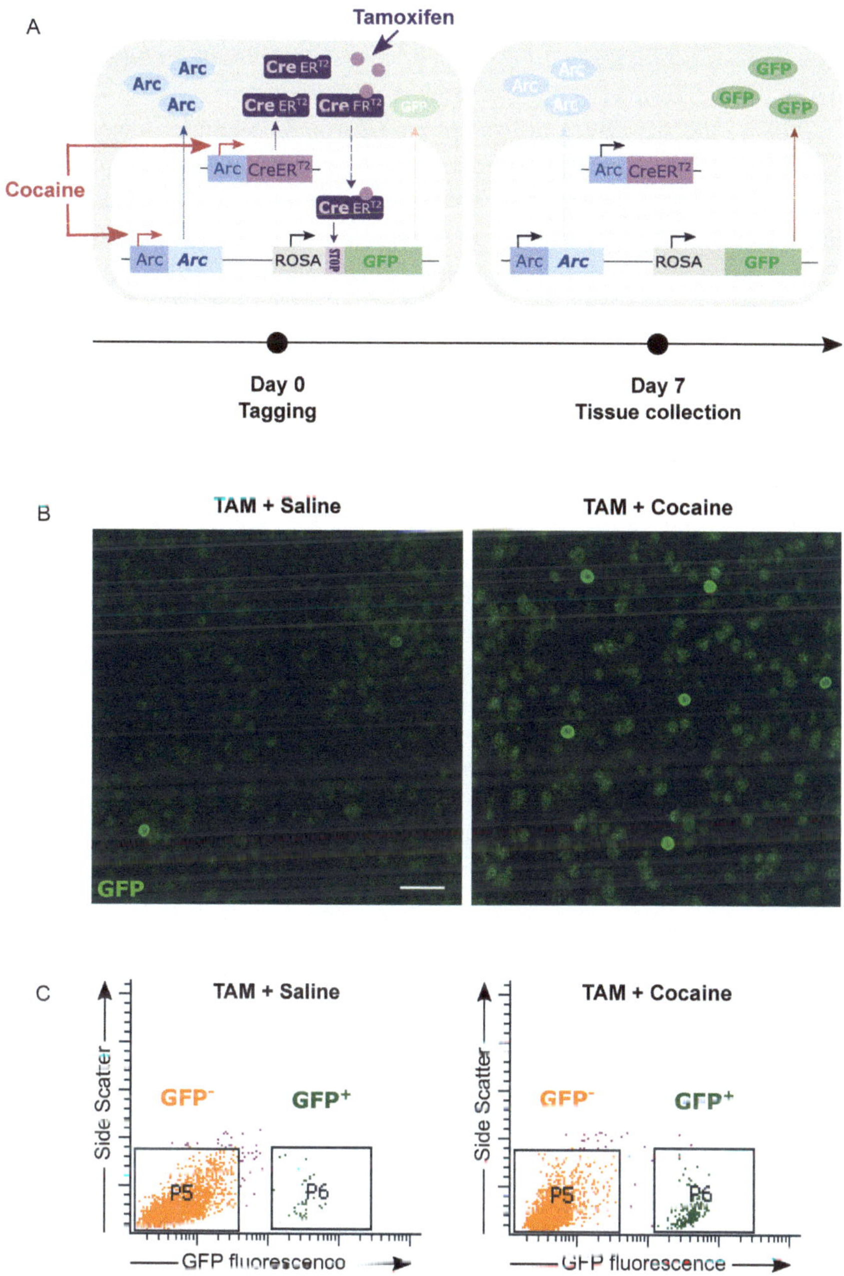

Fig. 1 See figure legend on opposite page.

of neuronal populations activated during specific behavioral tasks through recombination of a second Cre-dependent tag-expressing transgene (Allen et al., 2017; Denny et al., 2014; Wall et al., 2019).

These tools have been utilized to tag neuronal ensembles activated during memory formation and further track and manipulate their activity at later stages of memory expression, with most of the focus being on the acquisition and retrieval of contextual fear memory (Minatohara et al., 2016). Using TetTag mice, (Reijmers et al., 2007) first demonstrated that an amygdala Fos+ensemble activated during the learning phase of fear conditioning is reactivated during the retrieval of that fear memory. The level of reactivation correlated with the freezing fear response, indicating that this reactivated ensemble might represent the neural trace of the associative memory (Reijmers & Mayford, 2009). To evaluate their causal role, these activated and reactivated cells were later manipulated by expressing optogenetic (Channelrhodopsin ChR2, Archaerhodopsin ArchT) or chemogenetic (designer receptors exclusively activated by designer drugs or DREADDs) tags. In the dentate gyrus (DG), the optogenetic reactivation of a ChR2-tagged Fos+ensemble recruited during contextual fear conditioning training was sufficient for the later expression of fear memory (Liu et al., 2012). Reciprocally, the inactivation of hippocampal CA1 Fos+ ensemble activated during the conditioning session altered the retrieval

Fig. 1 Permanent tagging of cocaine-activated cells in NAc of Arc-CreER^{T2} mice. Arc-CreER^{T2} mice were crossed with a GFP reporter line to induce stable GFP expression in activated Arc+ neurons. (A) Schematic representation of the Arc-CreERT2 strategy applied to cocaine-activated cell tagging. On the day of tagging (day 0), animals are injected concomitantly with cocaine and tamoxifen. Cocaine triggers the activation of both the endogenous and artificially-expressed *Arc* promoters controlling, respectively, endogenous *Arc* and *CreER*^{T2} transcription. This leads to increased expression of both Arc and CreER^{T2} proteins in activated Arc+ cells. Upon tamoxifen binding, CreER^{T2} enters the nucleus where the Cre-dependent removal of a floxed-STOP cassette triggers GFP expression. The persistent expression of GFP in cells activated initially by cocaine allows for their visualization at any future time (e.g., 7 days). (B–C) On day 0, Arc-CreER^{T2} mice were treated concomitantly with tamoxifen + cocaine or tamoxifen + saline as a control. Tissue was collected on day 7 post-tagging to visualize cells previously activated by cocaine. TAM = Tamoxifen. (B) Representative confocal images of GFP immunostaining in the NAc at day 7 post-tagging showing a higher number of activated cells in the cocaine-treated group. Scalebar = 50 μm. (C) Fluorescence-activated nuclei sorting (FANS) strategy to isolate GFP+ nuclei from NAc punches at day 7 post-tagging. Cocaine-treated group shows a larger population of activated (GFP+) cells in comparison to saline-treated group.

of conditioned fear memory (Tanaka et al., 2014). The manipulation of Arc+ ensembles in the DG also controlled fear memory retrieval (Denny et al., 2014). These seminal studies were fundamental in demonstrating the causal role of IEG ensembles in several brain regions in memory retrieval and were followed by many others well reviewed elsewhere (Frankland, Josselyn, & Köhler, 2019; Liu, Ramirez, et al., 2014; Tonegawa, Morrissey, & Kitamura, 2018).

Together, this work provides direct evidence for specific reactivation during memory expression of neuronal ensembles that are initially activated during memory encoding and that such reactivation is both necessary and sufficient for memory expression. The sparse neuronal populations that meet these requirements—activated during memory encoding, reactivated during memory retrieval and both necessary and sufficient for memory expression—have been referred to as memory engram cells, and to date are thought to represent the neuronal substrate of the memory engram (Denny et al., 2017; Josselyn & Tonegawa, 2020; Tonegawa, Liu, Ramirez, & Redondo, 2015).

3.2 Tagging and manipulating neuronal ensembles in addiction

The robustness and persistence of associations formed between contextual information and the rewarding properties of drugs of abuse is proof of the strength of associative learning processes at play in the development of addiction (Robbins, Ersche, & Everitt, 2008). These memories are thought to be driven by a potent and enduring remodeling of reward-processing brain circuits during and after drug exposure (Lüscher & Malenka, 2011). As mentioned, these persistent adaptations are likely to occur in the sparse neuronal ensembles first activated during the early stages of addiction and whose later reactivation could account for the expression of drug-associated memories.

Most efforts towards characterizing neuronal ensembles in addiction have focused on the causal role of drug-activated Fos+ensembles in behavioral alterations across several addiction models (Cruz et al., 2015; Whitaker & Hope, 2018). Correlative studies described above indicate that Fos+ensembles respond to drugs or their associated cues (Cruz et al., 2015). However, the fact that Fos is induced at both early and late phases of drug-related paradigms raises the question of whether the same subset of neurons is recruited at different time points. From data on contextual fear conditioning, one can hypothesize that ensemble reactivation mediates the consolidation of the drug-associated engram and subsequent response to the drug itself or contextual cues. The earliest supporting evidence came from a study that took advantage of ΔFosB accumulation after chronic cocaine treatment to infer the past activation of those neurons (Mattson et al., 2008). Through co-labeling for recently induced *Fos* and remotely induced ΔFosB, the authors visualized the two waves of activation simultaneously and showed that 80% of the neurons recruited by chronic cocaine exposure (ΔFosB+) in a locomotor sensitization protocol are reactivated (*Fos*+) in response to a challenge injection in the cocaine-associated context. The causal role of these chronically activated Fos+ ensembles in drug memory encoding has been assessed using a transgenic rat line expressing *LacZ*—coding for ß-galactosidase (ß-gal)—under the control of the *Fos* promoter. In *Fos*-LacZ transgenic rats, selective inactivation of Fos expressing neurons can be achieved via the local injection of the prodrug Daun02 that inactivates ß-gal-expressing cells, i.e., Fos+cells (Koya et al., 2009, 2016). In a locomotor sensitization paradigm, the selective inactivation of NAc Fos+ neuronal ensembles activated in a cocaine-paired context severely impaired the conditioned locomotor response during re-exposure to the same context. Importantly, the behavioral response was not altered when the authors inactivated the cells activated by a second environment different from the drug-paired one (Koya et al., 2009). These findings support the idea that the drug-context associations are indeed encoded in a sparse and context-specific population of NAc neurons, whose activity is required for the expression of this associative memory, akin to the way contextual fear memories have been proposed to be encoded in the hippocampus and amygdala (Josselyn & Tonegawa, 2020). This scheme was further confirmed in an operant paradigm: selective inactivation of NAc shell neuronal ensembles activated by context-induced drug-seeking prevents the subsequent seeking during another re-exposure to the context (Cruz et al., 2014). Again, inactivation of a non-specific subset of neurons activated in a control context failed to alter context-induced drug seeking, and so did the inactivation of NAc core—not shell—ensembles, suggesting that context-induced drug-seeking is mediated by a context- and subregion-specific ensemble. The same approach was then used to identify medial PFC and orbitofrontal cortex (OFC) ensembles involved in heroin seeking following context (Bossert et al., 2011) or cue (Fanous et al., 2012) re-exposure, and dorsomedial striatum, central nucleus of amygdala and infralimbic cortex ensembles in the incubation of methamphetamine craving (Caprioli et al., 2017), alcohol dependence (de Guglielmo et al., 2016) and alcohol seeking (Pfarr et al., 2015), respectively. It is interesting to note that, across these studies, the proportion of neurons activated and subsequently manipulated is very low (5–10%), suggesting that drug memories are encoded in sparse neuronal populations, a hint at how precise and selective engram allocation mechanisms might be.

3.3 From a drug engram to a drug engram circuit?

Besides the *Fos*-LacZ mouse, other tools have been occasionally applied to addiction models. The TetTag mouse was used to analyze the encoding of a cocaine-associated spatial memory in hippocampal CA1 ensembles (Trouche et al., 2016). Through the optogenetic silencing of a CA1 Fos+ neuronal ensemble associated with a specific environment, the authors were able to shift the representation of this spatial context to a different hippocampal ensemble. They recoded the engram representing the cocaine-paired environment and thereby reversed cocaine-induced CPP (Trouche et al., 2016). A cocaine-context memory engram was also found in the lateral nucleus of amygdala (LA) through the manipulation of a CREB-expressing neuronal population (Hsiang et al., 2014). This approach, previously used to characterize LA neuronal ensembles involved in fear memory (Han et al., 2007, 2009), showed that the artificial overexpression of CREB in a sparse population of LA neurons during contextual conditioning is sufficient to increase their incorporation into an engram encoding the drug memory. While this approach does not directly manipulate the cells activated during encoding of drug memory, it demonstrates that activation of a given population of neurons during memory encoding is sufficient for it to become incorporated into the engram and to drive the expression of the corresponding memory.

Given that neuronal ensembles activated by drug exposure appear to emerge in multiple brain regions, one key question is whether these distributed engram cells are preferentially interconnected across brain regions. Recent but still limited data seem to support that statement. First, anatomically connected ventral CA1 (vCA1) and NAc core ensembles were shown to be concomitantly activated during cocaine CPP training and exhibit preferential synaptic strengthening with conditioning (Zhou et al., 2019). Second, a retrograde tracing study found a similar preferential strengthening of synaptic connections between cocaine-activated neurons from the

OFC projecting to cocaine-activated neurons in the dorsal striatum (Wall et al., 2019). In both cases, the manipulation of the coordinated activity of engram cells across regions modulated drug-induced behavioral plasticity. This has led to the proposal that the "cocaine engram" might actually be a "cocaine engram circuit" (Zhou et al., 2019) with preferential connectivity between engram cells of each region.

The broad distribution of sparse activated networks associated with a specific memory also suggests the co-existence within brain regions of neuronal ensembles associated with different experiences. Recently, this was confirmed by the identification of two distinct PFC ensembles either activated by events of positive (cocaine exposure) or negative (foot shock) valence, respectively. The cells also differed in their molecular phenotype and long-range wiring—with positive valence-encoding and negative valence-encoding PFC cells preferentially projecting to the NAc and lateral habenula, respectively—confirming that different experiences can be represented in divergent and specific networks of activated neurons within a given brain region (Ye et al., 2016). Functionally, the reactivation of these cocaine- or shock-associated ensembles in a real-time preference assay increased preference or aversion, respectively (Ye et al., 2016). Similarly, the two different memory traces related to two successive phases of a given paradigm—acquisition and then extinction of food (Warren et al., 2016) or cocaine (Warren et al., 2019) self-administration - were shown to be encoded in distinct non-overlapping neuronal ensembles of the ventral medial PFC. These distinct ensembles also have different outputs, with the self-administration ensembles projecting to the NAc Core and the extinction ensembles projecting to the NAc Shell, putatively reflecting the role of these two ensembles in, respectively, promoting or inhibiting cocaine-seeking (Warren et al., 2019). These studies (Wall et al., 2019; Warren et al., 2016; Warren et al., 2019; Ye et al., 2016; Zhou et al., 2019), all based on activity-dependent and permanent cell tagging methods, emphasize once again the importance of monitoring and modulating the activity of cells recruited at the early stages of drug exposure, i.e., during memory encoding. It is of course also true that the manipulation of ensembles associated with the expression of an already sensitized/learned response has greatly improved our understanding of the encoding of drug associations. Still, our ability to track and eventually modulate the fate of the originally activated ensemble remains a critical step in finding and characterizing a drug memory engram.

4. Cellular and molecular characteristics of neuronal ensembles

Drugs of abuse affect neuronal physiology in part by increasing dopamine neurotransmission and thereby activating dopamine-evoked signaling cascades throughout the brain reward circuitry (Di Chiara & Imperato, 1988). The resulting rapid cellular changes, including activity-dependent transcription of IEGs, are thought to then set the stage for more persistent adaptations within activity-defined neuronal networks (Nestler & Lüscher, 2019). However, the different time courses of these mechanisms limits our ability to assess whether lasting changes actually happen as a consequence of the initial activation of a given neuron. The permanent tagging of IEG expressing cells hence stands as a powerful tool to address these shortcomings, as it offers the possibility to subsequently question the neuronal properties and causal role of the populations targeted initially. This approach is particularly relevant in addiction models where the persistence of behavioral alterations is proposed to depend on the strengthening of neuronal alterations built up since the earliest stages of drug exposure. Given the possibility that at least part if not a majority of the several plasticity mechanisms implicated in the pathophysiology of addiction might be restricted to sparse neuronal ensembles, the cellular and molecular characterization of the ensemble cells becomes especially critical to reconcile with the decades of evidence for plastic changes detected in bulk tissue analyses. Efforts toward this goal are twofold: first, the identification of intrinsic properties shared by neurons from the same ensemble that would reflect their preferential recruitment based on their cell type or expression of specific molecular markers and, second, the dissection of acquired properties that would reflect coordinated adaptations developed in cells as they become part of the drug engram.

4.1 Cell type specificity of drug-activated neuronal ensembles

Much evidence regarding the preferential recruitment of specific cell types in drug responses comes from the cellular mapping of IEGs, which highlight a dramatic dichotomy between D1- and D2-MSNs of the NAc (Chandra & Lobo, 2017). These two striatal subpopulations, which have distinct or even opposite effects on drug-related behaviors, also diverge in their cellular and transcriptional profiles in both basal and drug-exposed conditions

(Calipari et al., 2016; Heiman et al., 2008; Lobo et al., 2010; Lobo, Karsten, Gray, Geschwind, & Yang, 2006; Salery, Trifilieff, Caboche, & Vanhoutte, 2020). Several IEGs, including *Fos, FosB, Egr1* and *Arc*, are induced in D1-MSNs specifically in response to drugs of abuse (Bertran-Gonzalez et al., 2008; Chandra et al., 2015; Chandra & Lobo, 2017; Heiman et al., 2008; Lobo et al., 2013). Consistently, Fos+ensembles activated by acute and chronic cocaine isolated via fluorescence-activated cell sorting (FACS) were shown to express higher levels of the D1-MSN marker prodynorphin and lower levels of the D2 receptor itself as well as the D2-MSN marker *Adora2a* (Guez-Barber et al., 2011), indicating a predominant activation of D1-MSNs. Likewise, all drugs of abuse after chronic exposure induce ΔFosB protein in D1-MSNs only, except for opioids which induce it equally in D1- and D2-MSNs (Lobo et al., 2013). This D1-D2 MSN dichotomy holds for ΔFosB in operant (i.e., self-administration) paradigms (Lobo et al., 2013), although less so for Fos: both D1- and D2-MSNs appear to be recruited in Fos+ensembles in the dorsomedial striatum, NAc shell, ventromedial PFC and OFC associated with incubation of methamphetamine craving (Caprioli et al., 2017), context-induced reinstatement of cocaine seeking (Cruz et al., 2014) and heroin seeking (Bossert et al., 2011) and incubation of heroin craving (Fanous et al., 2012), respectively. A contribution of both D1- and D2-MSNs to contextually guided drug seeking is consistent with previous reports of context-specific regulation of Fos expression in D1- and D2-MSNs (Badiani et al., 1999). Preferential recruitment of D1-MSNs in drug memory encoding and retrieval was further confirmed in a study showing that Fos+ensembles activated in the NAc core during both the acquisition and expression of cocaine CPP were mainly composed of D1-MSNs (Zhou et al., 2019). The D1 engram neurons are preferentially targeted by afferents from vCA1 cocaine-activated neuronal ensembles, which are thought to provide contextual information for cocaine CPP memory (Zhou et al., 2019). This D1-MSN engram appears critical in integrating and encoding drug-context memory since manipulation of vCA1 ensembles connecting to the D1-MSN engram cells was further shown to mediate the retrieval of cocaine CPP memory (Zhou et al., 2019). Consistent with the idea of D1-expressing NAc engram cells encoding drug associations, silencing D1-MSNs suppresses cocaine CPP, while activation of D1- or D2-MSNs promoted and impaired retrieval of this memory, respectively (Lobo et al., 2010; Zhou et al., 2019). However, these studies manipulated D1- and D2-MSNs populations as a whole and did not specifically target the activated D1- or D2-MSNs ensembles. While much indirect evidence supports the existence of a predominant D1 engram (Guez-Barber et al., 2011; Zhou et al., 2019), we still lack a comprehensive understanding of the specific contribution of D1- vs. D2-expressing engram cells. For instance, a similarly sparse D2-MSNs population could take part in the encoding of drug-associated memories through opposite dopamine-dependent regulatory mechanisms, and could thereby modulate the recruitment of the drug engram by regulating the signal to noise ratio in these circuits.

4.2 Synaptic adaptations in drug engram cells

The strengthened connectivity between broadly distributed activated neurons discussed above is mediated by synaptic adaptations. Upon cocaine CPP, the preferential recruitment of D1-MSNs is associated with synaptic structural (dendritic spine morphology) and electrophysiological (AMPA transmission, frequency of synaptic inputs and paired-pulse ratio) changes restricted to NAc D1-MSN engram cells compared to neighboring D1-MSN non-engram cells (Zhou et al., 2019). This was associated with a specific synaptic strengthening of vCA1 inputs onto NAc core D1-MSN engram cells compared to neighboring D1-MSN non-engram cells which was further shown to mediate the retrieval of cocaine CPP memory (Zhou et al., 2019). The investigation of similar engram-specific synaptic changes in cortico-striatal networks revealed a preferential connectivity between cocaine-activated cortical and striatal neurons which was associated with enhanced synaptic strength between these co-activated ensembles (Wall et al., 2019). In a cocaine locomotor sensitization paradigm, chronic cocaine specifically enhanced drug-activated OFC projections onto coactive dorsal striatal neurons as evidenced by increased AMPA/NMDA receptor ratios and smaller paired-pulse ratio in activated dorsal striatal neurons compared to non-activated neurons (Wall et al., 2019). Likewise, the silencing of the coactivated OFC-to-dorsal striatum network impaired the expression of cocaine locomotor sensitization. Plastic synaptic alterations were also reported for chronically activated NAc Fos+ensembles, as they formed more silent synapses—proposed to be the substrates of drug induced plasticity (Dong & Nestler, 2014)—than surrounding non-activated ensembles in animals expressing cocaine locomotor sensitization (Koya et al., 2012). This phenomenon was only observed in context-dependent cocaine sensitization indicating that it could also be restricted to neurons involved in the encoding of drug-context associations (Whitaker et al., 2016).

4.3 Molecular characteristics of drug engram cells

These synaptic adaptations presumably result from drug-evoked molecular and transcriptional adaptations. Genes involved in synaptic plasticity associated with glutamatergic transmission (*Homer1*, *Grin2A*, *Grin2B*) are for instance selectively increased in FACS-isolated Fos+ensembles of the dorsal striatum activated during context-induced reinstatement of cocaine seeking (Li et al., 2015; Rubio et al., 2015). Glutamatergic transmission plays an important role in drug-induced cue seeking, and high levels of glutamate release might expand the neuronal ensembles activated during cue-induced drug-seeking and precipitate relapse-like responses (Bobadilla et al., 2017). The transcriptional profiling of FACS-isolated NAc Fos+ensembles also revealed an increase in the expression of several IEGs including *Arc*, *FosB*, and *Nr4a3* in comparison with non-activated Fos- neurons (Guez-Barber et al., 2011). Similarly, PFC neuronal ensembles associated with cue-induced heroin seeking expressed higher levels of *Arc*, *Egr1* and *Egr2* (Fanous et al., 2013). Importantly, the magnitude of the increase compared to control groups was higher than previously reported in bulk tissue for the same genes in the same behavioral task (Koya et al., 2006; Kuntz, Patel, Grigson, Freeman, & Vrana, 2008), a strong argument defending the idea that changes detected in bulk are mostly driven by the changes engaged in activated cells. This was also demonstrated in methamphetamine-activated dorsostriatal Fos+ensembles, which exhibited a greater induction of *FosB* and *ΔFosB* than seen for total homogenates (Liu, Rubio, et al., 2014). Consistent with its major role in addiction (Lobo et al., 2010) and in cue-induced cocaine seeking (Graham et al., 2007; Grimm et al., 2003), the plasticity marker and neurotrophic factor Bdnf along with its receptor TrkB were also selectively increased in Fos+neurons during the incubation of methamphetamine (Li et al., 2015). In this same paradigm, the expression of genes encoding several epigenetic enzymes (e.g., *Hdac3, Hdac4, Hdac5, Ehmt1, Dnmt3a, Kdm1a*) was also affected, suggesting here again that various epigenetic mechanisms implicated in drug-induced plasticity at the bulk tissue level (LaPlant et al., 2010; Maze & Nestler, 2011; Renthal et al., 2008; Walker & Nestler, 2018) might occur specifically in drug-activated ensembles (Li et al., 2015). While the exploration of activity-regulated changes can inform cellular adaptations following drug exposure, recent evidence also suggests the existence of pre-existing molecular markers that define a neuronal population more likely to be allocated to the encoding of a specific memory (Ye et al., 2016). For instance, PFC neuronal ensembles encoding a positive valence experience preferentially expressing *Npas4* at baseline in comparison with negative valence-associated ensembles.

Across cell types, the segregation of neuronal populations based on their level of activation during specific behavioral tasks reveals the existence of complex patterns of gene expression specifically associated with the recruitment of a given cell in drug-activated neuronal ensembles. While D1-MSNs seem pivotal in encoding drug-context associations, the concomitant activation of D1- and D2 MSNs during re-exposure to the drug-paired context indicates that the definition of the cocaine engram could reside beyond cell type specificity. The co-induction of multiple IEGs in drug-activated ensembles suggests that they could be characterized by a transcriptional signature composed of the combination of specific activity-regulated genes. This hypothesis is corroborated by recent findings showing a tight correlation between the expression of different IEGs at the level of individual MSN neurons in the dorsal striatum after acute cocaine (Gonzales, Mukherjee, Ashwal-Fluss, Loewenstein, & Citri, 2020). The spatial segregation of IEG-expressing clusters was proposed by the authors to represent "super-ensembles" of neurons characterized by a coherent and robust expression of a specific set of IEGs. A more comprehensive molecular characterization of NAc populations after acute cocaine exposure was recently achieved using single-nucleus RNA sequencing (Savell et al., 2020). This approach identified a combinatorial cocaine-specific transcriptional program composed of distinct IEGs, and the coordinated manipulation of this set of genes using large-scale multiplexed CRISPR-dCAS9 potentiated cocaine locomotor sensitization (Savell et al., 2020). The implementation of transcriptional profiling of activated populations with single-cell resolution thus appears as a critical step to unmask subtle yet specific transcriptional alterations restricted to sparse neuronal populations involved in drug memory encoding, as well as intrinsic molecular markers that could determine a neuron's allocation to a drug memory engram. Applying these approaches to chronic drug exposure, in particular, to self-administration and relapse paradigms, is a high priority for the future.

5. Conclusion

From the study of bulk IEG regulation to the visualization and manipulation of IEG-expressing cells across several brain regions and learning paradigms, the exploration of activity-dependent transcription is a major tool to define behaviorally relevant networks at the molecular level. The recent finding that cocaine-activated IEG-expressing cells can form spatially defined clusters whose size is correlated with their level of activation (Gonzales et al., 2020) suggests that their pattern of induction could reflect complex regulation within brain regions and circuits during the encoding of specific information. At the single cell level, the consistent and coordinated induction of an IEG program in cocaine-activated cells provides an experience-specific transcriptional signature that is sufficient to recapitulate drug responses (Savell et al., 2020). While these studies confirm the relevance of studying IEG regulation, they also demonstrate the importance of more comprehensive approaches beyond focusing on a restricted set of genes to reveal experience-specific molecular signatures.

The mapping of neuronal ensembles recruited throughout the brain at different stages of addiction reveals a sparse but broad distribution of activated cells across brain regions. This suggests that different components of a given experience can be encoded in distinct but interconnected neuronal ensembles in brain regions involved in the processing of specific aspects of this experience. Reciprocally, the coexistence within a given brain region of neuronal ensembles encoding distinct experiences suggests complex patterns of intermingled ensembles and subtle mechanisms of cellular allocation to an ensemble, which highlights the importance of coupling permanent tagging of activated cells with wide-range tracing to achieve an extensive characterization of broadly distributed engrams.

Finally, while the study of neuronal ensembles in the addiction field has been fundamental for the identification of the small and specific neuronal populations involved in complex behavioral responses, we still lack a broad description of their cellular and molecular properties. Most molecular studies focusing on rapid changes in gene expression within activated ensembles indicate alterations in their transcriptional responses (Cruz et al., 2015; Koya et al., 2016; Whitaker & Hope, 2018). The exploration of stable molecular alterations in neuronal ensembles over long periods of withdrawal and relapse would also be extremely informative in regard to the persistence of addictive behaviors. Improving our ability to physically isolate neuronal ensembles using sorting techniques (Fig. 1) will facilitate the implementation of cutting edge epigenomic and transcriptomic techniques to this field and greatly expand our understanding of the complex transcriptional signature of activated cells at different stages of addiction.

Acknowledgments

This work was supported by the Boehringer Ingelheim Fonds (doctoral fellowship to AG) and National Institute of Health (Grant No. R01DA014133 [to EJN]).

Conflict of interest statement

The authors report no biomedical financial interests or potential conflicts of interest.

References

Alberini, C. M., & Kandel, E. R. (2015). The regulation of transcription in memory consolidation. *Cold Spring Harbor Perspectives in Biology*, 7(1), a021741. https://doi.org/10.1101/cshperspect.a021741.

Alibhai, I. N., Green, T. A., Potashkin, J. A., & Nestler, E. J. (2007). Regulation of fosB and ΔfosB mRNA expression: In vivo and in vitro studies. *Brain Research*, *1143*, 22–33. https://doi.org/10.1016/j.brainres.2007.01.069.

Allen, W. E., DeNardo, L. A., Chen, M. Z., Liu, C. D., Loh, K. M., Fenno, L. E., et al. (2017). Thirst-associated preoptic neurons encode an aversive motivational drive. *Science*, *357*(6356), 1149–1155. https://doi.org/10.1126/science.aan6747.

Ammon, S., Mayer, P., Riechert, U., Tischmeyer, H., & Höllt, V. (2003). Microarray analysis of genes expressed in the frontal cortex of rats chronically treated with morphine and after naloxone precipitated withdrawal. *Brain Research. Molecular Brain Research*, *112*(1–2), 113–125. https://doi.org/10.1016/s0169-328x(03)00057-3.

Badiani, A., Oates, M. M., Day, H. E. W., Watson, S. J., Akil, H., & Robinson, T. E. (1999). Environmental modulation of amphetamine-induced c-fos expression in D1 versus D2 striatal neurons. *Behavioural Brain Research*, *103*(2), 203–209. https://doi.org/10.1016/S0166-4328(99)00041-8.

Barbosa, F. F., Santos, J. R., Meurer, Y. S. R., Macêdo, P. T., Ferreira, L. M. S., Pontes, I. M. O., et al. (2013). Differential cortical c-Fos and Zif-268 expression after object and spatial memory processing in a standard or episodic-like object recognition task. *Frontiers in Behavioral Neuroscience*, 7, 112. https://doi.org/10.3389/fnbeh.2013.00112.

Bastle, R. M., Kufahl, P. R., Turk, M. N., Weber, S. M., Pentkowski, N. S., Thiel, K. J., et al. (2012). Novel cues reinstate cocaine-seeking behavior and induce fos protein expression as effectively as conditioned cues. *Neuropsychopharmacology*, *37*(9), 2109–2120. https://doi.org/10.1038/npp.2012.60.

Bertran-Gonzalez, J., Bosch, C., Maroteaux, M., Matamales, M., Hervé, D., Valjent, E., et al. (2008). Opposing patterns of signaling activation in dopamine D1 and D2 receptor-expressing striatal neurons in response to cocaine and haloperidol. *Journal of Neuroscience*, *28*(22), 5671–5685. https://doi.org/10.1523/JNEUROSCI.1039-08.2008.

Bhat, R. V., Cole, A. J., & Baraban, J. M. (1992a). Chronic cocaine treatment suppresses basal expression of zif268 in rat forebrain: In situ hybridization studies. *Journal of Pharmacology and Experimental Therapeutics*, *263*(1), 343–349.

Bhat, R. V., Cole, A. J., & Baraban, J. M. (1992b). Role of monoamine systems in activation of zif268 by cocaine. *Journal of Psychiatry and Neuroscience*, *17*(3), 94–102.

Bisagno, V., & Cadet, J. L. (2019). Expression of immediate early genes in brain reward circuitries: Differential regulation by psychostimulant and opioid drugs. *Neurochemistry International*, *124*, 10–18. https://doi.org/10.1016/j.neuint.2018.12.004.

Bloomer, W. A. C., VanDongen, H. M. A., & VanDongen, A. M. J. (2007). Activity-regulated cytoskeleton-associated protein Arc/Arg3.1 binds to spectrin and associates with nuclear promyelocytic leukemia (PML) bodies. *Brain Research*, *1153*, 20–33. https://doi.org/10.1016/j.brainres.2007.03.079.

Bobadilla, A.-C., Heinsbroek, J. A., Gipson, C. D., Griffin, W. C., Fowler, C. D., Kenny, P. J., et al. (2017). Chapter 4—Corticostriatal plasticity, neuronal ensembles, and regulation of drug-seeking behavior. In T. Calvey, & W. M. U. Daniels (Eds.), *Progress in brain research* (pp. 93–112). https://doi.org/10.1016/bs.pbr.2017.07.013.

Bossert, J. M., Stern, A. L., Theberge, F. R. M., Cifani, C., Koya, E., Hope, B. T., et al. (2011). Ventral medial prefrontal cortex neuronal ensembles mediate context-induced relapse to heroin. *Nature Neuroscience*, *14*(4), 420–422. https://doi.org/10.1038/nn.2758.

Brenhouse, H. C., & Stellar, J. R. (2006). C-Fos and deltaFosB expression are differentially altered in distinct subregions of the nucleus accumbens shell in cocaine-sensitized rats. *Neuroscience*, *137*(3), 773–780. https://doi.org/10.1016/j.neuroscience.2005.09.039.

Browne, C. J., Godino, A., Salery, M., & Nestler, E. J. (2020). Epigenetic mechanisms of opioid addiction. *Biological Psychiatry*, *87*(1), 22–33. https://doi.org/10.1016/j.biopsych.2019.06.027.

Calipari, E. S., Bagot, R. C., Purushothaman, I., Davidson, T. J., Yorgason, J. T., Peña, C. J., et al. (2016). In vivo imaging identifies temporal signature of D1 and D2 medium spiny neurons in cocaine reward. *Proceedings of the National Academy of Sciences of the United States of America*, *113*(10), 2726–2731. https://doi.org/10.1073/pnas.1521238113.

Cao, V. Y., Ye, Y., Mastwal, S., Ren, M., Coon, M., Liu, Q., et al. (2015). Motor learning consolidates arc-expressing neuronal ensembles in secondary motor cortex. *Neuron*, *86*(6), 1385–1392. https://doi.org/10.1016/j.neuron.2015.05.022.

Caprioli, D., Venniro, M., Zhang, M., Bossert, J. M., Warren, B. L., Hope, B. T., et al. (2017). Role of dorsomedial striatum neuronal ensembles in incubation of methamphetamine craving after voluntary abstinence. *The Journal of Neuroscience*, *37*(4), 1014–1027. https://doi.org/10.1523/JNEUROSCI.3091-16.2016.

Carpenter, M. D., Hu, Q., Bond, A. M., Lombroso, S. I., Czarnecki, K. S., Lim, C. J., et al. (2020). Nr4a1 suppresses cocaine-induced behavior via epigenetic regulation of homeostatic target genes. *Nature Communications*, *11*(1), 504. https://doi.org/10.1038/s41467-020-14331-y.

Chandra, R., Francis, T. C., Konkalmatt, P., Amgalan, A., Gancarz, A. M., Dietz, D. M., et al. (2015). Opposing role for Egr3 in nucleus accumbens cell subtypes in cocaine action. *The Journal of Neuroscience*, *35*(20), 7927–7937. https://doi.org/10.1523/JNEUROSCI.0548-15.2015.

Chandra, R., & Lobo, M. K. (2017). Beyond neuronal activity markers: Select immediate early genes in striatal neuron subtypes functionally mediate psychostimulant addiction. *Frontiers in Behavioral Neuroscience*, *11*, 112. https://doi.org/10.3389/fnbeh.2017.00112.

Chen, J., Nye, H. E., Kelz, M. B., Hiroi, N., Nakabeppu, Y., Hope, B. T., et al. (1995). Regulation of delta FosB and FosB-like proteins by electroconvulsive seizure and cocaine treatments. *Molecular Pharmacology*, *48*(5), 880–889.

Chen, J., Kelz, M. B., Hope, B. T., Nakabeppu, Y., & Nestler, E. J. (1997). Chronic Fos-related antigens: Stable variants of ΔFosB induced in brain by chronic treatments. *Journal of Neuroscience*, *17*(13), 4933–4941. https://doi.org/10.1523/JNEUROSCI.17-13-04933.1997.

Chowdhury, S., Shepherd, J. D., Okuno, H., Lyford, G., Petralia, R. S., Plath, N., et al. (2006). Arc/Arg3.1 interacts with the endocytic machinery to regulate AMPA receptor trafficking. *Neuron*, *52*(3), 445–459. https://doi.org/10.1016/j.neuron.2006.08.033.

Colby, C. R., Whisler, K., Steffen, C., Nestler, E. J., & Self, D. W. (2003). Striatal cell type-specific overexpression of ΔFosB enhances incentive for cocaine. *Journal of Neuroscience*, *23*(6), 2488–2493. https://doi.org/10.1523/JNEUROSCI.23-06-02488.2003.

Cole, A. J., Saffen, D. W., Baraban, J. M., & Worley, P. F. (1989). Rapid increase of an immediate early gene messenger RNA in hippocampal neurons by synaptic NMDA receptor activation. *Nature*, *340*(6233), 474–476. https://doi.org/10.1038/340474a0.

Crombag, H. S., Jedynak, J. P., Redmond, K., Robinson, T. E., & Hope, B. T. (2002). Locomotor sensitization to cocaine is associated with increased Fos expression in the accumbens, but not in the caudate. *Behavioural Brain Research*, *136*(2), 455–462. https://doi.org/10.1016/S0166-4328(02)00196-1.

Cruz, F. C., Babin, K. R., Leao, R. M., Goldart, E. M., Bossert, J. M., Shaham, Y., et al. (2014). Role of nucleus accumbens shell neuronal ensembles in context-induced reinstatement of cocaine-seeking. *Journal of Neuroscience*, *34*(22), 7437–7446. https://doi.org/10.1523/JNEUROSCI.0238-14.2014.

Cruz, F. C., Rubio, F. J., & Hope, B. T. (2015). Using c-fos to study neuronal ensembles in corticostriatal circuitry of addiction. *Brain Research*, *1628*, 157–173. https://doi.org/10.1016/j.brainres.2014.11.005.

Daberkow, D. P., Riedy, M. D., Kesner, R. P., & Keefe, K. A. (2007). Arc mRNA induction in striatal efferent neurons associated with response learning. *European Journal of Neuroscience*, *26*(1), 228–241. https://doi.org/10.1111/j.1460-9568.2007.05630.x.

Daunais, J. B., & McGinty, J. F. (1995). Cocaine binges differentially alter striatal preprodynorphin and zif/268 mRNAs. *Molecular Brain Research*, *29*(2), 201–210. https://doi.org/10.1016/0169-328X(94)00246-B.

DeNardo, L., & Luo, L. (2017). Genetic strategies to access activated neurons. *Current Opinion in Neurobiology*, *45*, 121–129. https://doi.org/10.1016/j.conb.2017.05.014.

Denny, C. A., Kheirbek, M. A., Alba, E. L., Tanaka, K. F., Brachman, R. A., Laughman, K. B., et al. (2014). Hippocampal memory traces are differentially modulated by experience, time, and adult neurogenesis. *Neuron*, *83*(1), 189–201. https://doi.org/10.1016/j.neuron.2014.05.018.

Denny, C. A., Lebois, E., & Ramirez, S. (2017). From engrams to pathologies of the brain. *Frontiers in Neural Circuits*, *11*, 23. https://doi.org/10.3389/fncir.2017.00023.

Di Chiara, G., & Imperato, A. (1988). Drugs abused by humans preferentially increase synaptic dopamine concentrations in the mesolimbic system of freely moving rats. *Proceedings of the National Academy of Sciences*, *85*(14), 5274–5278. https://doi.org/10.1073/pnas.85.14.5274.

Dong, Y., & Nestler, E. J. (2014). The neural rejuvenation hypothesis of cocaine addiction. *Trends in Pharmacological Sciences*, *35*(8), 374–383. https://doi.org/10.1016/j.tips.2014.05.005.

Dong, Y., Taylor, J. R., Wolf, M. E., & Shaham, Y. (2017). Circuit and synaptic plasticity mechanisms of drug relapse. *Journal of Neuroscience*, *37*(45), 10867–10876. https://doi.org/10.1523/JNEUROSCI.1821-17.2017.

Duclot, F., & Kabbaj, M. (2017). The role of early growth response 1 (EGR1) in brain plasticity and neuropsychiatric disorders. *Frontiers in Behavioral Neuroscience*, *11*, 35. https://doi.org/10.3389/fnbeh.2017.00035.

Fanous, S., Goldart, E. M., Theberge, F. R. M., Bossert, J. M., Shaham, Y., & Hope, B. T. (2012). Role of orbitofrontal cortex neuronal ensembles in the expression of incubation of heroin craving. *Journal of Neuroscience*, *32*(34), 11600–11609. https://doi.org/10.1523/JNEUROSCI.1914-12.2012.

Fanous, S., Guez-Barber, D. H., Goldart, E. M., Schrama, R., Theberge, F. R. M., Shaham, Y., et al. (2013). Unique gene alterations are induced in FACS-purified Fos-positive neurons activated during cue-induced relapse to heroin seeking. *Journal of Neurochemistry*, *124*(1), 100–108. https://doi.org/10.1111/jnc.12074.

Flavell, S. W., & Greenberg, M. E. (2008). Signaling mechanisms linking neuronal activity to gene expression and plasticity of the nervous system. *Annual Review of Neuroscience*, *31*, 563–590. https://doi.org/10.1146/annurev.neuro.31.060407.125631.

Fosnaugh, J. S., Bhat, R. V., Yamagata, K., Worley, P. F., & Baraban, J. M. (1995). Activation of arc, a putative "effector" immediate early gene, by cocaine in rat brain. *Journal of Neurochemistry*, *64*(5), 2377–2380. https://doi.org/10.1046/j.1471-4159.1995.64052377.x.

Frankland, P. W., Josselyn, S. A., & Köhler, S. (2019). The neurobiological foundation of memory retrieval. *Nature Neuroscience*, *22*(10), 1576–1585. https://doi.org/10.1038/s41593-019-0493-1.

Freeman, W. M., Lull, M. E., Patel, K. M., Brucklacher, R. M., Morgan, D., Roberts, D. C., et al. (2010). Gene expression changes in the medial prefrontal cortex and nucleus accumbens following abstinence from cocaine self-administration. *BMC Neuroscience*, *11*(1), 29. https://doi.org/10.1186/1471-2202-11-29.

Freeman, W. M., Patel, K. M., Brucklacher, R. M., Lull, M. E., Erwin, M., Morgan, D., et al. (2008). Persistent alterations in mesolimbic gene expression with abstinence from cocaine self-administration. *Neuropsychopharmacology: Official Publication of the American College of Neuropsychopharmacology*, *33*(8), 1807–1817. https://doi.org/10.1038/sj.npp.1301577.

Fujiyama, K., Kajii, Y., Hiraoka, S., & Nishikawa, T. (2003). Differential regulation by stimulants of neocortical expression of mrt1, arc, and homer1a mRNA in the rats treated with repeated methamphetamine. *Synapse (New York, N.Y.)*, *49*(3), 143–149. https://doi.org/10.1002/syn.10220.

Fumagalli, F., Bedogni, F., Frasca, A., Pasquale, L. D., Racagni, G., & Riva, M. A. (2006). Corticostriatal up-regulation of activity-regulated cytoskeletal-associated protein expression after repeated exposure to cocaine. *Molecular Pharmacology*, *70*(5), 1726–1734. https://doi.org/10.1124/mol.106.026302.

Gallo, F. T., Katche, C., Morici, J. F., Medina, J. H., & Weisstaub, N. V. (2018). Immediate early genes, memory and psychiatric disorders: Focus on c-Fos, Egr1 and Arc. *Frontiers in Behavioral Neuroscience*, *12*. https://doi.org/10.3389/fnbeh.2018.00079.

Gao, M., Sossa, K., Song, L., Errington, L., Cummings, L., Hwang, H., et al. (2010). A specific requirement of Arc/Arg3.1 for visual experience-induced homeostatic synaptic plasticity in mouse primary visual cortex. *Journal of Neuroscience*, *30*(21), 7168–7178. https://doi.org/10.1523/JNEUROSCI.1067-10.2010.

Garner, A. R., & Mayford, M. (2012). New approaches to neural circuits in behavior. *Learning & Memory (Cold Spring Harbor, N.Y.)*, *19*(9), 385–390. https://doi.org/10.1101/lm.025049.111.

Garner, A. R., Rowland, D. C., Hwang, S. Y., Baumgaertel, K., Roth, B. L., Kentros, C., et al. (2012). Generation of a synthetic memory trace. *Science (New York, N.Y.)*, *335*(6075), 1513–1516. https://doi.org/10.1126/science.1214985.

Gonzales, B. J., Mukherjee, D., Ashwal-Fluss, R., Loewenstein, Y., & Citri, A. (2020). Subregion-specific rules govern the distribution of neuronal immediate-early gene induction. *Proceedings of the National Academy of Sciences*, *117*(38), 23304–23310. https://doi.org/10.1073/pnas.1913658116.

Graham, D. L., Edwards, S., Bachtell, R. K., DiLeone, R. J., Rios, M., & Self, D. W. (2007). Dynamic BDNF activity in nucleus accumbens with cocaine use increases self-administration and relapse. *Nature Neuroscience*, *10*(8), 1029–1037. https://doi.org/10.1038/nn1929.

Graybiel, A. M., Moratalla, R., & Robertson, H. A. (1990). Amphetamine and cocaine induce drug-specific activation of the c-fos gene in striosome-matrix compartments and limbic subdivisions of the striatum. *Proceedings of the National Academy of Sciences*, *87*(17), 6912–6916.

Greenberg, M., Ziff, E., & Greene, L. (1986). Stimulation of neuronal acetylcholine receptors induces rapid gene transcription. *Science*, *234*(4772), 80–83. https://doi.org/10.1126/science.3749894.

Grimm, J. W., Lu, L., Hayashi, T., Hope, B. T., Su, T.-P., & Shaham, Y. (2003). Time-dependent increases in brain-derived neurotrophic factor protein levels within the mesolimbic dopamine system after withdrawal from cocaine: Implications for incubation of cocaine craving. *The Journal of Neuroscience: The Official Journal of the Society for Neuroscience, 23*(3), 742–747.

Grueter, B. A., Robison, A. J., Neve, R. L., Nestler, E. J., & Malenka, R. C. (2013). ΔFosB differentially modulates nucleus accumbens direct and indirect pathway function. *Proceedings of the National Academy of Sciences of the United States of America, 110*(5), 1923–1928. https://doi.org/10.1073/pnas.1221742110.

Guenthner, C. J., Miyamichi, K., Yang, H. H., Heller, H. C., & Luo, L. (2013). Permanent genetic access to transiently active neurons via trap: targeted recombination in active populations. *Neuron, 78*(5), 773–784. https://doi.org/10.1016/j.neuron.2013.03.025.

Guez-Barber, D., Fanous, S., Golden, S. A., Schrama, R., Koya, E., Stern, A. L., et al. (2011). FACS identifies unique cocaine-induced gene regulation in selectively activated adult striatal neurons. *Journal of Neuroscience, 31*(11), 4251–4259. https://doi.org/10.1523/JNEUROSCI.6195-10.2011.

de Guglielmo, G., Crawford, E., Kim, S., Vendruscolo, L. F., Hope, B. T., Brennan, M., et al. (2016). Recruitment of a neuronal ensemble in the central nucleus of the amygdala is required for alcohol dependence. *Journal of Neuroscience, 36*(36), 9446–9453. https://doi.org/10.1523/JNEUROSCI.1395-16.2016.

Guzowski, J. F., Knierim, J. J., & Moser, E. I. (2004). Ensemble dynamics of hippocampal regions CA3 and CA1. *Neuron, 44*(4), 581–584. https://doi.org/10.1016/j.neuron.2004.11.003.

Guzowski, J. F., Lyford, G. L., Stevenson, G. D., Houston, F. P., McGaugh, J. L., Worley, P. F., et al. (2000). Inhibition of activity-dependent arc protein expression in the rat hippocampus impairs the maintenance of long-term potentiation and the consolidation of long-term memory. *Journal of Neuroscience, 20*(11), 3993–4001. https://doi.org/10.1523/JNEUROSCI.20-11-03993.2000.

Guzowski, J. F., McNaughton, B. L., Barnes, C. A., & Worley, P. F. (1999a). Environment-specific expression of the immediate-early gene Arc in hippocampal neuronal ensembles. *Nature Neuroscience, 2*(12), 1120–1124. https://doi.org/10.1038/16046.

Guzowski, J. F., McNaughton, B. L., Barnes, C. A., & Worley, P. F. (2001). Imaging neural activity with temporal and cellular resolution using FISH. *Current Opinion in Neurobiology, 11*(5), 579–584. https://doi.org/10.1016/S0959-4388(00)00252-X.

Guzowski, J. F., Setlow, B., Wagner, E. K., & McGaugh, J. L. (2001). Experience-dependent gene expression in the rat hippocampus after spatial learning: A comparison of the immediate-early genes Arc, c-fos, and zif268. *Journal of Neuroscience, 21*(14), 5089–5098. https://doi.org/10.1523/JNEUROSCI.21-14-05089.2001.

Guzowski, J. F., Timlin, J. A., Roysam, B., McNaughton, B. L., Worley, P. F., & Barnes, C. A. (2005). Mapping behaviorally relevant neural circuits with immediate-early gene expression. *Current Opinion in Neurobiology, 15*(5), 599–606. https://doi.org/10.1016/j.conb.2005.08.018.

Hall, J., Thomas, K. L., & Everitt, B. J. (2001). Cellular imaging of zif268 expression in the hippocampus and amygdala during contextual and cued fear memory retrieval: Selective activation of hippocampal CA1 neurons during the recall of contextual memories. *Journal of Neuroscience, 21*(6), 2186–2193. https://doi.org/10.1523/JNEUROSCI.21-06-02186.2001.

Hamlin, A. S., Clemens, K. J., & McNally, G. P. (2008). Renewal of extinguished cocaine-seeking. *Neuroscience, 151*(3), 659–670. https://doi.org/10.1016/j.neuroscience.2007.11.018.

Han, J.-H., Kushner, S. A., Yiu, A. P., Cole, C. J., Matynia, A., Brown, R. A., et al. (2007). Neuronal competition and selection during memory formation. *Science (New York, N.Y.), 316*(5823), 457–460. https://doi.org/10.1126/science.1139438.

Han, J.-H., Kushner, S. A., Yiu, A. P., Hsiang, H.-L.(. L.)., Buch, T., Waisman, A., et al. (2009). Selective erasure of a fear memory. *Science, 323*(5920), 1492–1496. https://doi.org/10.1126/science.1164139.

Hayward, M. D., Duman, R. S., & Nestler, E. J. (1990). Induction of the c-fos proto-oncogene during opiate withdrawal in the locus coeruleus and other regions of rat brain. *Brain Research, 525*(2), 256–266. https://doi.org/10.1016/0006-8993(90)90872-9.

Hearing, M. C., Schwendt, M., & McGinty, J. F. (2011). Suppression of activity-regulated cytoskeleton-associated gene expression in the dorsal striatum attenuates extinction of cocaine-seeking. *The International Journal of Neuropsychopharmacology/Official Scientific Journal of the Collegium Internationale Neuropsychopharmacologicum (CINP), 14*(6), 784–795. https://doi.org/10.1017/S1461145710001173.

Heiman, M., Schaefer, A., Gong, S., Peterson, J. D., Day, M., Ramsey, K. E., et al. (2008). A translational profiling approach for the molecular characterization of CNS cell types. *Cell, 135*(4), 738–748. https://doi.org/10.1016/j.cell.2008.10.028.

Hope, B. T., Kosofsky, B., Hyman, S. E., & Nestler, E. J. (1992). Regulation of immediate early gene expression and AP-1 binding in the rat nucleus accumbens by chronic cocaine. *Proceedings of the National Academy of Sciences, 89*(13), 5764–5768. https://doi.org/10.1073/pnas.89.13.5764.

Hope, B. T., Nye, H. E., Kelz, M. B., Self, D. W., Iadarola, M. J., Nakabeppu, Y., et al. (1994). Induction of a long-lasting AP-1 complex composed of altered Fos-like proteins in brain by chronic cocaine and other chronic treatments. *Neuron, 13*(5), 1235–1244. https://doi.org/10.1016/0896-6273(94)90061-2.

Hope, B. T., Simmons, D. E., Mitchell, T. B., Kreuter, J. D., & Mattson, B. J. (2006). Cocaine-induced locomotor activity and Fos expression in nucleus accumbens are sensitized for 6 months after repeated cocaine administration outside the home cage. *European Journal of Neuroscience, 24*(3), 867–875. https://doi.org/10.1111/j.1460-9568.2006.04969.x.

Hsiang, H.-L.(. L.)., Epp, J. R., van den Oever, M. C., Yan, C., Rashid, A. J., Insel, N., et al. (2014). Manipulating a "cocaine engram" in mice. *The Journal of Neuroscience, 34*(42), 14115–14127. https://doi.org/10.1523/JNEUROSCI.3327-14.2014.

Hyman, S. E., Malenka, R. C., & Nestler, E. J. (2006). Neural mechanisms of addiction: The role of reward-related learning and memory. *Annual Review of Neuroscience, 29*, 565–598. https://doi.org/10.1146/annurev.neuro.29.051605.113009.

Josselyn, S. A., & Tonegawa, S. (2020). Memory engrams: Recalling the past and imagining the future. *Science, 367*(6473), eaaw4325. https://doi.org/10.1126/science.aaw4325.

Kandel, E. R. (2001). The molecular biology of memory storage: A dialogue between genes and synapses. *Science, 294*(5544), 1030–1038. https://doi.org/10.1126/science.1067020.

Kandel, E. R., Dudai, Y., & Mayford, M. R. (2014). The molecular and systems biology of memory. *Cell, 157*(1), 163–186. https://doi.org/10.1016/j.cell.2014.03.001.

Kelley, A. E. (2004). Memory and addiction: Shared neural circuitry and molecular mechanisms. *Neuron, 44*(1), 161–179. https://doi.org/10.1016/j.neuron.2004.09.016.

Kelly, M. P., & Deadwyler, S. A. (2002). Acquisition of a novel behavior induces higher levels of Arc mRNA than does overtrained performance. *Neuroscience, 110*(4), 617–626. https://doi.org/10.1016/S0306-4522(01)00605-4.

Kelly, M. P., & Deadwyler, S. A. (2003). Experience-dependent regulation of the immediate-early gene arc differs across brain regions. *The Journal of Neuroscience: The Official Journal of the Society for Neuroscience, 23*(16), 6443–6451.

Kelz, M. B., Chen, J., Carlezon, W. A., Whisler, K., Gilden, L., Beckmann, A. M., et al. (1999). Expression of the transcription factor ΔFosB in the brain controls sensitivity to cocaine. *Nature*, *401*(6750), 272–276. https://doi.org/10.1038/45790.

Kodama, M., Akiyama, K., Ujike, H., Shimizu, Y., Tanaka, Y., & Kuroda, S. (1998). A robust increase in expression of arc gene, an effector immediate early gene, in the rat brain after acute and chronic methamphetamine administration. *Brain Research*, *796*(1), 273–283. https://doi.org/10.1016/S0006-8993(98)00349-7.

Korb, E., & Finkbeiner, S. (2011). Arc in synaptic plasticity: From gene to behavior. *Trends in Neurosciences*, *34*(11), 591–598. https://doi.org/10.1016/j.tins.2011.08.007.

Korb, E., Wilkinson, C. L., Delgado, R. N., Lovero, K. L., & Finkbeiner, S. (2013). Arc in the nucleus regulates PML-dependent GluA1 transcription and homeostatic plasticity. *Nature Neuroscience*, *16*(7), 874–883. https://doi.org/10.1038/nn.3429.

Koya, E., Cruz, F. C., Ator, R., Golden, S. A., Hoffman, A. F., Lupica, C. R., et al. (2012). Silent synapses in selectively activated nucleus accumbens neurons following cocaine sensitization. *Nature Neuroscience*, *15*(11), 1556–1562. https://doi.org/10.1038/nn.3232.

Koya, E., Golden, S. A., Harvey, B. K., Guez, D. H., Berkow, A., Simmons, D. E., et al. (2009). Targeted disruption of cocaine-activated accumbens neurons prevents context-specific sensitization. *Nature Neuroscience*, *12*(8), 1069–1073. https://doi.org/10.1038/nn.2364.

Koya, E., Margetts-Smith, G., & Hope, B. T. (2016). Daun02 inactivation of behaviorally activated Fos-expressing neuronal ensembles. *Current Protocols in Neuroscience*, *76*, 8.36.1–8.36.17. https://doi.org/10.1002/cpns.2.

Koya, E., Spijker, S., Voorn, P., Binnekade, R., Schmidt, E. D., Schoffelmeer, A. N. M., et al. (2006). Enhanced cortical and accumbal molecular reactivity associated with conditioned heroin, but not sucrose-seeking behaviour. *Journal of Neurochemistry*, *98*(3), 905–915. https://doi.org/10.1111/j.1471-4159.2006.03917.x.

Kubik, S., Miyashita, T., & Guzowski, J. F. (2007). Using immediate-early genes to map hippocampal subregional functions. *Learning & Memory*, *14*(11), 758–770. https://doi.org/10.1101/lm.698107.

Kufahl, P. R., Zavala, A. R., Singh, A., Thiel, K. J., Dickey, E. D., Joyce, J. N., et al. (2009). C-Fos expression associated with reinstatement of cocaine-seeking behavior by response-contingent conditioned cues. *Synapse (New York, N.Y.)*, *63*(10), 823–835. https://doi.org/10.1002/syn.20666.

Kuntz, K. L., Patel, K. M., Grigson, P. S., Freeman, W. M., & Vrana, K. E. (2008). Heroin self-administration: II. CNS gene expression following withdrawal and cue-induced drug-seeking behavior. *Pharmacology Biochemistry and Behavior*, *90*(3), 349–356. https://doi.org/10.1016/j.pbb.2008.03.019.

Lanahan, A., & Worley, P. (1998). Immediate-early genes and synaptic function. *Neurobiology of Learning and Memory*, *70*(1–2), 37–43. https://doi.org/10.1006/nlme.1998.3836.

LaPlant, Q., Vialou, V., Covington, H. E., Dumitriu, D., Feng, J., Warren, B. L., et al. (2010). Dnmt3a regulates emotional behavior and spine plasticity in the nucleus accumbens. *Nature Neuroscience*, *13*(9), 1137–1143. https://doi.org/10.1038/nn.2619.

Lee, K.-W., Kim, Y., Kim, A. M., Helmin, K., Nairn, A. C., & Greengard, P. (2006). Cocaine-induced dendritic spine formation in D1 and D2 dopamine receptor-containing medium spiny neurons in nucleus accumbens. *Proceedings of the National Academy of Sciences*, *103*(9), 3399–3404. https://doi.org/10.1073/pnas.0511244103.

Li, X., Rubio, F. J., Zeric, T., Bossert, J. M., Kambhampati, S., Cates, H. M., et al. (2015). Incubation of methamphetamine craving is associated with selective increases in expression of Bdnf and Trkb, glutamate receptors, and epigenetic enzymes in Cue-activated Fos-expressing dorsal striatal neurons. *Journal of Neuroscience*, *35*(21), 8232–8244. https://doi.org/10.1523/JNEUROSCI.1022-15.2015.

Link, W., Konietzko, U., Kauselmann, G., Krug, M., Schwanke, B., Frey, U., et al. (1995). Somatodendritic expression of an immediate early gene is regulated by synaptic activity. *Proceedings of the National Academy of Sciences*, *92*(12), 5734–5738. https://doi.org/10.1073/pnas.92.12.5734.

Liu, Q.-R., Rubio, F. J., Bossert, J. M., Marchant, N. J., Fanous, S., Hou, X., et al. (2014). Detection of molecular alterations in methamphetamine-activated Fos-expressing neurons from a single rat dorsal striatum using fluorescence-activated cell sorting (FACS). *Journal of Neurochemistry*, *128*(1), 173–185. https://doi.org/10.1111/jnc.12381.

Liu, X., Ramirez, S., Pang, P. T., Puryear, C. B., Govindarajan, A., Deisseroth, K., et al. (2012). Optogenetic stimulation of a hippocampal engram activates fear memory recall. *Nature*, *484*(7394), 381–385. https://doi.org/10.1038/nature11028.

Liu, X., Ramirez, S., Redondo, R. L., & Tonegawa, S. (2014). Identification and Manipulation of Memory Engram Cells. *Cold Spring Harbor Symposia on Quantitative Biology*, *79*, 59–65. https://doi.org/10.1101/sqb.2014.79.024901.

Lobo, M. K., Covington, H. E., Chaudhury, D., Friedman, A. K., Sun, H., Damez-Werno, D., et al. (2010). Cell type–specific loss of BDNF signaling mimics optogenetic control of cocaine reward. *Science*, *330*(6002), 385–390. https://doi.org/10.1126/science.1188472.

Lobo, M. K., Karsten, S. L., Gray, M., Geschwind, D. H., & Yang, X. W. (2006). FACS-array profiling of striatal projection neuron subtypes in juvenile and adult mouse brains. *Nature Neuroscience*, *9*(3), 443–452. https://doi.org/10.1038/nn1654.

Lobo, M. K., Zaman, S., Damez-Werno, D. M., Koo, J. W., Bagot, R. C., DiNieri, J. A., et al. (2013). ΔFosB induction in striatal medium spiny neuron subtypes in response to chronic pharmacological, emotional, and optogenetic stimuli. *The Journal of Neuroscience: The Official Journal of the Society for Neuroscience*, *33*(47), 18381–18395. https://doi.org/10.1523/JNEUROSCI.1875-13.2013.

Lüscher, C., & Malenka, R. C. (2011). Drug-evoked synaptic plasticity in addiction: From molecular changes to circuit remodeling. *Neuron*, *69*(4), 650–663. https://doi.org/10.1016/j.neuron.2011.01.017.

Lv, X.-F., Xu, Y., Han, J.-S., & Cui, C.-L. (2011). Expression of activity-regulated cytoskeleton-associated protein (Arc/Arg3.1) in the nucleus accumbens is critical for the acquisition, expression and reinstatement of morphine-induced conditioned place preference. *Behavioural Brain Research*, *223*(1), 182–191. https://doi.org/10.1016/j.bbr.2011.04.029.

Lyford, G. L., Yamagata, K., Kaufmann, W. E., Barnes, C. A., Sanders, L. K., Copeland, N. G., et al. (1995). Arc, a growth factor and activity-regulated gene, encodes a novel cytoskeleton-associated protein that is enriched in neuronal dendrites. *Neuron*, *14*(2), 433–445. https://doi.org/10.1016/0896-6273(95)90299-6.

Manning, C. E., Williams, E. S., & Robison, A. J. (2017). Reward network immediate early gene expression in mood disorders. *Frontiers in Behavioral Neuroscience*, *11*, 77. https://doi.org/10.3389/fnbeh.2017.00077.

Marie-Claire, C., Courtin, C., Roques, B. P., & Noble, F. (2004). Cytoskeletal genes regulation by chronic morphine treatment in rat striatum. *Neuropsychopharmacology*, *29*(12), 2208–2215. https://doi.org/10.1038/sj.npp.1300513.

Mattson, B. J., Koya, E., Simmons, D. E., Mitchell, T. B., Berkow, A., Crombag, H. S., et al. (2008). Context-specific sensitization of cocaine-induced locomotor activity and associated neuronal ensembles in rat nucleus accumbens. *European Journal of Neuroscience*, *27*(1), 202–212. https://doi.org/10.1111/j.1460-9568.2007.05984.x.

Maze, I., & Nestler, E. J. (2011). The epigenetic landscape of addiction. *Annals of the New York Academy of Sciences*, *1216*, 99–113. https://doi.org/10.1111/j.1749-6632.2010.05893.x.

McClung, C. A., & Nestler, E. J. (2003). Regulation of gene expression and cocaine reward by CREB and ΔFosB. *Nature Neuroscience, 6*(11), 1208–1215. https://doi.org/10.1038/nn1143.

Minatohara, K., Akiyoshi, M., & Okuno, H. (2016). Role of immediate-early genes in synaptic plasticity and neuronal ensembles underlying the memory trace. *Frontiers in Molecular Neuroscience, 8*, 78. https://doi.org/10.3389/fnmol.2015.00078.

Miyashita, T., Kubik, S., Lewandowski, G., & Guzowski, J. F. (2008). Networks of neurons, networks of genes: An integrated view of memory consolidation. *Neurobiology of Learning and Memory, 89*(3), 269–284. https://doi.org/10.1016/j.nlm.2007.08.012.

Moga, D. E., Calhoun, M. E., Chowdhury, A., Worley, P., Morrison, J. H., & Shapiro, M. L. (2004). Activity-regulated cytoskeletal-associated protein is localized to recently activated excitatory synapses. *Neuroscience, 125*(1), 7–11. https://doi.org/10.1016/j.neuroscience.2004.02.004.

Montag-Sallaz, M., Welzl, H., Kuhl, D., Montag, D., & Schachner, M. (1999). Novelty-induced increased expression of immediate-early genes c-fos and arg 3.1 in the mouse brain. *Journal of Neurobiology, 38*(2), 234–246.

Moratalla, R., Robertson, H. A., & Graybiel, A. M. (1992). Dynamic regulation of NGFI-A (zif268, egr1) gene expression in the striatum. *The Journal of Neuroscience: The Official Journal of the Society for Neuroscience, 12*(7), 2609–2622.

Moratalla, R., Vickers, E. A., Robertson, H. A., Cochran, B. H., & Graybiel, A. M. (1993). Coordinate expression of c-fos and jun B is induced in the rat striatum by cocaine. *The Journal of Neuroscience: The Official Journal of the Society for Neuroscience, 13*(2), 423–433.

Morgan, J. I., Cohen, D. R., Hempstead, J. L., & Curran, T. (1987). Mapping patterns of c-fos expression in the central nervous system after seizure. *Science, 237*(4811), 192–197. https://doi.org/10.1126/science.3037702.

Morgan, J. I., & Curran, T. (1989). Stimulus-transcription coupling in neurons: Role of cellular immediate-early genes. *Trends in Neurosciences, 12*(11), 459–462. https://doi.org/10.1016/0166-2236(89)90096-9.

Neisewander, J. L., Baker, D. A., Fuchs, R. A., Tran-Nguyen, L. T. L., Palmer, A., & Marshall, J. F. (2000). Fos protein expression and cocaine-seeking behavior in rats after exposure to a cocaine self-administration environment. *Journal of Neuroscience, 20*(2), 798–805. https://doi.org/10.1523/JNEUROSCI.20-02-00798.2000.

Nestler, E. J. (2001). Molecular basis of long-term plasticity underlying addiction. *Nature Reviews Neuroscience, 2*(2), 119–128. https://doi.org/10.1038/35053570.

Nestler, E. J. (2013). Cellular basis of memory for addiction. *Dialogues in Clinical Neuroscience, 15*(4), 431–443.

Nestler, E. J., & Huganir, R. L. (2019). Paul Greengard (1925–2019). *Cell, 177*(6), 1365–1366. https://doi.org/10.1016/j.cell.2019.05.020.

Nestler, E. J., Kelz, M. B., & Chen, J. (1999). ΔFosB: A molecular mediator of long-term neural and behavioral plasticity1Published on the World Wide Web on 27 November 1998.1. *Brain Research, 835*(1), 10–17. https://doi.org/10.1016/S0006-8993(98)01191-3.

Nestler, E. J., & Lüscher, C. (2019). The molecular basis of drug addiction: Linking epigenetic to synaptic and circuit mechanisms. *Neuron, 102*(1), 48–59. https://doi.org/10.1016/j.neuron.2019.01.016.

Nordquist, R. E., Vanderschuren, L. J. M. J., Jonker, A. J., Bergsma, M., de Vries, T. J., Pennartz, C. M. A., et al. (2008). Expression of amphetamine sensitization is associated with recruitment of a reactive neuronal population in the nucleus accumbens core. *Psychopharmacology, 198*(1), 113–126. https://doi.org/10.1007/s00213-008-1100-4.

Norman, A. B., Lu, S. Y., Klug, J. M., & Norgren, R. B. (1993). Sensitization of c-fos expression in rat striatum following multiple challenges with D-amphetamine. *Brain Research*, *603*(1), 125–128. https://doi.org/10.1016/0006-8993(93)91308-f.

Perrotti, L. I., Weaver, R. R., Robison, B., Renthal, W., Maze, I., Yazdani, S., et al. (2008). Distinct patterns of ΔFosB induction in brain by drugs of abuse. *Synapse (New York, N.Y.)*, *62*(5), 358–369. https://doi.org/10.1002/syn.20500.

Pfarr, S., Meinhardt, M. W., Klee, M. L., Hansson, A. C., Vengeliene, V., Schönig, K., et al. (2015). Losing control: Excessive alcohol seeking after selective inactivation of cue-responsive neurons in the infralimbic cortex. *Journal of Neuroscience*, *35*(30), 10750–10761. https://doi.org/10.1523/JNEUROSCI.0684-15.2015.

Ramirez, S., Liu, X., Lin, P.-A., Suh, J., Pignatelli, M., Redondo, R. L., et al. (2013). Creating a false memory in the hippocampus. *Science*, *341*(6144), 387–391. https://doi.org/10.1126/science.1239073.

Ramirez, S., Liu, X., MacDonald, C. J., Moffa, A., Zhou, J., Redondo, R. L., et al. (2015). Activating positive memory engrams suppresses depression-like behaviour. *Nature*, *522*(7556), 335–339. https://doi.org/10.1038/nature14514.

Ramirez, S., Tonegawa, S., & Liu, X. (2014). Identification and optogenetic manipulation of memory engrams in the hippocampus. *Frontiers in Behavioral Neuroscience*, 7, 226. https://doi.org/10.3389/fnbeh.2013.00226.

Ramírez-Amaya, V., Vazdarjanova, A., Mikhael, D., Rosi, S., Worley, P. F., & Barnes, C. A. (2005). Spatial exploration-induced arc mRNA and protein expression: evidence for selective, network-specific reactivation. *Journal of Neuroscience*, *25*(7), 1761–1768. https://doi.org/10.1523/JNEUROSCI.4342-04.2005.

Reijmers, L. G., & Mayford, M. (2009). Genetic control of active neural circuits. *Frontiers in Molecular Neuroscience*, *2*, 27. https://doi.org/10.3389/neuro.02.027.2009.

Reijmers, L. G., Perkins, B. L., Matsuo, N., & Mayford, M. (2007). Localization of a stable neural correlate of associative memory. *Science (New York, N.Y.)*, *317*(5842), 1230–1233. https://doi.org/10.1126/science.1143839.

Renthal, W., Carle, T. L., Maze, I., Covington, H. E., Truong, H.-T., Alibhai, I., et al. (2008). Delta FosB mediates epigenetic desensitization of the c-fos gene after chronic amphetamine exposure. *The Journal of Neuroscience: The Official Journal of the Society for Neuroscience*, *28*(29), 7344–7349. https://doi.org/10.1523/JNEUROSCI.1043-08.2008.

Robbins, T. W., Ersche, K. D., & Everitt, B. J. (2008). Drug addiction and the memory systems of the brain. *Annals of the New York Academy of Sciences*, *1141*(1), 1–21. https://doi.org/10.1196/annals.1441.020.

Robertson, H. A., Paul, M. L., Moratalla, R., & Graybiel, A. M. (1991). Expression of the immediate early gene c-fos in basal ganglia: Induction by dopaminergic drugs. *The Canadian Journal of Neurological Sciences. Le Journal Canadien Des Sciences Neurologiques*, *18*(3 Suppl), 380–383. https://doi.org/10.1017/s0317167100032480.

Robison, A. J., & Nestler, E. J. (2011). Transcriptional and epigenetic mechanisms of addiction. *Nature Reviews Neuroscience*, *12*(11), 623–637. https://doi.org/10.1038/nrn3111.

Robison, A. J., Vialou, V., Mazei-Robison, M., Feng, J., Kourrich, S., Collins, M., et al. (2013). Behavioral and structural responses to chronic cocaine require a feedforward loop involving ΔFosB and calcium/calmodulin-dependent protein kinase II in the nucleus accumbens shell. *The Journal of Neuroscience*, *33*(10), 4295–4307. https://doi.org/10.1523/JNEUROSCI.5192-12.2013.

Rosen, J. B., Chuang, E., & Iadarola, M. J. (1994). Differential induction of Fos protein and a Fos-related antigen following acute and repeated cocaine administration. *Molecular Brain Research*, *25*(1), 168–172. https://doi.org/10.1016/0169-328X(94)90295-X.

Rosen, J. B., Fanselow, M. S., Young, S. L., Sitcoske, M., & Maren, S. (1998). Immediate-early gene expression in the amygdala following footshock stress and contextual fear conditioning. *Brain Research, 796*(1–2), 132–142. https://doi.org/10.1016/S0006-8993(98)00294-7.

Rubio, F. J., Liu, Q.-R., Li, X., Cruz, F. C., Leão, R. M., Warren, B. L., et al. (2015). Context-induced reinstatement of methamphetamine seeking is associated with unique molecular alterations in fos-expressing dorsolateral striatum neurons. *Journal of Neuroscience, 35*(14), 5625–5639. https://doi.org/10.1523/JNEUROSCI.4997-14.2015.

Rubio, F. J., Quintana-Feliciano, R., Warren, B. L., Li, X., Witonsky, K. F. R., del Valle, F. S., et al. (2019). Prelimbic cortex is a common brain area activated during cue-induced reinstatement of cocaine and heroin seeking in a polydrug self-administration rat model. *European Journal of Neuroscience, 49*(2), 165–178. https://doi.org/10.1111/ejn.14203.

Salery, M., Dos Santos, M., Saint-Jour, E., Moumné, L., Pagès, C., Kappès, V., et al. (2017). Activity-regulated cytoskeleton-associated protein accumulates in the nucleus in response to cocaine and acts as a brake on chromatin remodeling and long-term behavioral alterations. *Biological Psychiatry, 81*(7), 573–584. https://doi.org/10.1016/j.biopsych.2016.05.025.

Salery, M., Trifilieff, P., Caboche, J., & Vanhoutte, P. (2020). From signaling molecules to circuits and behaviors: Cell-type–specific adaptations to psychostimulant exposure in the striatum. *Biological Psychiatry, 87*(11), 944–953. https://doi.org/10.1016/j.biopsych.2019.11.001.

Samaha, A.-N., Mallet, N., Ferguson, S. M., Gonon, F., & Robinson, T. E. (2004). The rate of cocaine administration alters gene regulation and behavioral plasticity: Implications for addiction. *Journal of Neuroscience, 24*(28), 6362–6370. https://doi.org/10.1523/JNEUROSCI.1205-04.2004.

Savell, K. E., Tuscher, J. J., Zipperly, M. E., Duke, C. G., Phillips, R. A., Bauman, A. J., et al. (2020). A dopamine-induced gene expression signature regulates neuronal function and cocaine response. *Science Advances, 6*(26), eaba4221. https://doi.org/10.1126/sciadv.aba4221.

Sheng, M., & Greenberg, M. E. (1990). The regulation and function of c-fos and other immediate early genes in the nervous system. *Neuron, 4*(4), 477–485. https://doi.org/10.1016/0896-6273(90)90106-P.

Shepherd, J. D., & Bear, M. F. (2011). New views of Arc, a master regulator of synaptic plasticity. *Nature Neuroscience, 14*(3), 279–284. https://doi.org/10.1038/nn.2708.

Shepherd, J. D., Rumbaugh, G., Wu, J., Chowdhury, S., Plath, N., Kuhl, D., et al. (2006). Arc/Arg3.1 mediates homeostatic synaptic scaling of AMPA receptors. *Neuron, 52*(3), 475–484. https://doi.org/10.1016/j.neuron.2006.08.034.

Steward, O., Wallace, C. S., Lyford, G. L., & Worley, P. F. (1998). Synaptic activation causes the mRNA for the IEG Arc to localize selectively near activated postsynaptic sites on dendrites. *Neuron, 21*(4), 741–751. https://doi.org/10.1016/S0896-6273(00)80591-7.

Tan, A., Moratalla, R., Lyford, G. L., Worley, P., & Graybiel, A. M. (2000). The activity-regulated cytoskeletal-associated protein arc is expressed in different striosome-matrix patterns following exposure to amphetamine and cocaine. *Journal of Neurochemistry, 74*(5), 2074–2078. https://doi.org/10.1046/j.1471-4159.2000.0742074.x.

Tanaka, K. Z., Pevzner, A., Hamidi, A. B., Nakazawa, Y., Graham, J., & Wiltgen, B. J. (2014). Cortical representations are reinstated by the hippocampus during memory retrieval. *Neuron, 84*(2), 347–354. https://doi.org/10.1016/j.neuron.2014.09.037.

Taniguchi, M., Carreira, M. B., Cooper, Y. A., Bobadilla, A.-C., Heinsbroek, J. A., Koike, N., et al. (2017). HDAC5 and its target gene, Npas4, function in the nucleus accumbens to regulate cocaine-conditioned behaviors. *Neuron*, *96*(1), 130–144.e6. https://doi.org/10.1016/j.neuron.2017.09.015.

Thomas, K. L., Arroyo, M., & Everitt, B. J. (2003). Induction of the learning and plasticity-associated gene Zif268 following exposure to a discrete cocaine-associated stimulus. *European Journal of Neuroscience*, *17*(9), 1964–1972. https://doi.org/10.1046/j.1460-9568.2003.02617.x.

Tischmeyer, W., & Grimm, R. (1999). Activation of immediate early genes and memory formation. *Cellular and Molecular Life Sciences: CMLS*, *55*(4), 564–574. https://doi.org/10.1007/s000180050315.

Tonegawa, S., Liu, X., Ramirez, S., & Redondo, R. (2015). Memory engram cells have come of age. *Neuron*, *87*(5), 918–931. https://doi.org/10.1016/j.neuron.2015.08.002.

Tonegawa, S., Morrissey, M. D., & Kitamura, T. (2018). The role of engram cells in the systems consolidation of memory. *Nature Reviews Neuroscience*, *19*(8), 485–498. https://doi.org/10.1038/s41583-018-0031-2.

Torres, O. V., McCoy, M. T., Ladenheim, B., Jayanthi, S., Brannock, C., Tulloch, I., et al. (2015). CAMKII-conditional deletion of histone deacetylase 2 potentiates acute methamphetamine-induced expression of immediate early genes in the mouse nucleus accumbens. *Scientific Reports*, *5*(1), 13396. https://doi.org/10.1038/srep13396.

Trouche, S., Perestenko, P. V., van de Ven, G. M., Bratley, C. T., McNamara, C. G., Campo-Urriza, N., et al. (2016). Recoding a cocaine-place memory engram to a neutral engram in the hippocampus. *Nature Neuroscience*, *19*(4), 564–567. https://doi.org/10.1038/nn.4250.

Unal, C. T., Beverley, J. A., Willuhn, I., & Steiner, H. (2009). Long-lasting dysregulation of gene expression in corticostriatal circuits after repeated cocaine treatment in adult rats: Effects on zif 268 and homer 1a. *The European Journal of Neuroscience*, *29*(8), 1615–1626. https://doi.org/10.1111/j.1460-9568.2009.06691.x.

Valjent, E., Aubier, B., Corbillé, A.-G., Brami-Cherrier, K., Caboche, J., Topilko, P., et al. (2006). Plasticity-associated gene Krox24/Zif268 is required for long-lasting behavioral effects of cocaine. *Journal of Neuroscience*, *26*(18), 4956–4960. https://doi.org/10.1523/JNEUROSCI.4601-05.2006.

Vann, S. D., Brown, M. W., Erichsen, J. T., & Aggleton, J. P. (2000). Fos imaging reveals differential patterns of hippocampal and parahippocampal subfield activation in rats in response to different spatial memory tests. *Journal of Neuroscience*, *20*(7), 2711–2718. https://doi.org/10.1523/JNEUROSCI.20-07-02711.2000.

Vazdarjanova, A., & Guzowski, J. F. (2004). Differences in hippocampal neuronal population responses to modifications of an environmental context: Evidence for distinct, yet complementary, functions of CA3 and CA1 ensembles. *Journal of Neuroscience*, *24*(29), 6489–6496. https://doi.org/10.1523/JNEUROSCI.0350-04.2004.

Vazdarjanova, A., McNaughton, B. L., Barnes, C. A., Worley, P. F., & Guzowski, J. F. (2002). Experience-dependent coincident expression of the effector immediate-early genes arc and Homer 1a in hippocampal and neocortical neuronal networks. *The Journal of Neuroscience: The Official Journal of the Society for Neuroscience*, *22*(23), 10067–10071.

Walker, D. M., Cates, H. M., Loh, Y.-H. E., Purushothaman, I., Ramakrishnan, A., Cahill, K. M., et al. (2018). Cocaine self-administration alters transcriptome-wide responses in the brain's reward circuitry. *Biological Psychiatry*, *84*(12), 867–880. https://doi.org/10.1016/j.biopsych.2018.04.009.

Walker, D. M., & Nestler, E. J. (2018). Neuroepigenetics and addiction. *Handbook of Clinical Neurology*, *148*, 747–765. https://doi.org/10.1016/B978-0-444-64076-5.00048-X.

Wall, N. R., Neumann, P. A., Beier, K. T., Mokhtari, A. K., Luo, L., & Malenka, R. C. (2019). Complementary genetic targeting and monosynaptic input mapping reveal recruitment and refinement of distributed corticostriatal ensembles by cocaine. *Neuron*, *104*(5), 916–930.e5. https://doi.org/10.1016/j.neuron.2019.10.032.

Wang, K. H., Majewska, A., Schummers, J., Farley, B., Hu, C., Sur, M., et al. (2006). In vivo two-photon imaging reveals a role of arc in enhancing orientation specificity in visual cortex. *Cell*, *126*(2), 389–402. https://doi.org/10.1016/j.cell.2006.06.038.

Warren, B. L., Kane, L., Venniro, M., Selvam, P., Quintana-Feliciano, R., Mendoza, M. P., et al. (2019). Separate vmPFC ensembles control cocaine self-administration versus extinction in rats. *Journal of Neuroscience*, *39*(37), 7394–7407. https://doi.org/10.1523/JNEUROSCI.0918-19.2019.

Warren, B. L., Mendoza, M. P., Cruz, F. C., Leao, R. M., Caprioli, D., Rubio, F. J., et al. (2016). Distinct Fos-expressing neuronal ensembles in the ventromedial prefrontal cortex mediate food reward and extinction memories. *Journal of Neuroscience*, *36*(25), 6691–6703. https://doi.org/10.1523/JNEUROSCI.0140-16.2016.

Waung, M. W., Pfeiffer, B. E., Nosyreva, E. D., Ronesi, J. A., & Huber, K. M. (2008). Rapid translation of Arc/Arg3.1 selectively mediates mGluR-dependent LTD through persistent increases in AMPAR endocytosis rate. *Neuron*, *59*(1), 84–97. https://doi.org/10.1016/j.neuron.2008.05.014.

West, A. E., & Greenberg, M. E. (2011). Neuronal activity–regulated gene transcription in synapse development and cognitive function. *Cold Spring Harbor Perspectives in Biology*, *3*(6), a005744. https://doi.org/10.1101/cshperspect.a005744.

Whitaker, L. R., Carneiro de Oliveira, P. E., McPherson, K. B., Fallon, R. V., Planeta, C. S., Bonci, A., et al. (2016). Associative learning drives the formation of silent synapses in neuronal ensembles of the nucleus accumbens. *Biological Psychiatry*, *80*(3), 246–256. https://doi.org/10.1016/j.biopsych.2015.08.006.

Whitaker, L. R., & Hope, B. T. (2018). Chasing the addicted engram: Identifying functional alterations in Fos-expressing neuronal ensembles that mediate drug-related learned behavior. *Learning & Memory*, *25*(9), 455–460. https://doi.org/10.1101/lm.046698.117.

Wolf, M. E. (2016). Synaptic mechanisms underlying persistent cocaine craving. *Nature Reviews. Neuroscience*, *17*(6), 351–365. https://doi.org/10.1038/nrn.2016.39.

Xu, M. (2008). C-Fos is an intracellular regulator of cocaine-induced long-term changes. *Annals of the New York Academy of Sciences*, *1139*, 1–9. https://doi.org/10.1196/annals.1432.049.

Yap, E.-L., & Greenberg, M. E. (2018). Activity-regulated transcription: bridging the gap between neural activity and behavior. *Neuron*, *100*(2), 330–348. https://doi.org/10.1016/j.neuron.2018.10.013.

Ye, L., Allen, W. E., Thompson, K. R., Tian, Q., Hsueh, B., Ramakrishnan, C., et al. (2016). Wiring and molecular features of prefrontal ensembles representing distinct experiences. *Cell*, *165*(7), 1776–1788. https://doi.org/10.1016/j.cell.2016.05.010.

Young, S. T., Porrino, L. J., & Iadarola, M. J. (1991). Cocaine induces striatal c-fos-immunoreactive proteins via dopaminergic D1 receptors. *Proceedings of the National Academy of Sciences of the United States of America*, *88*(4), 1291–1295. https://doi.org/10.1073/pnas.88.4.1291.

Yuferov, V., Kroslak, T., Laforge, K. S., Zhou, Y., Ho, A., & Kreek, M. J. (2003). Differential gene expression in the rat caudate putamen after "binge" cocaine administration: Advantage of triplicate microarray analysis. *Synapse (New York, N.Y.)*, *48*(4), 157–169. https://doi.org/10.1002/syn.10198.

Zachariou, V., Bolanos, C. A., Selley, D. E., Theobald, D., Cassidy, M. P., Kelz, M. B., et al. (2006). An essential role for ΔFosB in the nucleus accumbens in morphine action. *Nature Neuroscience*, *9*(2), 205–211. https://doi.org/10.1038/nn1636.

Zavala, A. R., Biswas, S., Harlan, R. E., & Neisewander, J. L. (2007). Fos and glutamate AMPA receptor subunit coexpression associated with cue-elicited cocaine-seeking behavior in abstinent rats. *Neuroscience*, *145*(2), 438–452. https://doi.org/10.1016/j.neuroscience.2006.12.038.

Zavala, A. R., Osredkar, T., Joyce, J. N., & Neisewander, J. L. (2008). Upregulation of Arc mRNA expression in the prefrontal cortex following cue-induced reinstatement of extinguished cocaine-seeking behavior. *Synapse (New York, N.Y.)*, *62*(6), 421–431. https://doi.org/10.1002/syn.20502.

Zhang, G.-C., Mao, L.-M., Liu, X.-Y., Parelkar, N. K., Arora, A., Yang, L., et al. (2007). In vivo regulation of homer1a expression in the striatum by cocaine. *Molecular Pharmacology*, *71*(4), 1148–1158. https://doi.org/10.1124/mol.106.028399.

Zhou, Y., Zhu, H., Liu, Z., Chen, X., Su, X., Ma, C., et al. (2019). A ventral CA1 to nucleus accumbens core engram circuit mediates conditioned place preference for cocaine. *Nature Neuroscience*, *22*(12), 1986–1999. https://doi.org/10.1038/s41593-019-0524-y.

Ziółkowska, B., Korostyński, M., Piechota, M., Kubik, J., & Przewłocki, R. (2012). Effects of morphine on immediate-early gene expression in the striatum of C57BL/6J and DBA/2J mice. *Pharmacological Reports: PR*, *64*(5), 1091–1104. https://doi.org/10.1016/s1734-1140(12)70906-4.

CHAPTER NINE

NAPE-specific phospholipase D regulates LRRK2 association with neuronal membranes

Francesca Palese[a,b], Silvia Pontis[a], Natalia Realini[a], and Daniele Piomelli[b,*]

[a]Department of Drug Discovery and Development, Istituto Italiano di Tecnologia, Genoa, Italy
[b]Departments of Anatomy and Neurobiology, Pharmacology and Biological Chemistry, University of California, Irvine, CA, United States
[*]Corresponding author: e-mail address: piomelli@uci.edu

Contents

Abstract

N-acylphosphatidylethanolamines (NAPEs) are glycerophospholipid precursors for bioactive lipid amides and potential regulators of membrane function. They are hydrolyzed by NAPE-specific phospholipase D (NAPE-PLD) and have been implicated in neurodegenerative disorders such as Parkinson's disease. Here, we used siRNA-mediated silencing of NAPE-PLD in human SH-SY5Y cells and NAPE-PLD$^{-/-}$ mice to determine whether NAPEs influence the membrane association of LRRK2, a multifunctional protein kinase that is frequently mutated in persons with sporadic Parkinson's disease. NAPE-PLD deletion caused a significant accumulation of non-metabolized NAPEs, which was accompanied by a shift of LRRK2 from membrane to cytosol and a reduction in total LRRK2

Advances in Pharmacology, Volume 90
ISSN 1054-3589
https://doi.org/10.1016/bs.apha.2020.09.003

content. Conversely, exposure of intact SH-SY5Y cells to bacterial PLD lowered NAPE levels and enhanced LRRK2 association with membranes. The results suggest that NAPE-PLD activity may contribute to the control of LRRK2 localization by regulating membrane NAPE levels.

Abbreviations

1,2-DAG	1,2-diacylglycerol
BCA	bicinchoninic acid
COR	C-terminal of Roc
DMEM	Dulbecco's Modified Eagle's Medium
ECL	electrochemical luminescence
FAE	fatty-acid ethanolamide
HPRT	hypoxanthine phosphoribosyltransferase 1
IHC	immunohistochemical
LC/MS	liquid chromatography/mass spectrometry
LRR	leucine-rich repeat region
LRRK2	leucine-rich repeat kinase
MRM	multiple reaction monitoring
NAPE	*N*-acylphosphatidylethanolamine
NAPE-PLD	NAPE-specific phospholipase D
NMDA	*N*-methyl-D-aspartate
OEA	oleoylethanolamide
PA	phosphatidic acid
PAF	paraformaldehyde
PBS	phosphate-buffered saline
PC	phosphatidylcholine
PD	Parkinson's disease
PE	phosphatidylethanolamine
PEA	palmitoylethanolamide
PLA2A4E	phospholipase A_2 ε isoform
PLD	phospholipase D
ROC	Ras of Complex
TBS	tris-buffered saline

1. Introduction

N-acylphosphatidylethanolamines (NAPEs) are a class of signaling glycerophospholipids that are normally present at relatively low concentrations in the membranes of neurons and other cells (Cadas, Di Tomaso, & Piomelli, 1997), but can be quickly generated in a stimulus-dependent manner via transfer of an acyl group from the *sn*-1 position of phosphatidylcholine (PC) to the free amino group of phosphatidylethanolamine (PE) (Natarajan, Reddy, Schmid, & Schmid, 1982). NAPE biosynthesis is catalyzed by a calcium-dependent *N*-acyltransferase activity (Cadas, Gaillet, Beltramo, Venance, & Piomelli, 1996; Cadas, Schinelli, & Piomelli, 1996; Cadas et al., 1997), which was identified as the ε isoform of cytosolic phospholipase A_2 (PLA2A4E) (Ogura, Parsons, Kamat, & Cravatt, 2016). As PLA2A4E activity is not selective with regard to the chain length or degree of unsaturation in the acyl chain transferred (Sugiura et al., 1996), the molecular composition of cellular NAPEs predominantly reflects the *sn*-1 substituent in donor PC. Thus, the N-acyl group is generally dominated by saturated or monounsaturated fatty acids [palmitic (16:0), stearic (18:0) or oleic (18:1)], but can also contain polyunsaturated fatty acids [such as arachidonic (20:4) and docosahexaenoic acid (22.6)], albeit in much lower amounts (Astarita & Piomelli, 2009; Jung et al., 2012). The NAPEs are substrates for multiple phospholipases, including a unique NAPE-specific phospholipase D (NAPE-PLD) (Magotti et al., 2015; Okamoto, Morishita, Tsuboi, Tonai, & Ueda, 2004), which cleaves the *N*-linked chain of NAPEs to release fatty-acid ethanolamides (FAEs) and phosphatidic acid. The FAEs are a class of lipid-derived mediators that includes endogenous agonists for cannabinoid receptors [e.g., arachidonoylethanolamide (anandamide)], nuclear peroxisome proliferator-activated receptor type-α [e.g., oleoylethanolamide (OEA) and palmitoylethanolamide (PEA)] and possibly ligand-activated ion channels (Hansen, Moesgaard, Petersen, & Hansen, 2002).

The biological functions served by the FAEs in the control of pain, inflammation and energy balance have been the object of intense investigation (DiPatrizio & Piomelli, 2015; Piomelli, 2013; Piomelli & Sasso, 2014; Skaper et al., 2015). Given the diverse and important roles played by these lipid mediators, research on NAPEs has been mostly focused on their role as FAE precursors. Nevertheless, there is evidence that NAPEs may also have effects that are independent of their ability to generate FAEs. For example, biophysical experiments suggest that NAPEs may contribute to cell-membrane dynamics, for example by stabilizing the lipid bilayer through their embedded *N*-acyl chains (Lafrance, Blochet, & Pezolet, 1997; Swamy, Tarafdar, & Kamlekar, 2010) or by supporting calcium-dependent membrane fusion (Shangguan, Pak, Ali, Janoff, & Meers, 1998). Moreover, similarly to phosphoinositides (Zoncu et al., 2007), NAPEs might regulate the association of intracellular proteins to the internal facet of the membrane bilayer (Mileykovskaya & Dowhan, 2005). Consistent with roles in cell function, the production of NAPEs is controlled by a variety of physiological (Cadas et al., 1997; Fu et al., 2007; Gillum et al., 2008) and pathological stimuli (Hansen, Ikonomidou, Bittigau, Hansen, & Hansen, 2001; Natarajan, Schmid, & Schmid, 1986), including activation of glutamate *N*-methyl-D-aspartate (NMDA) receptors (Hansen et al., 1997) and exposure to the dopaminergic neurotoxin 6-hydroxydopamine (Basit, Pontis, Piomelli, & Armirotti, 2016).

Leucine-rich repeat kinase (LRRK2) is a ubiquitous, multi-domain protein kinase that belongs to the ROCO family of proteins (Tsika & Moore, 2013). It contains two catalytic domains: a Ras of Complex (Roc) GTPase domain that is separated by a C-terminal of Roc (COR) domain (Cookson, 2010) from a serine/threonine-directed protein kinase domain. LRRK2 also features several protein-protein interaction regions flanking the Roc-COR-kinase catalytic core, such as an armadillo repeat region, ankyrin-like repeat region, a leucine-rich repeat region (LRR), and a WD40 domain (Cookson, 2010). This molecular architecture has led to suggest that LRRK2 may serve as a scaffold for the assembly of intracellular protein complexes (Cookson, 2010). LRRK2 predominantly exists as a homodimeric protein, whose two interacting units are linked through their Roc-COR tandem domains (Civiero et al., 2012; Greggio et al., 2008). Moreover, LRRK2 dimers are enriched in cell membranes and display higher levels of kinase activity than do LRRK2 monomers (Berger, Smith, & Lavoie, 2010; Greggio et al., 2009; Sen, Webber, & West, 2009). Despite the important role of membrane association in regulating LRRK2 function, the mechanism through which this protein binds to membranes is still unclear.

Evidence indicates that LRRK2 participates in cellular processes, such as cytoskeletal dynamics, mitochondrial function and autophagy (Cookson, 2010), which are known to be dysregulated in neurodegenerative processes. Indeed, LRRK2 is the most frequently mutated gene in familial Parkinson's disease and variations at the LRRK2 locus are associated with increased risk of developing the more common non-familial form of the disease (Nalls et al., 2014). Because NAPEs have also been implicated in neurodegeneration (Hansen, Hansen, Schousboe, & Hansen, 2000; Hansen et al., 2001; Hansen, Moesgaard, Hansen, & Petersen, 2000; Natarajan et al., 1986), in the present study we examined whether NAPE-PLD might be involved in regulating the association of LRRK2 with neuronal cell membranes. Our results show that genetic NAPE-PLD deletion simultaneously increases NAPE levels and decreases LRRK2 association with membranes as well as total LRRK2 levels. Conversely, exposure to a bacterial PLD exerts opposite effects. The results suggest that NAPE-PLD-driven NAPE hydrolysis may participate in the control of LRRK2 localization in neuronal cells.

2. Materials and methods

2.1 Animals

All procedures were performed in accordance with the Ethical Guidelines of the European Union (directive 2010/63/EU of 22 September 2010) and the Italian Ministry of Health. C57BL6J NAPE-PLD$^{-/-}$ mice were generated as previously described (Leung, Saghatelian, Simon, & Cravatt, 2006). All mice were group-housed in ventilated cages and had free access to food and water. They were maintained under a 12h light/dark cycle (lights on at 8:00 am) at controlled temperature (21 ± 1 °C) and relative humidity ($55\% \pm 10\%$). All efforts were made to minimize animal suffering and to use the minimal number of animals required to produce reliable results.

2.2 Chemicals

Chloral hydrate, paraformaldehyde (PAF) and phospholipase D (PLD) (*Streptomyces chromofuscus*, $\geq$50,000 units/mL) were purchased from Sigma Aldrich (Milan, Italy). NAPE standards and internal standards were synthetized in the lab as previously described (Basit et al., 2016).

2.3 Cell cultures

SH-SY5Y cells (Sigma Aldrich) and LRRK2 deficient Raw 264.7 cells (ATCC, Manassas, USA) were cultured at 37 °C and 5% CO_2 in Dulbecco's Modified Eagle's Medium (DMEM) (Euroclone, Milan, Italy) supplemented with 10% fetal bovine serum (FBS, Thermo Fisher, Waltham, MA, USA), L-glutamine (2mM) and antibiotics (Euroclone). Cells were treated with *S. chromofuscus* PLD (25 U/mL) or vehicle (100mM Tris/HCl, pH 8.0, 10% glycerol and 0.1% Triton X-100) for 15 or 30min.

2.4 NAPE-PLD silencing

siRNA experiments were performed using a *Napepld*-specific 27mer siRNA duplex (Origene, Rockville, MD, USA). A siRNA duplex carrying TYE-563 fluorescence was used to monitor transfection. A siRNA duplex carrying a 27-mer sequence targeting the hypoxanthine phosphoribosyltransferase 1 (HPRT) gene was used as positive control. Scrambled siRNA was included in each experiment as negative control. NAPE-PLD siRNA complexes (10 nM) were formed by mixing siRNA with lipofectamine (Invitrogen, Carlsbad, CA, USA) for 10 min at room temperature and then added to SH-SY5Y cells cultured with 1% FBS Optimem medium (Gibco, Waltham, MA, USA). After 6 h, the cell medium was changed to fresh full growth medium and cells were further incubated for 18 h before being harvested.

2.5 Lipid extraction and liquid chromatography/mass spectrometry (LC/MS) analysis

NAPE and FAE levels in cells and tissues were measured as described (Basit et al., 2016). Briefly, snap-frozen cell pellets or pre-weighed tissues were homogenized in a chloroform: methanol mixture (1:2 (v/v), 2 mL) containing 18:0–22:6–17:0 NAPE [synthetized in the lab (Basit et al., 2016)], [$^2H^4$]-PEA, [$^2H^4$]-OEA and [$^2H^3$]-SEA (Cayman Chemical, Ann Arbor, MI), as internal standards. Lipids were extracted twice with chloroform (0.6 mL) and the organic phases were washed with water (0.6 mL), collected, and dried under N_2. The organic extracts from cells were reconstituted in a mix of methanol/chloroform (9:1 (v/v), 0.1 mL). The organic extracts from tissues were fractionated by silica gel column chromatography (Astarita & Piomelli, 2009) and NAPEs were eluted with chloroform/methanol (1:1, v/v), while FAEs were eluted with chloroform/methanol (9:1, v/v). Organic phases were evaporated under N_2 and reconstituted in 0.1 mL of methanol/chloroform (9:1, v/v). LC/MS analyses were conducted on a Xevo TQ LC-MS/MS system equipped with a reversed-phase HSS T3 column (2.1 × 50 mm) (Waters, Milford MA), using gradient elution (1 min 95% A and 5% B followed by 7 min 100% B and again 2 min 95% A and 5% B) at a flow rate of 0.4 mL/min. The mobile phase consisted of solvent A containing acetonitrile and 10 mM ammonium formate in water (60:40, v/v) and solvent B containing acetonitrile and 10 mM ammonium formate in isopropyl alcohol (10:90, v/v). Multiple reaction monitoring (MRM) transitions for all the analytes are reported in Table 1. The capillary voltage was set at 3 kV. The cone voltage was 25 V. The source temperature was 120 °C. Desolvation gas and cone gas (N_2) flow were set to 800 and 20 L/h, respectively. Desolvation temperature was 450 °C. Detection and analysis were controlled by Waters MassLynx software version 4.1.

Table 1 MRM transitions and MS parameters for the NAPE and FAE species investigated in the present study. P = plasmalogen.

NAPE	Parent ion *(m/z)*	Daughter ion *(m/z)*	Cone voltage (V)	Collision energy (V)
P40:6-N16:0	1014.8	282.3/635.5	25	20
P38:6-N18:0	1014.8	310.3/607.5	25	20
40:6-N16:0	1030.8	282.3/651.5	25	20
38:6-N18:0	1030.8	310.3/623.5	25	20
38:4-N18:0	1034.8	310.3/627.5	25	20
P40:6-N18:0	1042.8	310.3/635.5	25	20
40:6-N18:0	1058.8	310.3/651.5	25	20
40:6-N17:0	1044.6	296.4/651.5	25	20
PEA	300	62	20	30
OEA	326	62	20	30
SEA	328	62	20	30
[$^2H^4$]-PEA	304	66	20	30
[$^2H^4$]-OEA	330	66	20	30
[$^2H^3$]-SEA	331	62	20	30

2.6 Immunocytochemistry

Cells were grown on sterile coverslips, fixed with PAF [4% in PBS, 2 ml] for 10 min and then quickly washed with phosphate-buffered saline (PBS). Immunostaining was performed by sequential incubation with previously validated anti-LRRK2 antibodies (1:500; Ab133474, Abcam) (Manzoni et al., 2016; Rassu et al., 2017; Zhou et al., 2016), followed by secondary Alexa Fluor 488 antibodie (both at 1:1000; Invitrogen). Images were collected using a Nikon A1 confocal microscope with a 60 × 1.4 numerical aperture objective lens.

2.7 Western blot analyses

Cell pellets or midbrain tissue fragments were dissected under microscope control, and homogenized in 150 μL of a radioimmunoprecipitation assay buffer (RIPA), consisting of 50 mM Tris-HCI (pH 7.4), 1% NP40, 0.5%

sodium-deoxycholate, 0.1% sodium dodecyl sulfate, 150 mM sodium chloride and 2 mM EDTA. Protein concentrations were measured using the bicinchoninic acid (BCA) method, following manufacturer's instructions (Thermo Fisher Scientific). Detection of LRRK2 was performed on membrane-enriched and cytosol fractions. Brain tissue from control or lesioned hemisphere, or control and silenced SHSY5Y cells were homogenized in five volumes of a buffer consisting of 10 mM HEPES-potassium hydroxide (pH 7.4), 0.25 M sucrose and proteinase inhibitor cocktail (Sigma, Saint Louis, MO, USA). Homogenates were centrifuged at 900 × *g* for 10 min. Pellets were homogenized again and centrifuged at 900 × *g* for 10 min. The pellets were collected as nuclear fraction. Supernatants were centrifuged at 12,000 × *g* for 15 min obtaining a synaptosome-enriched pellet. Supernatants were further ultracentrifuged at 46,000 × *g* for 1 h; the obtained pellets were collected as membrane fraction, while supernatants were collected as cytosolic fraction. Proteins (30 μg) were denatured in SDS (8%) and β-mercaptoethanol (5%) at 95 °C for 5 min. After separation by SDS-PAGE on a 4–15% gel (for NAPE-PLD), or on a 3–8% Tris Acetate gel (for LRRK2) under denaturing conditions, the proteins were electrotransferred to nitrocellulose membranes. The membranes were blocked with 5% non-fat dry milk in tris-buffered saline (TBS) and incubated overnight with primary antibodies (anti-LRRK2 antibody and anti-NAPE-PLD antibody, Abcam, 1:5000 and 1:200, respectively) and anti-GAPDH antibody (1:2000; Abcam) in 1% milk-TBS containing 0.1% Tween-20, followed by incubation with horseradish peroxidase-linked anti-rabbit IgG antibody (1:5000, Millipore, Darmstadt, Germany) in TBS containing 0.1% Tween-20 at room temperature for 1 h. Finally, proteins were visualized using an electrochemical luminescence (ECL) kit (Bio-Rad, Hercules, CA, USA) and the images were obtained using a LAS-4000 lumino-image analyzer system (Fujifilm, Tokyo, Japan).

2.8 Real-time quantitative PCR

Total RNA was prepared from cell pellets (2.5×10^5 cells) using the Ambion PureLink RNA minikit (Life Technologies, Carlsbad, CA, USA) as directed by the supplier. Samples were treated with DNase (PureLink DNase, Life Technologies) and cDNA synthesis was carried out using the SuperScript VILO cDNA synthesis kit (Life Technologies) according to the manufacturer's protocol using purified RNA (0.5–1 μg). First-strand cDNA was amplified using the TaqMan 5′ nuclease activity from the

TaqMan Universal PCR Master Mix, fluorogenic probes, and oligonucleotide primers. Copy numbers of cDNA targets were quantified by the point during cycling when the PCR product was first detected. Gene-specific primers for Taqman assays were purchased from Life Technologies. Quantitative PCR was performed in a 96-well PCR plate and run at 95 °C for 10 min, followed by 40 cycles, each cycle consisting of 15 s at 95 °C and 1 min at 60 °C, using a ViiA7 instrument (ViiATM 7 real-time PCR system, Life Technologies). The BestKeeper software (Pfaffl, Tichopad, Prgomet, & Neuvians, 2004) was used to determine expression stability and geometric mean of 2 different housekeeping genes (HMBS and HPRT). ΔCt values were calculated by subtracting the Ct value of the geometric mean of these housekeeping genes from the Ct value for the genes of interest. The relative quantity of genes of interest was calculated by the expression 2-ΔΔCt. Data are reported as fold induction over control.

2.9 Statistical analyses

Data were analyzed as described using GraphPad Prism version 5 for Windows (La Jolla, California, USA). Parametric statistical analysis was performed using the two-tailed Student's *t*-test for two groups or one-way analysis of variance (ANOVA) was applied for multiple comparisons with Bonferroni post hoc analysis for data meeting homogeneity of variance. Differences between groups were considered statistically significant at values of $P < 0.05$. Results are expressed as mean ± S.E.M.

3. Results

We silenced the *Napepld* gene in human catecholaminergic SH-SY5Y cells using a selective 27-mer siRNA duplex. After 6 h incubation followed by a 18 h washout period, siRNA-treated cells showed ≈60% down regulation in *Napepld* transcription (Fig. 1A), which was accompanied by ≈75% reduction in the levels of NAPE-PLD protein, when compared to cells that had been exposed to a scrambled 27-mer control (Fig. 1B and C). As expected from previous studies (Magotti et al., 2015), NAPE-PLD was present in both cytosol and membrane fractions (Fig. 1B and C).

Recent experiments have shown that pharmacological inhibition of NAPE-PLD activity in intact Hek-293 cells results in a significant accumulation of non-metabolized NAPEs, with no alteration in FAE levels (Castellani et al., 2017). This result is consistent with the non-rate limiting role of NAPE-PLD in FAE formation, which is primarily driven by

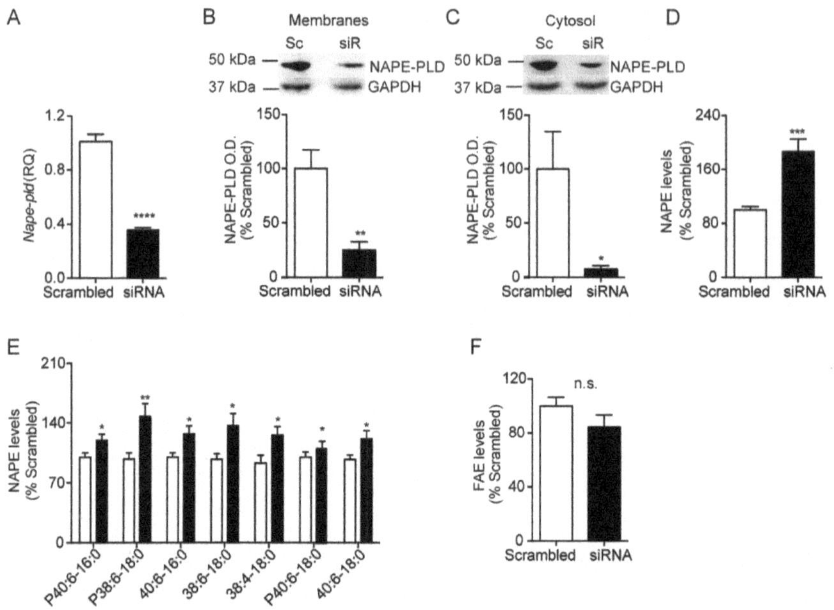

Fig. 1 NAPE-PLD silencing increases NAPE levels in human catecholaminergic SH-SY5Y cells. (A) NAPE-PLD transcription levels in NAPE-PLD-silenced SH-SY5Y cells (closed bars) compared to control cells incubated with scrambled siRNA (open bars); (B–C) Western blot quantification of NAPE-PLD levels in membrane (B) and cytosolic (C) fractions of NAPE-PLD-silenced SH-SY5Y cells compared to control cells: top, representative blot; bottom, densitometric quantification. Glyceraldehyde 3-phosphate dehydrogenase (GAPDH) was used for normalization ($n = 3$–5 independent experiments); (D–E) NAPE-PLD silencing increases total (D) and individual (E) NAPE levels. (F) NAPE-PLD silencing does not alter baseline FAE levels ($n = 14$). $^{*}P < 0.05$, $^{**}P < 0.01$ $^{***}P < 0.001$, $^{****}P < 0.0001$ two-tailed Student's *t*-test.

calcium-dependent NAPE biosynthesis (Cadas et al., 1997; Cadas, Gaillet, et al., 1996; Cadas, Schinelli, & Piomelli, 1996; Ogura et al., 2016). Similarly, in the present experiments we found that siRNA-mediated NAPE-PLD silencing in SH-SY5Y cells was accompanied by a ≈twofold increase in total NAPE content (Fig. 1D), but no significant changes in FAE levels (Fig. 1F). NAPEs involved in the response primarily included species containing saturated fatty acyl chains – either palmitic (16:0) or stearic (18:0)—linked to the amino group of acyl or alkyl PE (Fig. 1E and Table 1).

Next, we examined the impact of siRNA-mediated NAPE-PLD deletion and consequent NAPE accrual on the localization of endogenous LRRK2 in SH-SY5Y cells (Häbig, Walter, Poths, Riess, & Bonin, 2008; Liu et al., 2016; Saez-Atienzar et al., 2014). Immunohistochemical (IHC)

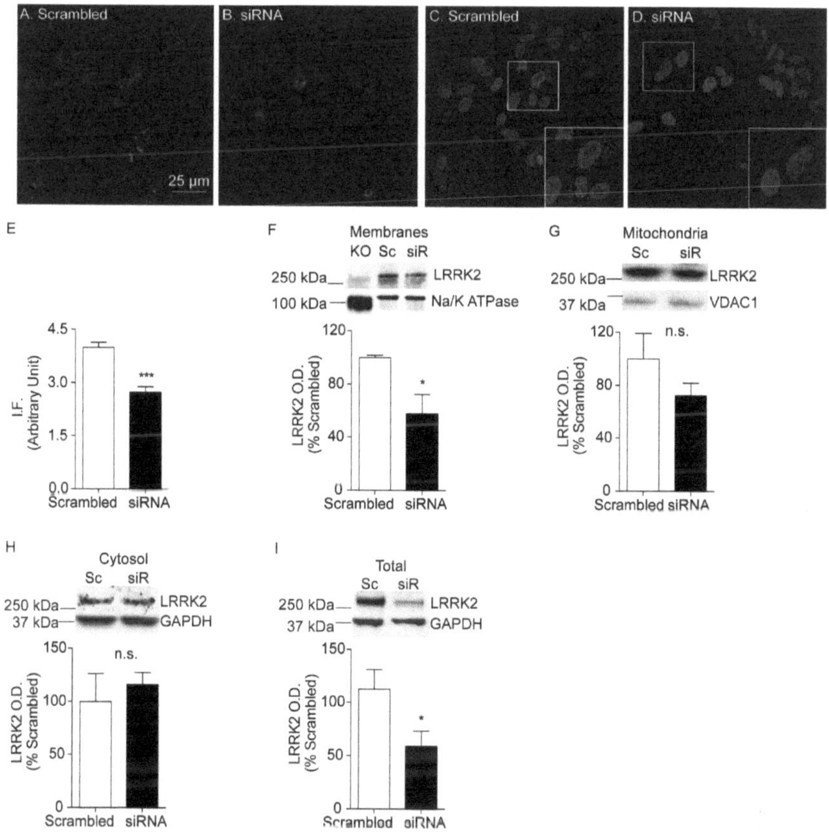

Fig. 2 NAPE-PLD silencing alters LRRK2 localization in SH-SY5Y cells. (A–D) Immunofluorescence images of LRRK2 (green) in control (scrambled, A, C) or NAPE-PLD silenced (siRNA, B, D) SH-SY5Y cells. Highlighted squares are magnified in the insets. Cell nuclei were stained with DAPI. Calibration bar: 25 μm. (E) Intensity of fluorescence staining for LRRK2 ($n = 5$). (F–I) Western blot quantification of LRRK2 levels in membrane fraction (F), mitochondrial fraction (G), cytosolic fraction (H) or total extract (I) from control (Sc) or NAPE-PLD-silenced (siR) SH-SY5Y cells. LRRK2-deficient RAW 264.7 cells (KO) were used as negative control. Top, representative blot; bottom, densitometric quantification. Normalization was performed using α1-Sodium/Potassium ATPase (Na/K ATPase, membrane fraction), voltage-dependent anion-selective channel 1 (VDAC1, mitochondrial fraction) and glyceraldehyde 3-phosphate dehydrogenase (GAPDH, cytosolic fraction or total extracts) ($n = 5$–8). *$P < 0.05$, ***$P < 0.001$ two-tailed Student's *t*-test.

studies illustrated in Fig. 2 showed that removal of NAPE-PLD was associated with a significant decrease in LRRK2 levels in SH-SY5Y cells (Fig. 2A–E). Consistent with these observations, immunoblot analyses revealed a reduction in LRRK2 levels in membrane fractions, but not in cytosolic or mitochondrial fractions of SH-SY5Y cells (Fig. 2F–H). The total amount of LRRK2 was also reduced (Fig. 2I), which is suggestive of a role for NAPE-PLD in regulating both membrane association and overall levels of LRRK2 in SH-SY5Y cells. LRRK2-deficient RAW 264.7 cells were used as control for antibody specificity (Fig. 2F).

To further test this possibility, we asked whether LRRK2 distribution might be altered in brain tissue of NAPE-PLD$^{-/-}$ mice (Leung et al., 2006). As previously reported, brain extracts from these mutants contained vanishingly low levels of NAPE-PLD protein, compared to extracts from wild-type littermate controls (Fig. 3Aand B) (Zhu et al., 2011). Moreover, total and individual NAPE levels were substantially elevated in NAPE-PLD$^{-/-}$ mice relative to controls (Fig. 3C and D).

Previous work has demonstrated that LRRK2 is expressed throughout the mouse brain (Higashi et al., 2007; West et al., 2014). Consistent with

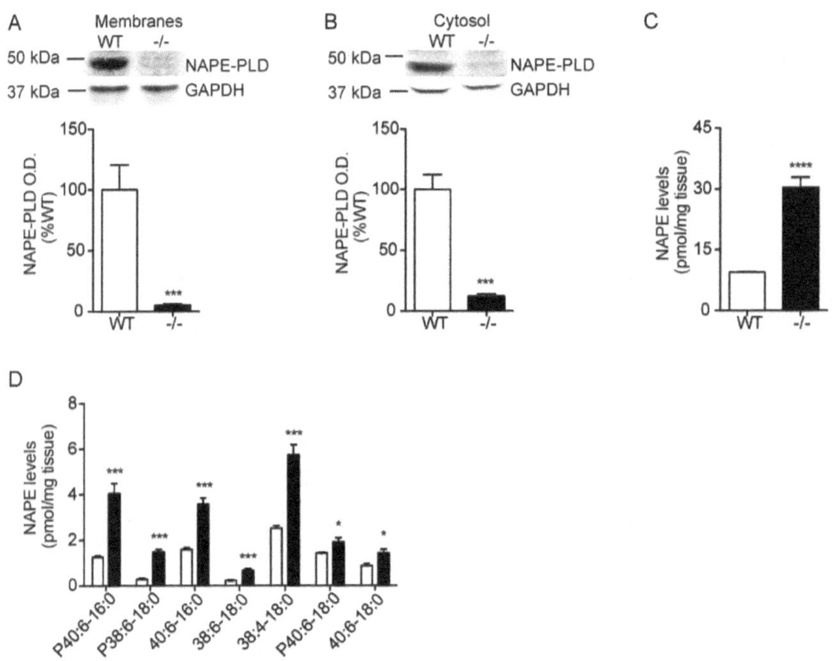

Fig. 3 NAPE-PLD deletion increases NAPE levels in mouse brain. (A–B) Western blot quantification of NAPE-PLD in membrane (A) and cytosolic (B) fractions from wild-type mice (open bars) or NAPE-PLD$^{-/-}$ mice (closed bars) mice: top, representative blot; bottom, densitometric quantification. Glyceraldehyde 3-phosphate dehydrogenase (GAPDH) was used for normalization (n = 4–6). (C–D) NAPE levels in brain tissue from wild-type mice compared to NAPE-PLD$^{-/-}$ mice (n = 6–7). $^{*}P < 0.05$, $^{***}P < 0.001$, $^{****}P < 0.0001$ two-tailed Student's t-test.

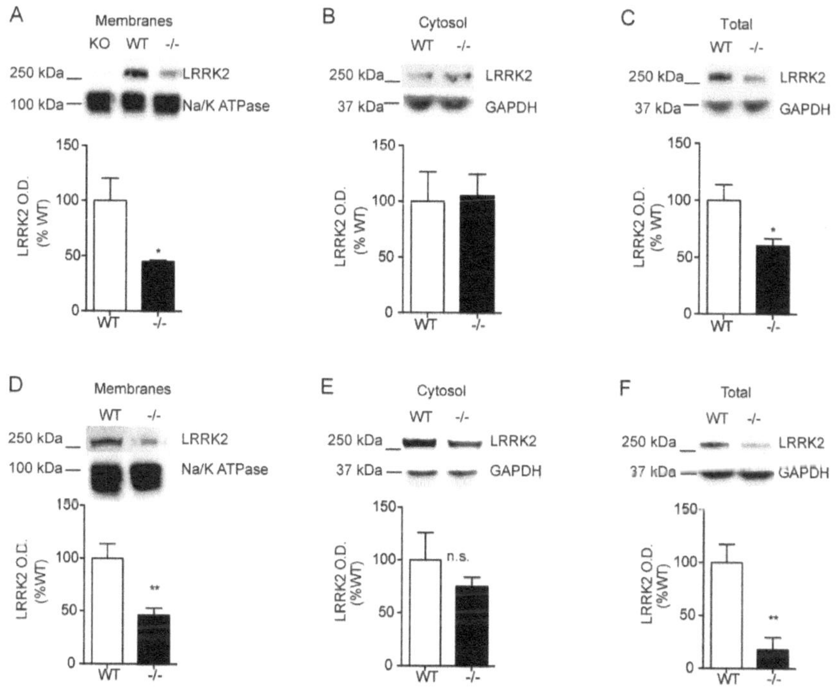

Fig. 4 NAPE-PLD deletion alters LRRK2 localization in mouse brain. (A–F) Western blot quantification of LRRK2 levels in membrane fraction (A,D), cytosolic fraction (B,E) or total extract (C,F) from wild-type (WT) and NAPE-PLD$^{-/-}$ (−/−) mouse brain (A–C) or midbrain (D–F) extracts; LRRK2-deficient RAW 264.7 cells (KO) were used as negative control: top, representative blot; bottom densitometric quantification. Normalization was performed using α1 Sodium/Potassium ATPase (Na/K ATPase, membrane fraction) and glyceraldehyde 3-phosphate dehydrogenase (GAPDH, cytosolic fraction or total extracts) (n = 4–5). *$P < 0.05$, **$P < 0.01$, two-tailed Student's t-test.

these results, we detected LRRK2 in both total brain and midbrain extracts of wild type and NAPE-PLD$^{-/-}$ mice (Fig. 4A; LRRK2-deficient RAW 264.7 cells were used as control for antibody specificity). As seen in SH-SY5Y cells, membrane LRRK2 levels were significantly lower in both total brain and midbrain extracts of NAPE-PLD$^{-/-}$ mice, compared to wild-type animals (Fig. 4A, D). By contrast, no such effect was observed in the cytosolic fraction (Fig. 4B, E). In both cases, the apparent dissociation of LRRK2 from membranes was accompanied by a decrease in total LRRK2 content (Fig. 4C, F).

Finally, as an independent strategy to modify NAPE levels in situ, we incubated intact SH-SY5Y cells with purified PLD from the gram-positive bacterium *S. chromofuscus* (15 or 30 min at 37 °C). Earlier studies in intact primary cultures of rat brain neurons have shown that this bacterial PLD

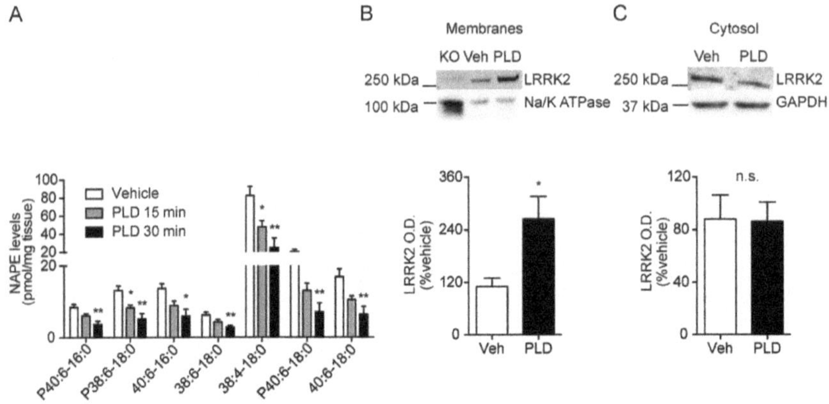

Fig. 5 Effect of exogenous PLD administration on LRRK2 localization in SH-SY5Y cells. (A) Incubation with PLD (25 U/mL, 15–30 min, *S. Chromofuscus*) lowers NAPE levels in SH-SY5Y cells ($n = 4$). (B, C) Western blot quantification of LRRK2 levels in the membrane (B) orcytosolic (C) fraction from SH-SY5Y cells treated with *S. Chromofuscus* PLD or vehicle; LRRK2-deficient RAW 264.7 cells (KO) were used as negative control: top, representative blots; bottom, densitometric quantification. Normalization was performed using α1-Sodium/Potassium ATPase (Na/K ATPase, membrane fraction) and glyceraldehyde 3-phosphate dehydrogenase (GAPDH, cytosolic fraction) ($n = 6$). $^*P < 0.05$, $^{**}P < 0.01$ two-tailed Student's *t*-test or one-way ANOVA followed by Bonferroni post-test.

lowers neuronal NAPE levels in a time-dependent manner without accessing the cellular interior (Cadas, Gaillet, et al., 1996; Cadas, Schinelli, & Piomelli, 1996). A similar result was obtained in SH-SY5Y cells (Fig. 5A). Levels of all NAPE species detectable by our LC/MS-MS assay were significantly decreased in cells incubated for 15 or 30 min in the presence of bacterial PLD, compared to control vehicle-treated cells. This reduction in NAPE content was accompanied by a significant increase in the level of LRRK2 associated with membranes (Fig. 5B). By contrast, no change in LRRK2 levels was observed in cytosolic fractions. The results suggest that PLD-catalyzed NAPE hydrolysis facilitates the association of LRRK2 to membranes in SH-SY5Y cells.

4. Discussion

In the present study, we report that genetic ablation of the NAPE-hydrolyzing enzyme, NAPE-PLD, results in the accumulation of saturated NAPE species, such as N-palmitoyl- and N-stearoyl-PE, in SH-SY5Y cells. This is accompanied by a dissociation of the multifunctional protein kinase, LRRK2, from membranes and a reduction in total LRRK2 levels. We further show that a short-lasting (15–30 min) exposure to a bacterial PLD lowers NAPE content in intact SH-SY5Y cells and concomitantly increases the association of LRRK2 to membranes. The results point to a previously unrecognized role for NAPE-PLD-driven NAPE hydrolysis in the control of LRRK2 localization in neuronal cells.

NAPE biosynthesis is catalyzed by the calcium-activated N-acyltransferase, PLA2A4E (Ogura et al., 2016). Newly formed NAPEs give rise to bioactive FAEs, such as the endocannabinoid messenger, anandamide (Cadas et al., 1997; Di Marzo et al., 1994), and the endogenous PPAR-α agonists, OEA and PEA (Fu et al., 2007). In addition to this role as FAE precursors, emerging evidence suggests that NAPEs may also regulate cell-membrane dynamics (Coulon, Faure, Salmon, Wattelet, & Bessoule, 2012) and subcellular localization of intracellular proteins (Mileykovskaya & Dowhan, 2005). Such dual role as signaling molecule and precursor for other signals is not uncommon among glycerophospholipids. For example, phosphatidylinositol-4, 5-bisphosphate is known to serve both as a precursor for the second messengers, 1,3,4-inositol-trisphosphate and 1,2-diacylglycerol (1,2-DAG), and as tether for membrane protein anchoring (Zoncu et al., 2007). Likewise, phosphatidic acid may act both as a precursor for 1,2-DAG and as second-messenger regulator of protein kinase and ion channel activities (Hite, Butterwick, & MacKinnon, 2014; Piomelli, Astarita, & Rapaka, 2007). In this context, it is worth noting that a variety of physiological and pathological stimuli are able to trigger calcium-dependent NAPE biosynthesis. Early studies have demonstrated that NAPEs accumulate in infarcted canine myocardium (Epps, Natarajan, Schmid, & Schmid, 1980; Natarajan et al., 1982) and ischemic rat brain (Natarajan et al., 1986). More recent work has shown that neurotransmitters such as glutamate (Hansen, Lauritzen, Strand, Moesgaard, & Frandsen, 1995) or neurotoxins such as sodium azide (Hansen, Hansen, et al., 2000; Hansen, Moesgaard, et al., 2000) and 6-hydroxydopamine (Basit et al., 2016; Palese, Pontis, Realini, & Piomelli, 2019) stimulate the production of NAPEs and FAEs in neurons. The present results suggest that stimulus-dependent NAPE biosynthesis may be not only involved in FAE production, but also in modulating intracellular signaling by regulating the association of LRRK2 with membranes.

How may NAPE-PLD activity influence LRRK2 localization? The available data do not allow us to answer this question firmly. In addition to hydrolyzing NAPEs, NAPE-PLD may also cleave lyso-NAPEs and glycerophospho-*N*-acylethanolamines (Tsuboi et al., 2011), which might contribute to the effect produced by NAPE-PLD deletion. Moreover,

S. chromofuscus PLD is not selective for NAPEs and can thus generate phosphatidic acid (PA) also from other glycerophospholipids (Wang et al., 2006). PA may anchor various proteins to membranes, such as Raf1 or mTOR, regulating their activity (Stace & Ktistakis, 2006). We cannot exclude that the effect observed here is due, at least in part, to the production of PA, whose content was not quantified in the present study. However, the fact that exogenous PLD, which is not able to enter the intact cell membrane, influences LRRK2 localization at the membrane is an indicator of the involvement of lipid molecules rather than direct regulation of protein binding by NAPE-PLD.

LRRK2 is a large multidomain protein containing a ROC-GTPase domain, a serine/threonine protein kinase domain, protein-protein interactions domains (Greggio et al., 2009). This complex architecture reflects its involvement in a wide variety of biological processes such as protein translation, cytoskeletal processes, vesicular dynamics, neurite extension, mitochondrial function, autophagy and ubiquitin-proteasome system (Wallings, Manzoni, & Bandopadhyay, 2015). When it is recruited to the membrane, LRRK2 serves as a scaffold protein in many signaling pathways (Berwick & Harvey, 2012), participates in cytoskeleton organization (Gandhi, Chen, & Wilson-Delfosse, 2009), mediates kinase activity through the formation of dimers (Berger et al., 2010), and interacts with small GTPases such as Rac1 favoring its activation (Chan, Citro, Cordy, Shen, & Wolozin, 2011). In this regard, we recently observed that NAPE-PLD$^{-/-}$ mice lack Rac1 activation when exposed to the neurotoxin, 6-hydroxy-dopamine (Palese et al., 2019). It is tempting to speculate that the decrease of LRRK2 in membranes of NAPE-PLD-deficient mice might suppress Rac1 activation. Further experimentation is needed to test this possibility.

Several mechanisms have been hypothesized for the association of LRRK2 with the lipid bilayer (Cookson, 2016). These include direct interactions with lipid components of membranes as well as binding to membrane-associated proteins, such as Rab proteins, which have been identified as LRRK2 kinase-substrates (Steger et al., 2016; Tsika & Moore, 2013). Our findings suggest that NAPE-PLD activity may play an important role in the control of LRRK2 association with membranes. Previous studies have suggested that LRRK2 may interact with lipid rafts (Hatano et al., 2007), membrane micro-domains that are enriched in cholesterol and sphingomyelin (Brown & London, 1998). Interestingly, biophysical experiments indicate that NAPEs can prevent the formation of ordered cholesterol- and sphingomyelin-rich domains (Li, Ramakrishnan, Brockman, Brown, & Swamy, 2002), raising the intriguing possibility that NAPE-PLD activity might influence LRRK2 association to membranes by lowering membrane NAPE content and thus favoring lipid raft formation. Alternatively, NAPEs might act indirectly, for example by influencing other LRRK2 interactors such as the chaperone complexes BAG2-HCS70 (Fukuzono, Pastuhov, Fukushima, Li, & Hattori, 2016) or the Rab family of proteins (Steger et al., 2016). Testing those alternative hypotheses will require, of course, additional work. Surprisingly, our results show that genetic NAPE-PLD deletion was also accompanied by an overall decrease in cellular LRRK2 levels, which might be accounted by proteolysis of membrane-dissociated LRRK2 and/or compensatory changes in LRRK2 expression.

LRRK2 mutations are relatively frequent in both sporadic and familiar form of PD (Nalls et al., 2014), but the possible roles played by such mutations in this neurodegenerative disorder remain unclear. Since the most common LRRK2 mutation, G2019S, causes an increase in LRRK2-associated kinase activity, attention has primarily focused on the effects of pharmacological inhibition or genetic deletion of LRRK2. The results obtained thus far have not lead, however, to univocal conclusions. For example, whereas genetic LRRK2 ablation protects mice from α-synuclein-induced dopaminergic neurodegeneration (Daher, Volpicelli-Daley, Blackburn, Moehle, & West, 2014), double deletion of LRRK1 and LRRK2 genes causes an age-dependent loss of dopaminergic neurons (Giaime et al., 2017). Similarly, LRRK2 inhibition is protective against the G2019S mutation in vitro (Smith et al., 2016) and in vivo (Daher et al., 2015; Liu et al., 2011), but causes disruption of mitochondrial morphology and imbalance in reactive oxygen species in SH-SY5Y cells (Saez-Atienzar et al., 2016). Despite these uncertainties, the present results are consistent with an involvement of LRRK2 in neurodegeneration. As noted above, there is substantial evidence that calcium-dependent NAPE biosynthesis is enhanced by neurotoxic and pro-degenerative stimuli (Hansen, Hansen, et al., 2000; Hansen, Moesgaard, et al., 2000). It will be interesting to test whether NAPE-PLD activity and NAPE accrual participate in the response to neuronal cell damage, at least in part, by regulating the subcellular localization of LRRK2 and its consequences on intracellular signaling events.

Acknowledgments

We are grateful to Abdul Basit for help with NAPE analysis and Alessandra Misto for help with breeding of NAPE-PLD$^{-/-}$ mice.

Conflict of interests statement

The authors declare no competing interests.

References

Astarita, G., & Piomelli, D. (2009). Lipidomic analysis of endocannabinoid metabolism in biological samples. *Journal of Chromatography B: Analytical Technologies in the Biomedical and Life Sciences*. Retrieved from https://doi.org/10.1016/j.jchromb.2009.01.008.

Basit, A., Pontis, S., Piomelli, D., & Armirotti, A. (2016). Ion mobility mass spectrometry enhances low-abundance species detection in untargeted lipidomics. *Metabolomics*. Retrieved from https://doi.org/10.1007/s11306-016-0971-3.

Berger, Z., Smith, K. A., & Lavoie, M. J. (2010). Membrane localization of LRRK2 is associated with increased formation of the highly active lrrk2 dimer and changes in its phosphorylation. *Biochemistry*. Retrieved from https://doi.org/10.1021/bi100157u.

Berwick, D. C., & Harvey, K. (2012). LRRK2 functions as a wnt signaling scaffold, bridging cytosolic proteins and membrane-localized LRP6. *Human Molecular Genetics*. Retrieved from https://doi.org/10.1093/hmg/dds342.

Brown, D. A., & London, E. (1998). Structure and origin of ordered lipid domains in biological membranes. *Journal of Membrane Biology*. Retrieved from https://doi.org/10.1007/s002329900397.

Cadas, H., Gaillet, S., Beltramo, M., Venance, L., & Piomelli, D. (1996). Biosynthesis of an endogenous cannabinoid precursor in neurons and its control by calcium and cAMP. In *J.Neurosci*.

Cadas, H., Schinelli, S., & Piomelli, D. (1996). Membrane localization of N-acylphosphatidylethanolamine in central neurons: Studies with exogenous phospholipases. *Journal of Lipid Mediators and Cell Signalling*. Retrieved from https://doi.org/10.1016/0929-7855(96)00510-X.

Cadas, H., Di Tomaso, E., & Piomelli, D. (1997). Occurrence and biosynthesis of endogenous cannabinoid precursor, N-arachidonoyl phosphatidylethanolamine, in rat brain. *The Journal of Neuroscience*, *17*, 1226–1242.

Castellani, B., Diamanti, E., Pizzirani, D., Tardia, P., Maccesi, M., Realini, N., et al. (2017). Synthesis and characterization of the first inhibitor of: N -acylphosphatidylethanolamine phospholipase D (NAPE-PLD). *Chemical Communications*. Retrieved from https://doi.org/10.1039/c7cc07582k.

Chan, D., Citro, A., Cordy, J. M., Shen, G. C., & Wolozin, B. (2011). Rac1 protein rescues neurite retraction caused by G2019s leucine-rich repeat kinase 2 (LRRK2). *Journal of Biological Chemistry*. Retrieved from https://doi.org/10.1074/jbc.M111.234005.

Civiero, L., Vancraenenbroeck, R., Belluzzi, E., Beilina, A., Lobbestael, E., Reyniers, L., et al. (2012). Biochemical characterization of highly purified leucine-rich repeat kinases 1 and 2 demonstrates formation of homodimers. *PLoS One*. Retrieved from https://doi.org/10.1371/journal.pone.0043472.

Cookson, M. R. (2010). The role of leucine-rich repeat kinase 2 (LRRK2) in Parkinson's disease. *Nature Reviews Neuroscience*. Retrieved from https://doi.org/10.1038/nrn2935.

Cookson, M. R. (2016). Cellular functions of LRRK2 implicate vesicular trafficking pathways in Parkinson's disease. *Biochemical Society Transactions*. Retrieved from https://doi.org/10.1042/BST20160228.

Coulon, D., Faure, L., Salmon, M., Wattelet, V., & Bessoule, J. J. (2012). Occurrence, biosynthesis and functions of N-acylphosphatidylethanolamines (NAPE): Not just precursors of N-acylethanolamines (NAE). *Biochimie*. Retrieved from https://doi.org/10.1016/j.biochi.2011.04.023.

Daher, J. P. L., Abdelmotilib, H. A., Hu, X., Volpicelli-Daley, L. A., Moehle, M. S., Fraser, K. B., et al. (2015). LRRK2 pharmacological inhibition abates α-Synuclein induced neurodegeneration. *The Journal of Biological Chemistry*, *290*(32), 19433–19444. Retrieved from https://doi.org/10.1074/jbc.M115.660001.

Daher, J. P. L., Volpicelli-Daley, L. A., Blackburn, J. P., Moehle, M. S., & West, A. B. (2014). Abrogation of -synuclein-mediated dopaminergic neurodegeneration in LRRK2-deficient rats. *Proceedings of the National Academy of Sciences of the United States of America*. Retrieved from https://doi.org/10.1073/pnas.1403215111.

Di Marzo, V., Fontana, A., Cadas, H., Schinelli, S., Cimino, G., Schwartz, J. C., et al. (1994). Formation and inactivation of endogenous cannabinoid anandamide in central neurons. *Nature*, *372*(6507), 686–691. Retrieved from https://doi.org/10.1038/372686a0.

DiPatrizio, N. V., & Piomelli, D. (2015). Intestinal lipid'derived signals that sense dietary fat. *Journal of Clinical Investigation*. Retrieved from https://doi.org/10.1172/JCI76302.

Epps, D. E., Natarajan, V., Schmid, P. C., & Schmid, H. H. O. (1980). Accumulation of N-acylethanolamine glycerophospholipids in infarcted myocardium. *Biochimica et Biophysica Acta (BBA)/Lipids and Lipid Metabolism*. Retrieved from https://doi.org/10.1016/0005-2760(80)90260-X.

Fu, J., Astarita, G., Gaetani, S., Kim, J., Cravatt, B. F., Mackie, K., et al. (2007). Food intake regulates oleoylethanolamide formation and degradation in the proximal small intestine. *Journal of Biological Chemistry*. Retrieved from https://doi.org/10.1074/jbc.M607809200.

Fukuzono, T., Pastuhov, S. I., Fukushima, O., Li, C., Hattori, A., Iemura, Shun-ichiro, … Hisamoto, N. (2016). Chaperone complex BAG2 HSC70 regulates localization of *Caenorhabditis elegans* leucine-rich repeat kinase LRK-1 to the Golgi. Genes to Cells. Retrieved from https://doi.org/10.1111/gtc.12338.

Gandhi, P. N., Chen, S. G., & Wilson-Delfosse, A. L. (2009). Leucine-rich repeat kinase 2 (LRRK2): A key player in the pathogenesis of Parkinson's disease. *Journal of Neuroscience Research*. Retrieved from https://doi.org/10.1002/jnr.21949.

Giaime, E., Tong, Y., Wagner, L. K., Yuan, Y., Huang, G., & Shen, J. (2017). Age-dependent dopaminergic neurodegeneration and impairment of the autophagy-lysosomal pathway in LRRK-deficient mice. *Neuron*. Retrieved from https://doi.org/10.1016/j.neuron.2017.09.036.

Gillum, M. P., Zhang, D., Zhang, X. M., Erion, D. M., Jamison, R. A., Choi, C., et al. (2008). N-acylphosphatidylethanolamine, a gut- derived circulating factor induced by fat ingestion, inhibits food intake. *Cell*. Retrieved from https://doi.org/10.1016/j.cell.2008.10.043.

Greggio, E., Taymans, J. M., Zhen, E. Y., Ryder, J., Vancraenenbroeck, R., Beilina, A., et al. (2009). The Parkinson's disease kinase LRRK2 autophosphorylates its GTPase domain at multiple sites. *Biochemical and Biophysical Research Communications*. Retrieved from https://doi.org/10.1016/j.bbrc.2009.08.163.

Greggio, E., Zambrano, I., Kaganovich, A., Beilina, A., Taymans, J. M., Daniëls, V., et al. (2008). The Parkinson disease-associated leucine-rich repeat kinase 2 (LRRK2) is a dimer that undergoes intramolecular autophosphorylation. *Journal of Biological Chemistry*. Retrieved from https://doi.org/10.1074/jbc.M708718200.

Hübig, K., Walter, M., Poths, S., Riess, O., & Bonin, M. (2008). RNA interference of LRRK2-microarray expression analysis of a Parkinson's disease key player. *Neurogenetics*. Retrieved from https://doi.org/10.1007/s10048-007-0114-0.

Hansen, H. H., Hansen, S. H., Schousboe, A., & Hansen, H. S. (2000). Determination of the phospholipid precursor of anandamide and other N- acylethanolamine phospholipids before and after sodium azide-induced toxicity in cultured neocortical neurons. *Journal of Neurochemistry*. Retrieved from https://doi.org/10.1046/j.1471-4159.2000.0750861.x.

Hansen, H. H., Ikonomidou, C., Bittigau, P., Hansen, S. H., & Hansen, H. S. (2001). Accumulation of the anandamide precursor and other N-acylethanolamine phospholipids in infant rat models of in vivo necrotic and apoptotic neuronal death. *Journal of Neurochemistry*. Retrieved from https://doi.org/10.1046/j.1471-4159.2001.00006.x.

Hansen, H. S., Lauritzen, L., Strand, A. M., Moesgaard, B., & Frandsen, A. (1995). Glutamate stimulates the formation of N-acylphosphatidylethanolamine and N-acylethanolamine in cortical neurons in culture. *Biochimica et Biophysica Acta*.

Hansen, H. S., Lauritzen, L., Strand, A. M., Vinggaard, A. M., Frandsen, A., & Schousboe, A. (1997). Characterization of glutamate-induced formation of N-acylphosphatidylethanolamine and N-acylethanolamine in cultured neocortical neurons. *Journal of Neurochemistry*.

Hansen, H. S., Moesgaard, B., Hansen, H. H., & Petersen, G. (2000). N-acylethanolamines and precursor phospholipids - relation to cell injury. *Chemistry and Physics of Lipids*. Retrieved from https://doi.org/10.1016/S0009-3084(00)00192-4.

Hansen, H. S., Moesgaard, B., Petersen, G., & Hansen, H. H. (2002). Putative neuroprotective actions of N-acyl-ethanolamines. *Pharmacology and Therapeutics*. Retrieved from https://doi.org/10.1016/S0163-7258(02)00251-6.

Hatano, T., Kubo, S.-I., Imai, S., Maeda, M., Ishikawa, K., Mizuno, Y., et al. (2007). Leucine-rich repeat kinase 2 associates with lipid rafts. *Human Molecular Genetics*. Retrieved from https://doi.org/10.1093/hmg/ddm013.

Higashi, S., Moore, D. J., Colebrooke, R. E., Biskup, S., Dawson, V. L., Arai, H., et al. (2007). Expression and localization of Parkinson's disease-associated leucine-rich repeat kinase 2 in the mouse brain. *Journal of Neurochemistry*. Retrieved from https://doi.org/10.1111/j.1471-4159.2006.04246.x.

Hite, R. K., Butterwick, J. A., & MacKinnon, R. (2014). Phosphatidic acid modulation of Kv channel voltage sensor function. *eLife*. Retrieved from https://doi.org/10.7554/eLife.04366.

Jung, K.-M., Astarita, G., Yasar, S., Vasilevko, V., Cribbs, D. H., Head, E., et al. (2012). An amyloid beta42-dependent deficit in anandamide mobilization is associated with cognitive dysfunction in Alzheimer's disease. *Neurobiology of Aging*. Retrieved from https://doi.org/10.1016/j.neurobiolaging.2011.03.012.

Lafrance, C.-P., Blochet, J.-E., & Pezolet, M. (1997). N-Acylphosphatidylethanolamines: Effect of the N-acyl chain length on its orientation. *Biophysical Journal*, *72*, 2559–2568. June. Retrieved from https://doi.org/10.1016/S0006-3495(97)78899-4.

Leung, D., Saghatelian, A., Simon, G. M., & Cravatt, B. F. (2006). Inactivation of N-acyl phosphatidylethanolamine phospholipase D reveals multiple mechanisms for the biosynthesis of endocannabinoids. *Biochemistry*, *45*(15), 4720–4726. Retrieved from https://doi.org/10.1021/bi060163l.

Li, X. M., Ramakrishnan, M., Brockman, H. L., Brown, R. E., & Swamy, M. J. (2002). N-myristoylated phosphatidylethanolamine: Interfacial behavior and interaction with cholesterol. *Langmuir*. Retrieved from https://doi.org/10.1021/la010937t.

Liu, S., Cui, B., Dai, Z. X., Shi, P. K., Wang, Z. H., & Guo, Y. Y. (2016). Long non-coding RNA HOTAIR promotes Parkinson's disease induced by MPTP through up-regulating the expression of LRRK2. *Current Neurovascular Research*, *13*(2), 115–120. Retrieved from https://doi.org/10.2174/1567202613666160316155228.

Liu, Z., Hamamichi, S., Lee, B. D., Yang, D., Ray, A., Caldwell, G. A., et al. (2011). Inhibitors of LRRK2 kinase attenuate neurodegeneration and Parkinson-like phenotypes in Caenorhabditis elegans and Drosophila Parkinson's disease models. *Human Molecular Genetics*. Retrieved from https://doi.org/10.1093/hmg/ddr312.

Magotti, P., Bauer, I., Igarashi, M., Babagoli, M., Marotta, R., Piomelli, D., et al. (2015). Structure of human NAPE-PLD: Regulation of fatty-acid ethanolamide biosynthesis by bile acids. *Structure (London, England: 1993)*, *23*(3), 598–604. Retrieved from https://doi.org/10.1016/j.str.2014.12.018.

Manzoni, C., Mamais, A., Roosen, D. A., Dihanich, S., Soutar, M. P. M., Plun-Favreau, H., et al. (2016). MTOR independent regulation of macroautophagy by leucine rich repeat kinase 2 via Beclin-1. *Scientific Reports*. Retrieved from https://doi.org/10.1038/srep35106.

Mileykovskaya, E., & Dowhan, W. (2005). Role of membrane lipids in bacterial division-site selection. *Current Opinion in Microbiology*. Retrieved from https://doi.org/10.1016/j.mib.2005.02.012.

Nalls, M. A., Pankratz, N., Lill, C. M., Do, C. B., Hernandez, D. G., Saad, M., et al. (2014). Large-scale meta-analysis of genome-wide association data identifies six new risk loci for Parkinson's disease. *Nature Genetics*. Retrieved from https://doi.org/10.1038/ng.3043.

Natarajan, V., Reddy, P. V., Schmid, P. C., & Schmid, H. H. O. (1982). N-acylation of ethanolamine phospholipids in canine myocardium. Biochimica et Biophysica Acta (BBA)/Lipids and Lipid Metabolism Retrieved from https://doi.org/10.1016/0005-2760(82)90352-6.

Natarajan, V., Schmid, P. C., & Schmid, H. H. O. (1986). N-Acylethanolamine phospholipid metabolism in normal and ischemic rat brain. *Biochimica et Biophysica Acta (BBA) - Lipids and Lipid Metabolism*. Retrieved from https://doi.org/10.1016/0005-2760(86)90341-3.

Ogura, Y., Parsons, W. H., Kamat, S. S., & Cravatt, B. F. (2016). A calcium-dependent acyltransferase that produces N-acyl phosphatidylethanolamines. *Nature Chemical Biology*. Retrieved from https://doi.org/10.1038/nchembio.2127.

Okamoto, Y., Morishita, J., Tsuboi, K., Tonai, T., & Ueda, N. (2004). Molecular characterization of a phospholipase D generating anandamide and its congeners. *Journal of Biological Chemistry*. Retrieved from https://doi.org/10.1074/jbc.M306642200.

Palese, F., Pontis, S., Realini, N., & Piomelli, D. (2019). A protective role for N-acylphosphatidylethanolamine phospholipase D in 6-OHDA-induced neurodegeneration. *Scientific Reports*. Retrieved from https://doi.org/10.1038/s41598-019-51799-1.

Pfaffl, M. W., Tichopad, A., Prgomet, C., & Neuvians, T. P. (2004). Determination of stable housekeeping genes, differentially regulated target genes and sample integrity: BestKeeper- -excel-based tool using pair-wise correlations. *Biotechnology Letters*, *26*(6), 509–515.

Piomelli, D. (2013). A fatty gut feeling. *Trends in Endocrinology and Metabolism*. Retrieved from https://doi.org/10.1016/j.tem.2013.03.001.

Piomelli, D., Astarita, G., & Rapaka, R. (2007). A neuroscientist's guide to lipidomics. *Nature Reviews Neuroscience*. Retrieved from https://doi.org/10.1038/nrn2233.

Piomelli, D., & Sasso, O. (2014). Peripheral gating of pain signals by endogenous lipid mediators. *Nature Neuroscience*. Retrieved from https://doi.org/10.1038/nn.3612.

Rassu, M., Del Giudice, M. G., Sanna, S., Taymans, J. M., Morari, M., Brugnoli, A., et al. (2017). Role of LRRK2 in the regulation of dopamine receptor trafficking. *PLoS One*. Retrieved from https://doi.org/10.1371/journal.pone.0179082.

Saez-Atienzar, S., Bonet-Ponce, L., Blesa, J. R., Romero, F. J., Murphy, M. P., Jordan, J., et al. (2014). The LRRK2 inhibitor GSK2578215A induces protective autophagy in SH-SY5Y cells: Involvement of Drp-1-mediated mitochondrial fission and mitochondrial-derived ROS signaling. *Cell Death and Disease*. Retrieved from https://doi.org/10.1038/cddis.2014.320.

Saez-Atienzar, S., Bonet-Ponce, L., da Casa, C., Perez-Dolz, L., Blesa, J. R., Nava, E., et al. (2016). Bcl-xL-mediated antioxidant function abrogates the disruption of mitochondrial dynamics induced by LRRK2 inhibition. *Biochimica et Biophysica Acta - Molecular Basis of Disease*, *1862*(1), 20–31. Retrieved from https://doi.org/10.1016/j.bbadis.2015.09.021.

Sen, S., Webber, P. J., & West, A. B. (2009). Dependence of leucine-rich repeat kinase 2 (LRRK2) kinase activity on dimerization. *Journal of Biological Chemistry*. Retrieved from https://doi.org/10.1074/jbc.M109.025437.

Shangguan, T., Pak, C. C., Ali, S., Janoff, A. S., & Meers, P. (1998). Cation-dependent fusogenicity of an N-acyl phosphatidylethanolamine. *Biochimica et Biophysica Acta - Biomembranes*. Retrieved from https://doi.org/10.1016/S0005-2736(97)00151-X.

Skaper, S. D., Facci, L., Barbierato, M., Zusso, M., Bruschetta, G., Impellizzeri, D., et al. (2015). N-Palmitoylethanolamine and Neuroinflammation: A novel therapeutic strategy of resolution. *Molecular Neurobiology*. Retrieved from https://doi.org/10.1007/s12035-015-9253-8.

Smith, G. A., Jansson, J., Rocha, E. M., Osborn, T., Hallett, P. J., & Isacson, O. (2016). Fibroblast biomarkers of sporadic Parkinson's disease and LRRK2 kinase inhibition. *Molecular Neurobiology*. Retrieved from https://doi.org/10.1007/s12035-015-9435-4.

Stace, C. L., & Ktistakis, N. T. (2006). Phosphatidic acid- and phosphatidylserine-binding proteins. *Biochimica et Biophysica Acta—Molecular and Cell Biology of Lipids*. Retrieved from https://doi.org/10.1016/j.bbalip.2006.03.006.

Steger, M., Tonelli, F., Ito, G., Davies, P., Trost, M., Vetter, M., et al. (2016). Phosphoproteomics reveals that Parkinson's disease kinase LRRK2 regulates a subset of Rab GTPases. *eLife*. Retrieved from https://doi.org/10.7554/eLife.12813.001.

Sugiura, T., Kondo, S., Sukagawa, A., Tonegawa, T., Nakane, S., Yamashita, A., et al. (1996). Enzymatic synthesis of anandamide, an endogenous cannabinoid receptor ligand, through N-acylphosphatidylethanolamine pathway in testis: Involvement of ca(2+)-dependent transacylase and phosphodiesterase activities. *Biochemical and Biophysical Research Communications*, *218*(1), 113–117. Retrieved from https://doi.org/10.1006/bbrc.1996.0020.

Swamy, M. J., Tarafdar, P. K., & Kamlekar, R. K. (2010). Structure, phase behaviour and membrane interactions of N-acylethanolamines and N-acylphosphatidylethanolamines. *Chemistry and Physics of Lipids*. Retrieved from https://doi.org/10.1016/j.chemphyslip.2010.01.002.

Tsika, E., & Moore, D. J. (2013). Contribution of GTPase activity to LRRK2-associated Parkinson disease. *Small GTPases*. Retrieved from https://doi.org/10.4161/sgtp.25130.

Tsuboi, K., Okamoto, Y., Ikematsu, N., Inoue, M., Shimizu, Y., Uyama, T., et al. (2011). Enzymatic formation of N-acylethanolamines from N-acylethanolamine plasmalogen through N-acylphosphatidylethanolamine-hydrolyzing phospholipase D-dependent and -independent pathways. *Biochimica et Biophysica Acta - Molecular and Cell Biology of Lipids*. Retrieved from https://doi.org/10.1016/j.bbalip.2011.07.009.

Wallings, R., Manzoni, C., & Bandopadhyay, R. (2015). Cellular processes associated with LRRK2 function and dysfunction. *FEBS Journal*. Retrieved from https://doi.org/10.1111/febs.13305.

Wang, J., Okamoto, Y., Morishita, J., Tsuboi, K., Miyatake, A., & Ueda, N. (2006). Functional analysis of the purified anandamide-generating phospholipase D as a member of the metallo-β-lactamase family. *Journal of Biological Chemistry*. Retrieved from https://doi.org/10.1074/jbc.M512359200.

West, A. B., Cowell, R. M., Daher, J. P. L., Moehle, M. S., Hinkle, K. M., Melrose, H. L., et al. (2014). Differential LRRK2 expression in the cortex, striatum, and substantia nigra in transgenic and nontransgenic rodents. *Journal of Comparative Neurology*. Retrieved from https://doi.org/10.1002/cne.23583.

Zhou, Q., Yen, A., Rymarczyk, G., Asai, H., Trengrove, C., Aziz, N., et al. (2016). Impairment of PARK14-dependent Ca2+signalling is a novel determinant of Parkinson's disease. *Nature Communications*. Retrieved from https://doi.org/10.1038/ncomms10332.

Zhu, C., Solorzano, C., Sahar, S., Realini, N., Fung, E., Sassone-Corsi, P., et al. (2011). Proinflammatory stimuli control NAPE-PLD expression in macrophages. *Molecular Pharmacology*, . https://doi.org/10.1124/mol.110.070201. Retrieved from.

Zoncu, R., Perera, R. M., Sebastian, R., Nakatsu, F., Chen, H., Balla, T., et al. (2007). Loss of endocytic clathrin-coated pits upon acute depletion of phosphatidylinositol 4,5-bisphosphate. *Proceedings of the National Academy of Sciences of the United States of America*. Retrieved from https://doi.org/10.1073/pnas.0611733104.

CHAPTER TEN

Amyloidogenic and anti-amyloidogenic properties of presenilin 1

Victor Bustos*, Maria V. Pulina, and Jose Ledo

Laboratory of Cellular and Molecular Neuroscience, Rockefeller University, New York, NY, United States

*Corresponding author: e-mail address: vbustos@rockefeller.edu

Contents

Abstract

Presenilin 1 (PS1) is an intramembrane protease, the active subunit of the γ-secretase complex. Its well-studied function is the amyloidogenic cleavage of the C-terminal fragment of the amyloid precursor protein, also known as C99, to produce the Abeta peptide. Recent findings from the Greengard laboratory suggest that PS1 also have anti-amyloidogenic activities, which reduce Abeta levels. First, it redirects APP-C99 toward autophagic degradation, lowering the amount that can be converted into Abeta. The protein kinase CK1γ2 phosphorylates PS1 at Ser367. Phosphorylated PS1 at this position interacts with Annexin A2, which, in turn, interacts with the lysosomal *N*-ethylmaleimide-sensitive factor attachment protein receptor (SNARE) Vamp8. Annexin A2 facilitates the binding of Vamp8 to the autophagosomal SNARE Syntaxin 17 to modulate the fusion of autophagosomes with lysosomes. Thus, PS1 phosphorylated at Ser367 has an anti-amyloidogenic function, promoting autophagosome-lysosome fusion and increasing C99 degradation.

Second, it enhances the ability of microglia to phagocyte and degrade extracellular Abeta oligomer, through regulating the expression of the lysosomal master regulator TFEB. Thus, PS1 has a role in both the production and the clearance of Abeta. Drugs

Advances in Pharmacology, Volume 90
ISSN 1054-3589
https://doi.org/10.1016/bs.apha.2020.09.010

designed to activate CK1γ2 and increase the level of PS1 phosphorylated at Ser367 should be useful in the treatment of Alzheimer's disease.

Abbreviations

Aβ amyloid beta
AD Alzheimer's disease
ANXA2 annexin A2
APP amyloid precursor protein
CK1 casein kinase 1
CK1γ2 casein kinase 1 gamma 2
CMA chaperone mediated autophagy
EOAD early onset Alzheimer's disease
ER endoplasmic reticulum
FACS fluorescence assisted cell sorting
FAD familial Alzheimer's disase
GWAS genetic wide association studies
PS presenilins
PS1 presenilin 1
PS2 presenilin 2
STX17 syntaxin 17
TFEB transcription factor EB
TMD transmembrane domain
VAMP8 vesicle associated membrane protein 8
WT wild type

1. Introduction

A working session with Paul Greengard started with the question "Why did you do that?" At the beginning, it was disconcerting, as you will think he should know the answer. It took me several working sessions to understand he feigned ignorance because he wanted to see if you understood the question you were trying to solve, and took a bottom up approach, building the problem from the beginning, and following a rigorous logic based on the results. "Why did you do that?" meant what was the problem to be solved and what was the approach you tried. In my case, the project of PS1 was rooted on results from the Greengard lab that the protein kinase CK1 modulates the levels of beta-amyloid (Flajolet et al., 2007) and the clinical observation that the protein kinase CK1 is highly expressed in Alzheimer's disease (Yasojima, Kuret, DeMaggio, McGeer, & McGeer, 2000). The surprising conclusion of our work, which we kept discussing until his passing, was that PS1 was as responsible for the creation of beta-amyloid as for its destruction, an emerging principle that has not being widely recognized. In the following pages, we will summarize the evidence for the anti-amyloidogenic activities of PS1, and the evolving role of PS1 in neurodegeneration.

2. Alzheimer's disease

Alzheimer's disease (AD) is the leading age-related dementia, affecting over 44 million people worldwide. Current therapies help mask the symptoms of AD, but do not treat the underlying disease. Several promising drug candidates have failed in late-stage clinical trials (Doody et al., 2013, 2014; Relkin et al., 2017; Salloway et al., 2014). Hence, there is an urgent need to improve our understanding of the basic mechanisms that drive the development of AD.

AD is characterized by intracellular and extracellular deposits of beta-amyloid (Gouras et al., 2000), Tau (Brion, Passareiro, Nunez, & Jacqueline Flament-Durand, 1985), and intracellular deposits of APP-C99 (Lauritzen et al., 2012; Pulina, Hopkins, Haroutunian, Greengard, & Bustos, 2020). The beta-Amyloid peptide is generated through sequential proteolysis of the Amyloid Precursor Protein (APP), first by the action of β-secretase, generating APP-C99 and then by the PS1 enzyme in the γ-secretase complex.

Mutations in the intramembrane protease PS1 are responsible for about 70% of the early onset familial AD cases. PS1 was first identified by genetic linkage of families with early onset Alzheimer's disease (Sherrington et al., 1995). In the first milestone, five mutations were detected that mapped to the gene coding for PS1. Shortly after, another gene linked to AD was identified that code for Presenilin 2 (PS2) (Levy-Lahad et al., 1995; Rogaev et al., 1995). In the year 2000, by using a covalent transition state analogue, Presenilin was shown to be the active subunit of the γ-secretase complex (Esler et al., 2000; Li et al., 2000). Presenilins have two homologs, PS1 and PS2, with 67% homology. PS1 and PS2 are multipass transmembrane proteins with nine TMDs (Doan et al., 1996; Laudon et al., 2005). Upon assembly of the heterotetramer in early biosynthetic compartments of the secretory pathway, the PS subunit undergoes autoproteolytic cleavage within the large loop between transmembrane domains 6 and 7, resulting in the active protease complex. These fragments form a stable heterodimer in a ratio of one to one (Selkoe & Wolfe, 2007).

3. How does PS1 produce Abeta species?

To date, 149 membrane proteins have been described as γ-secretase substrates (Güner & Lichtenthaler, 2020; Haapasalo & Kovacs, 2011). Nearly all of them require a prior cleavage, commonly by α- or β-secretases to yield a shorter fragment, before they can be subject to intramembrane proteolysis by γ-secretase. In the case of APP, it is first cleaved by β-secretase, giving rise to APP-C99. APP-C99 enters the active site, being cleaved at the called E site by the γ-secretase endopeptidase activity, which gives rise to Aβ peptides ranging in size from 37 to 49 residues. If cleaved at Aβ49, it follows a processive cleavage by γ-secretase carboxipeptidase activity, which by unwinding its helical transmembrane domain in a stepwise fashion can be further truncated by about three amino acids. Thus, if first cleaved at Aβ49, it will be processed to Aβ46, Aβ43, Aβ40 and Aβ37, whereas if it is first cleaved at Aβ48, it will be processed to Aβ45, Aβ42 and Aβ39 (Funamoto et al., 2004; Okochi et al., 2013).

Longer forms of Aβ, containing a longer hydrophobic transmembrane domain, might be more likely to be retained in the active site of the protease, whereas the shorter forms are more likely to be released (Szaruga et al., 2017).

To date, 316 mutations map to the PSEN1 gene, and 56 map to the PSEN2 gene ("Alzforum.org/mutations", 2020; Kelleher & Shen, 2017). A common consequence of a Presenilin associated EOAD mutation is an increase in the ratio of Aβ42/Aβ40. As the EOAD mutation lowers the proteolytic activity, it fails to progress to the more soluble species, destabilizing the interaction with the substrate, giving rise to more pathogenic, insoluble species and increasing the Aβ42/Aβ40 ratio.

4. Role of PS1 in neurodegeneration

One of the major gaps in our understanding of AD is how PS1 contributes to neurodegeneration.

To date, two leading opposing hypothesis are:

1. The Amyloid hypothesis, proposes that beta-amyloid is toxic to neurons. PS1 contributes to neurodegeneration by synthesizing the toxic peptide beta-amyloid (Hardy & Higgins, 1992; Hardy & Selkoe, 2002). Thus, PS1 causes neurodegeneration through a "gain of function" change in the proteolytic activity, which induces the synthesis of more beta-amyloid.

2. The Presenilin hypothesis, proposes that a loss of function of PS1 leads to neurodegeneration (Saura et al., 2004; Zhang et al., 2009). According to this hypothesis, PS1 is necessary for neuronal survival, and in the course of the disease, PS1 suffers a loss of function, which results in neuronal death.

If hypothesis 1 is true, drugs designed to inhibit PS1 catalytic activity and lower Abeta levels should be useful in the cure of AD. However, if hypothesis 2 is true, it could be expected that g-secretase inhibitors will worsen the disease.

For several years, pharmaceutical companies have been pursuing inhibitors or modulators of γ-secretase to decrease its catalytic activity (Coric et al., 2015; De Strooper, 2014). In all cases, clinical trials were stopped before completion because of unacceptable toxicity or did not achieve statistical significance in improving the symptoms (Coric et al., 2015; Doody et al., 2013). Hence, it is very important to understand fully the mechanism by which PS1 dysfunction leads to neurodegeneration.

5. Role of PS1 in autophagy

Besides its role as the catalytic subunit of the γ-secretase complex, PS1 has been shown to have non-catalytic functions. Here, we will review the evidence about its role in autophagy. Although autophagy was first described more than 50 years ago (De Duve, 1963), only recently the molecular mechanisms involved in its regulation have been successfully investigated including the Greengard lab (Hernandez et al., 2012; Klionsky & Emr, 2000; Liu, Zhi, & Zhong, 2015; Moreau, Renna, & Rubinsztein, 2013; Tian, Chang, Fan, Flajolet, & Greengard, 2013).

It is now broadly accepted that defects in autophagy are at the core of neurodegenerative diseases, and the last 10 years have seen a great increase in research devoted to understand the mechanisms leading to autophagy dysfunction (Hernandez et al., 2012; Liu et al., 2015; Neely, Green, & LaFerla, 2011; Tang et al., 2014; Wolfe et al., 2013).

Autophagy is an intracellular degradative system that delivers a variety of cellular components, organelles and pathogens for degradation and recycling into the lysosome (Klionsky & Emr, 2000). There are three types of autophagy. Macroautophagy, which refers to the delivery of autophagic cargo to lysosomes inside double membrane vesicles, known as autophagosomes, is the best characterized form. Stepwise maturation of autophagosomes culminates in the degradation of sequestered substrates in lysosomes. Recently, it has emerged that there is a selectivity to the autophagic degradation. For instance, a specific type of autophagy known as chaperone mediated autophagy (CMA), in which cytosolic proteins enter lysosomes for degradation through a protein translocation system at the lysosomal membrane.

Other examples of selective autophagy, also known as microphagy, is the uptake and degradation of specific organelles, like mitochondria (Mitophagy) (Youle & Narendra, 2011), lipophagy (Liu & Czaja, 2013), ribophagy (Ossareh-Nazari et al., 2010) and aggrephagy (Yamamoto & Simonsen, 2011). Little is known about the molecules mediating this selectivity.

The process of autophagy has been shown to be defective in AD (Boland et al., 2008; Mizushima, Levine, Cuervo, & Klionsky, 2008; Nixon et al., 2005; Wolfe et al., 2013; Wong & Cuervo, 2010; Yu et al., 2004).

It has been experimentally demonstrated that PS1 holoprotein helps to maintain lysosomal acidity by serving as a chaperone in the ER for the vATPase V0a1, a subunit of the proton pump responsible for the acidification of lysosomes (Lee et al., 2015, 2010). Binding of PS1 to V0a1 in the ER facilitates V0a1 glycosylation, a required modification for ER exit. In PS1-deficient cells the vATPase V01a subunit is poorly glycosylated and unstable, which prevents proper assembly and function of the multisubunit vATPase pump, resulting in reduced acidification of lysosomes and defective autophagy (Lee et al., 2015, 2010; Wolfe et al., 2013).

In agreement with these findings, several lysosomal defects and dysfunctional autophagy have been shown to associate with loss of presenilin or affected by FAD mutations (Boland et al., 2008; Bustos, Pulina, Bispo, et al., 2017; Neely et al., 2011; Nixon et al., 2005; Wong & Cuervo, 2010).

Taken together, these findings indicate that PS1 deletion or PS1 FAD mutations cause lysosomal and autophagy deficits that contribute to abnormal cellular calcium homeostasis.

We have uncovered a novel way in which PS1 affects autophagy. Our group found that phosphorylation of PS1-Ser367 serves as a switch to induce the autophagy-mediated degradation of APP-C99, which results in reduced Abeta levels.

When the protein kinase CK1γ2 phosphorylates PS1 at Ser367, it binds Annexin A2 (AnxA2), which then is able to bind the lysosomal Snare protein Vamp8, which in turn binds the autophagosomal Snare Stx17 to promote autophagosome/lysosome fusion, in a process that enhances the degradation of APP-C99. Thus, a potential mechanism by which a mutation

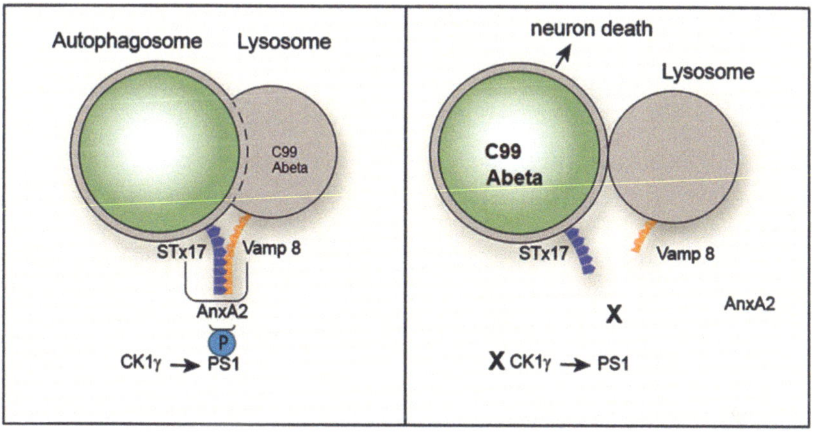

Fig. 1 PS1, phosphorylated at Ser367 by the protein kinase CK1γ2, interacts with AnxA2, which in turn promotes autophagosome/lysosome fusion through its interaction with Vamp8/Stx17. In absence of Ps1 phosphorylation, there is an increase in the levels of APP-C99 and Abeta.

in PS1 that affects autophagosome/lysosome fusion in partial or incomplete SNARE pair complex formation.

Loss of the scaffolding function of PS1 results in decreased autophagic degradation of beta-amyloid, leading to its accumulation. Together, the results suggest that the accumulation of beta-amyloid is the result of a dysfunctional autophagic pathway caused by the loss of PS1 phosphorylation.

Thus, the loss of autophagic function of PS1 induces a gain of a toxic function resulting in loss of lysosomal function, increased levels of APP-C99 and beta-amyloid, leading to neurodegeneration (Bustos, Pulina, Bispo, et al., 2017; Bustos, Pulina, Kelahmetoglu, et al., 2017) (Fig. 1).

If this hypothesis is true, then γ-secretase inhibitors directed at lowering the catalytic activity of PS1 would not address the underlying problem of a dysfunctional degradation pathway, and those drugs will not be disease modifying.

6. Role of PS1 in regulation of APP-C99 levels

PS1 cleaves APP-C99 to produce Abeta and directs APP-C99 toward autophagic degradation. Both activities have as outcome a reduction of APP-C99 levels. It appears that the main function of PS1 is to keep low levels of APP-C99, rather than producing Abeta. Indeed, findings from different laboratories, including ours, seem to suggest that APP-C99, rather than Abeta, may be the toxic species in Alzheimer's disease. In support of this hypothesis, it has been found that APP-C99 accumulates selectively in vulnerable neurons in postmortem brain samples of sporadic AD patients and in mouse models of genetic AD (Bourgeois et al., 2018; Kim et al., 2016; Kwart et al., 2019; Lauritzen et al., 2016). Interestingly, recent findings suggest that APP-C99 is responsible for lysosomal dysfunction in Down syndrome (Jiang et al., 2019).

7. Role of PS1 in microglial degradation of Abeta oligomers

GWAS and systems-biology approaches have identified an unexpected role of the microglial immune response as a dominant factor in AD risk. Several genes that increase the risk for AD are expressed mainly in microglia, for instance, TREM2, CD33, CR1 (Griciuc et al., 2013; Guerreiro et al., 2013; Hollingworth et al., 2011; Karch & Goate, 2015).

Microglia has an important role in the clearance of beta-amyloid plaques. Based on our results showing an effect of PS1 in lysosomal function, we decided to analyze the role of PS1 in microglial function. Microglia FACS sorted from wt and PS1-S367A mice were challenged with soluble Aβ oligomers to evaluate uptake and degradation of Aβ. While PS1-S367A derived microglia showed Aβ oligomer uptake rates similar to those seen in WT microglia, they displayed an impaired capacity for Aβ oligomer degradation. These effects correlated with an accumulation of lysosomes containing undigested material, elevated lysosomal pH and autophagic impairment (Ledo et al., 2020).

Next generation sequencing analysis revealed that many genes related to the autophagic-lysosomal pathway were perturbed by the PS1-S367A mutation. Interestingly, the TFEB, a master regulator of lysosome biogenesis and autophagy, was reduced. TFEB mRNA levels is decreased in PS1-Ser367A derived microglial cells compared to WT microglia. Therefore, we sought to rescue the phenotype by overexpressing TFEB in WT and PS1-Ser367A microglia and evaluate *v-ATP6v0a1* mRNA levels and lysosomal pH. Our data showed that the overexpression of TFEB in PS1-Ser367A microglia increased *v-ATP6v0a1* mRNA levels and normalized lysosomal pH. These results suggest that TFEB acts downstream of PS1 and regulates transcriptional changes related to v-atpases and consequently lysosomal acidification (Fig. 2). A recent report indicates that PS1 knock-out or FAD mutations downregulate TFEB function (Reddy et al., 2016), and a

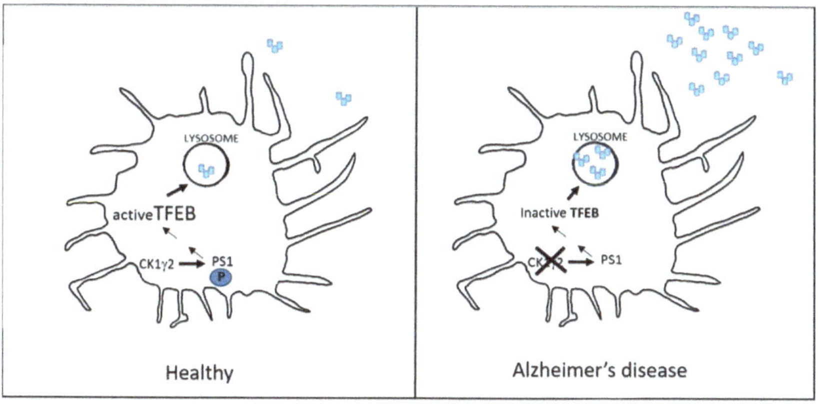

Fig. 2 CK1γ2 phosphorylates PS1 at Ser367. Phosphorylated PS1 induces, through an unknown mechanism, the expression of active TFEB. TFEB allows the lysosomal degradation of beta-amyloid oligomers, depicted as light blue cylinders. In pathological condition, PS1 fails to be phosphorylated, decreasing the levels of active TFEB, causing an accumulation of Abeta oligomers.

conditional TFEB knockout mouse developed increased Abeta and Tau levels (Reddy et al., 2016; Xu et al., 2020). The mechanism by which PS1 regulates TFEB remains to be elucidated.

8. Conclusion

The classical, well-studied amyloidogenic activity of PS1 cleaves APP-C99 to produce Abeta peptides of different lengths. In contrast, the anti-amyloidogenic activities of PS1 depend on its non-catalytic activities. On one hand, it facilitates the autophagic degradation of APP-C99, on a process that depends on phosphorylation at Ser367. This same phosphorylation is responsible for increasing the microglial clearance of soluble beta-amyloid oligomers, on a process dependent on modulation of the transcription factor TFEB. Both activities, the amyloidogenic and the autophagic induction of APP-C99 degradation, despite opposite effects on beta-amyloid levels have for effect reducing APP-C99 levels.

In summary, PS1 has an anti-amyloidogenic activity, manifested by its role in the degradation of C99 in a γ-secretase independent fashion and by modulation of the amyloid phagocytic activity of microglia.

Consideration of the effects of PS1 mutations in the anti-amyloidogenic activity of PS1 is necessary to obtain a complete picture of the role of PS1 in neurodegeneration. Future studies should analyze the effect of common early onset disease mutations on the anti-amyloidogenic activities of PS1.

Acknowledgments

We thank the Fisher Foundation for Alzheimer's research for funding this work, Ana Jedlicki for proofreading and editing and Dr. Ralph Nixon for critical reading and suggestions. This paper is dedicated to the memory of Paul Greengard.

Conflict of interest

No conflicts of interest are noted.

References

Alzforum.org/mutations. (2020). Retrieved from https://www.alzforum.org/mutations.

Boland, B., Kumar, A., Lee, S., Platt, F. M., Wegiel, J., Yu, W. H., et al. (2008). Autophagy induction and autophagosome clearance in neurons: Relationship to autophagic pathology in Alzheimer's disease. *The Journal of Neuroscience, 28*(27), 6926–6937. https://doi.org/10.1523/JNEUROSCI.0800-08.2008.

Bourgeois, A., Lauritzen, I., Lorivel, T., Bauer, C., Checler, F., & Pardossi-Piquard, R. (2018). Intraneuronal accumulation of C99 contributes to synaptic alterations, apathy-like behavior, and spatial learning deficits in 3ŨTgAD and 2ŨTgAD mice. *Neurobiology of Aging, 71*, 21–31.

Brion, J. P., Passareiro, H., Nunez, J., & Jacqueline Flament-Durand, J. (1985). Mise en évidence immunologique de la protéine tau au niveau des lésions de dégénérescence neurofibrillaires de la maladie d'Alzheimer. *Archieves de Biologie (Brux), 95*, 229–235.

Bustos, V., Pulina, M. V., Bispo, A., Lam, A., Flajolet, M., Gorelick, F. S., et al. (2017). Phosphorylated presenilin 1 decreases beta-amyloid by facilitating autophagosome-lysosome fusion. *Proceedings of the National Academy of Sciences of the United States of America, 114*(27), 7148–7153. https://doi.org/10.1073/pnas.1705240114.

Bustos, V., Pulina, M. V., Kelahmetoglu, Y., Sinha, S. C., Gorelick, F. S., Flajolet, M., et al. (2017). Bidirectional regulation of Aβ levels by Presenilin 1. *Proceedings of the National Academy of Sciences of the United States of America, 114*(27), 7142–7147.

Coric, V., Salloway, S., van Dyck, C. H., Dubois, B., Andreasen, N., Brody, M., et al. (2015). Targeting prodromal Alzheimer disease with avagacestat: A randomized clinical trial. *JAMA Neurology, 72*(11), 1324–1333.

De Duve, C. (1963). *Ciba foundation symposium: Lysosomes*. Little, Brown.

De Strooper, B. (2014). Lessons from a failed gamma-secretase Alzheimer trial. *Cell, 159*(4), 721–726. https://doi.org/10.1016/j.cell.2014.10.016.

Doan, A., Thinakaran, G., Borchelt, D. R., Slunt, H. H., Ratovitsky, T., Podlisny, M., et al. (1996). Protein topology of presenilin 1. *Neuron, 17*(5), 1023–1030.

Doody, R. S., Raman, R., Farlow, M., Iwatsubo, T., Vellas, B., Joffe, S., et al. (2013). A phase 3 trial of semagacestat for treatment of Alzheimer's disease. *New England Journal of Medicine, 369*(4), 341–350.

Doody, R. S., Thomas, R. G., Farlow, M., Iwatsubo, T., Vellas, B., Joffe, S., et al. (2014). Phase 3 trials of solanezumab for mild-to-moderate Alzheimer's disease. *The New England Journal of Medicine, 370*(4), 311–321. https://doi.org/10.1056/NEJMoa1312889.

Esler, W. P., Kimberly, W. T., Ostaszewski, B. L., Diehl, T. S., Moore, C. L., Tsai, J.-Y., et al. (2000). Transition-state analogue inhibitors of γ-secretase bind directly to presenilin-1. *Nature Cell Biology, 2*(7), 428–434.

Flajolet, M., He, G., Heiman, M., Lin, A., Nairn, A. C., & Greengard, P. (2007). Regulation of Alzheimer's disease amyloid-β formation by casein kinase I. *Proceedings of the National Academy of Sciences of the United States of America*, *104*(10), 4159–4164.

Funamoto, S., Morishima-Kawashima, M., Tanimura, Y., Hirotani, N., Saido, T. C., & Ihara, Y. (2004). Truncated carboxyl-terminal fragments of β-amyloid precursor protein are processed to amyloid β-proteins 40 and 42. *Biochemistry*, *43*(42), 13532–13540.

Gouras, G. K., Tsai, J., Naslund, J., Vincent, B., Edgar, M., Checler, F., et al. (2000). Intraneuronal Aβ42 accumulation in human brain. *The American Journal of Pathology*, *156*(1), 15–20.

Griciuc, A., Serrano-Pozo, A., Parrado, A. R., Lesinski, A. N., Asselin, C. N., Mullin, K., et al. (2013). Alzheimer's disease risk gene CD33 inhibits microglial uptake of amyloid beta. *Neuron*, *78*(4), 631–643.

Guerreiro, R., Wojtas, A., Bras, J., Carrasquillo, M., Rogaeva, E., Majounie, E., et al. (2013). TREM2 variants in Alzheimer's disease. *New England Journal of Medicine*, *368*(2), 117–127.

Güner, G., & Lichtenthaler, S. F. (2020). The substrate repertoire of γ-secretase/presenilin. In *Paper presented at the seminars in cell & developmental biology*.

Haapasalo, A., & Kovacs, D. M. (2011). The many substrates of presenilin/γ-secretase. *Journal of Alzheimer's Disease*, *25*(1), 3–28.

Hardy, J. A., & Higgins, G. A. (1992). Alzheimer's disease: The amyloid cascade hypothesis. *Science*, *256*(5054), 184.

Hardy, J., & Selkoe, D. J. (2002). The amyloid hypothesis of Alzheimer's disease: Progress and problems on the road to therapeutics. *Science*, *297*(5580), 353–356.

Hernandez, D., Torres, C. A., Setlik, W., Cebrian, C., Mosharov, E. V., Tang, G., et al. (2012). Regulation of presynaptic neurotransmission by macroautophagy. *Neuron*, *74*(2), 277–284. https://doi.org/10.1016/j.neuron.2012.02.020.

Hollingworth, P., Harold, D., Sims, R., Gerrish, A., Lambert, J.-C., Carrasquillo, M. M., et al. (2011). Common variants at ABCA7, MS4A6A/MS4A4E, EPHA1, CD33 and CD2AP are associated with Alzheimer's disease. *Nature Genetics*, *43*(5), 429–435.

Jiang, Y., Sato, Y., Im, E., Berg, M., Bordi, M., Darji, S., et al. (2019). Lysosomal dysfunction in Down syndrome is APP-dependent and mediated by APP-βCTF (C99). *Journal of Neuroscience*, *39*(27), 5255–5268.

Karch, C. M., & Goate, A. M. (2015). Alzheimer's disease risk genes and mechanisms of disease pathogenesis. *Biological Psychiatry*, 77(1), 43–51. https://doi.org/10.1016/j.biopsych.2014.05.006.

Kelleher, R. J., & Shen, J. (2017). Presenilin-1 mutations and Alzheimer's disease. *Proceedings of the National Academy of Sciences of the United States of America*, *114*(4), 629–631.

Kim, S., Sato, Y., Mohan, P. S., Peterhoff, C., Pensalfini, A., Rigoglioso, A., et al. (2016). Evidence that the rab5 effector APPL1 mediates APP-βCTF-induced dysfunction of endosomes in Down syndrome and Alzheimer's disease. *Molecular Psychiatry*, *21*(5), 707.

Klionsky, D. J., & Emr, S. D. (2000). Cell biology—Autophagy as a regulated pathway of cellular degradation. *Science*, *290*(5497), 1717–1721. https://doi.org/10.1126/science.290.5497.1717.

Kwart, D., Gregg, A., Scheckel, C., Murphy, E. A., Paquet, D., Duffield, M., et al. (2019). A large panel of isogenic APP and PSEN1 mutant human iPSC neurons reveals shared endosomal abnormalities mediated by APP β-CTFs, not Aβ. *Neuron*, *104*(2), 256–270. e255.

Laudon, H., Hansson, E. M., Melén, K., Bergman, A., Farmery, M. R., Winblad, B., et al. (2005). A nine-transmembrane domain topology for presenilin 1. *Journal of Biological Chemistry*, *280*(42), 35352–35360.

Lauritzen, I., Pardossi-Piquard, R., Bauer, C., Brigham, E., Abraham, J.-D., Ranaldi, S., et al. (2012). The β-secretase-derived C-terminal fragment of βAPP, C99, but not

Aβ, is a key contributor to early intraneuronal lesions in triple-transgenic mouse hippocampus. *Journal of Neuroscience*, *32*(46), 16243–16255.

Lauritzen, I., Pardossi-Piquard, R., Bourgeois, A., Pagnotta, S., Biferi, M.-G., Barkats, M., et al. (2016). Intraneuronal aggregation of the β-CTF fragment of APP (C99) induces Aβ-independent lysosomal-autophagic pathology. *Acta Neuropathologica*, *132*(2), 257–276.

Ledo, J. H., Liebmann, T., Zhang, R., Chang, J. C., Azevedo, E. P., Wong, E., et al. (2020). Presenilin 1 phosphorylation regulates amyloid-β degradation by microglia. *Molecular Psychiatry*, 1–16.

Lee, J. H., McBrayer, M. K., Wolfe, D. M., Haslett, L. J., Kumar, A., Sato, Y., et al. (2015). Presenilin 1 maintains lysosomal Ca(2+) homeostasis via TRPML1 by regulating vATPase-mediated lysosome acidification. *Cell Reports*, *12*(9), 1430–1444. https://doi.org/10.1016/j.celrep.2015.07.050.

Lee, J. H., Yu, W. H., Kumar, A., Lee, S., Mohan, P. S., Peterhoff, C. M., et al. (2010). Lysosomal proteolysis and autophagy require presenilin 1 and are disrupted by Alzheimer-related PS1 mutations. *Cell*, *141*(7), 1146–1158. https://doi.org/10.1016/j.cell.2010.05.008.

Levy-Lahad, E., Wasco, W., Poorkaj, P., Romano, D. M., Oshima, J., Pettingell, W. H., et al. (1995). Candidate gene for the chromosome 1 familial Alzheimer's disease locus. *Science*, *269*(5226), 973–977.

Li, Y.-M., Xu, M., Lai, M.-T., Huang, Q., Castro, J. L., DiMuzio-Mower, J., et al. (2000). Photoactivated γ-secretase inhibitors directed to the active site covalently label presenilin 1. *Nature*, *405*(6787), 689–694.

Liu, K., & Czaja, M. J. (2013). Regulation of lipid stores and metabolism by lipophagy. *Cell Death and Differentiation*, *20*(1), 3–11. https://doi.org/10.1038/cdd.2012.63.

Liu, R., Zhi, X., & Zhong, Q. (2015). ATG14 controls SNARE-mediated autophagosome fusion with a lysosome. *Autophagy*, *11*(5), 847–849. https://doi.org/10.1080/15548627.2015.1037549.

Mizushima, N., Levine, B., Cuervo, A. M., & Klionsky, D. J. (2008). Autophagy fights disease through cellular self-digestion. *Nature*, *451*(7182), 1069–1075. https://doi.org/10.1038/nature06639.

Moreau, K., Renna, M., & Rubinsztein, D. C. (2013). Connections between SNAREs and autophagy. *Trends in Biochemical Sciences*, *38*(2), 57–63. https://doi.org/10.1016/j.tibs.2012.11.004.

Neely, K. M., Green, K. N., & LaFerla, F. M. (2011). Presenilin is necessary for efficient proteolysis through the autophagy–lysosome system in a γ-secretase-independent manner. *Journal of Neuroscience*, *31*(8), 2781–2791.

Nixon, R. A., Wegiel, J., Kumar, A., Yu, W. H., Peterhoff, C., Cataldo, A., et al. (2005). Extensive involvement of autophagy in Alzheimer disease: An immuno-electron microscopy study. *Journal of Neuropathology & Experimental Neurology*, *64*(2), 113–122.

Okochi, M., Tagami, S., Yanagida, K., Takami, M., Kodama, T. S., Mori, K., et al. (2013). γ-Secretase modulators and presenilin 1 mutants act differently on presenilin/γ-secretase function to cleave Aβ42 and Aβ43. *Cell Reports*, *3*(1), 42–51.

Ossareh-Nazari, B., Bonizec, M., Cohen, M., Dokudovskaya, S., Delalande, F., Schaeffer, C., et al. (2010). Cdc48 and Ufd3, new partners of the ubiquitin protease Ubp3, are required for ribophagy. *EMBO Reports*, *11*(7), 548–554. https://doi.org/10.1038/embor.2010.74.

Pulina, M. V., Hopkins, M., Haroutunian, V., Greengard, P., & Bustos, V. (2020). C99 selectively accumulates in vulnerable neurons in Alzheimer's disease. *Alzheimer's & Dementia*, *16*(2), 9. https://doi.org/10.1016/j.jalz.2019.09.002.

Reddy, K., Cusack, C. L., Nnah, I. C., Khayati, K., Saqcena, C., Huynh, T. B., et al. (2016). Dysregulation of nutrient sensing and CLEARance in presenilin deficiency. *Cell Reports*, *14*(9), 2166–2179.

Relkin, N. R., Thomas, R. G., Rissman, R. A., Brewer, J. B., Rafii, M. S., van Dyck, C. H., et al. (2017). A phase 3 trial of IV immunoglobulin for Alzheimer disease. *Neurology*, *88*(18), 1768–1775. https://doi.org/10.1212/WNL.0000000000003904.

Rogaev, E., Sherrington, R., Rogaeva, E., Levesque, G., Ikeda, M., Liang, Y., et al. (1995). Familial Alzheimer's disease in kindreds with missense mutations in a gene on chromosome 1 related to the Alzheimer's disease type 3 gene. *Nature*, *376*(6543), 775–778.

Salloway, S., Sperling, R., Fox, N. C., Blennow, K., Klunk, W., Raskind, M., et al. (2014). Two phase 3 trials of bapineuzumab in mild-to-moderate Alzheimer's disease. *The New England Journal of Medicine*, *370*(4), 322–333. https://doi.org/10.1056/NEJMoa1304839.

Saura, C. A., Choi, S.-Y., Beglopoulos, V., Malkani, S., Zhang, D., Rao, B. S., et al. (2004). Loss of presenilin function causes impairments of memory and synaptic plasticity followed by age-dependent neurodegeneration. *Neuron*, *42*(1), 23–36.

Selkoe, D. J., & Wolfe, M. S. (2007). Presenilin: Running with scissors in the membrane. *Cell*, *131*(2), 215–221.

Sherrington, R., Rogaev, E., Liang, Y.a., Rogaeva, E., Levesque, G., Ikeda, M., et al. (1995). Cloning of a gene bearing missense mutations in early-onset familial Alzheimer's disease. *Nature*, *375*(6534), 754–760.

Szaruga, M., Munteanu, B., Lismont, S., Veugelen, S., Horré, K., Mercken, M., et al. (2017). Alzheimer's-causing mutations shift Aβ length by destabilizing γ-secretase-Aβn interactions. *Cell*, *170*(3), 443–456. e414.

Tang, G., Gudsnuk, K., Kuo, S. H., Cotrina, M. L., Rosoklija, G., Sosunov, A., et al. (2014). Loss of mTOR-dependent macroautophagy causes autistic-like synaptic pruning deficits. *Neuron*, *83*(5), 1131–1143. https://doi.org/10.1016/j.neuron.2014.07.040.

Tian, Y., Chang, J. C., Fan, E. Y., Flajolet, M., & Greengard, P. (2013). Adaptor complex AP2/PICALM, through interaction with LC3, targets Alzheimer's APP-CTF for terminal degradation via autophagy. *Proceedings of the National Academy of Sciences of the United States of America*, *110*(42), 17071–17076. https://doi.org/10.1073/pnas.1315110110.

Wolfe, D. M., Lee, J. H., Kumar, A., Lee, S., Orenstein, S. J., & Nixon, R. A. (2013). Autophagy failure in Alzheimer's disease and the role of defective lysosomal acidification. *The European Journal of Neuroscience*, *37*(12), 1949–1961. https://doi.org/10.1111/ejn.12169.

Wong, E., & Cuervo, A. M. (2010). Autophagy gone awry in neurodegenerative diseases. *Nature Neuroscience*, *13*(7), 805–811. https://doi.org/10.1038/nn.2575.

Xu, Y., Du, S., Marsh, J. A., Horie, K., Sato, C., Ballabio, A., et al. (2020). TFEB regulates lysosomal exocytosis of tau and its loss of function exacerbates tau pathology and spreading. *Molecular Psychiatry*, 1–15.

Yamamoto, A., & Simonsen, A. (2011). The elimination of accumulated and aggregated proteins: A role for aggrephagy in neurodegeneration. *Neurobiology of Disease*, *43*(1), 17–28. https://doi.org/10.1016/j.nbd.2010.08.015.

Yasojima, K., Kuret, J., DeMaggio, A. J., McGeer, E., & McGeer, P. L. (2000). Casein kinase 1 delta mRNA is upregulated in Alzheimer disease brain. *Brain Research*, *865*(1), 116–120.

Youle, R. J., & Narendra, D. P. (2011). Mechanisms of mitophagy. *Nature Reviews. Molecular Cell Biology*, *12*(1), 9–14. https://doi.org/10.1038/nrm3028.

Yu, W. H., Kumar, A., Peterhoff, C., Shapiro Kulnane, L., Uchiyama, Y., Lamb, B. T., et al. (2004). Autophagic vacuoles are enriched in amyloid precursor protein-secretase activities: Implications for β amyloid peptide over-production and localization in Alzheimer's disease. *The International Journal of Biochemistry & Cell Biology*, *36*(12), 2531–2540. https://doi.org/10.1016/j.biocel.2004.05.010.

Zhang, C., Wu, B., Beglopoulos, V., Wines-Samuelson, M., Zhang, D., Dragatsis, I., et al. (2009). Presenilins are essential for regulating neurotransmitter release. *Nature*, *460*(7255), 632–636.

CHAPTER ELEVEN

A review of the pharmacology and clinical profile of lumateperone for the treatment of schizophrenia

Gretchen L. Snyder*, Kimberly E. Vanover†, Robert E. Davis, Peng Li, Allen Fienberg, and Sharon Mates
Intra-Cellular Therapies, Inc., The Alexandria Center for Life Science, New York, NY, United States
*Corresponding author: e-mail address: gsnyder@itci-inc.com

Contents

Abstract

Schizophrenia is associated with a tremendous individual and societal burden. The disease is characterized by a complex set of symptoms including psychosis, hallucinations, delusions and related positive symptoms combined with social function deficits, cognitive disturbances and, often, devastating mood disorder, such as comorbid

† Current affiliation: Advan CNS LLC, Tulsa, OK 74137.

Advances in Pharmacology, Volume 90
ISSN 1054-3589
https://doi.org/10.1016/bs.apha.2020.09.001

depression. Management of the disease often requires lifelong pharmacotherapy. However, many pharmacotherapies do not improve all symptoms (e.g., social withdrawal, depression, cognitive deficits) and can be associated with intolerable side effects such as weight gain and metabolic disturbances, motor dysfunction and endocrine dysregulation. Lumateperone (ITI-007, CAPLYTA™) is a novel antipsychotic agent, discovered and developed by Intra-Cellular Therapies, Inc. (ITCI) and approved for treatment of schizophrenia in adults in December 2019. Lumateperone simultaneously modulates serotonin, dopamine and glutamate neurotransmission, three key neurotransmitters implicated in schizophrenia. It achieves efficacy with a favorable safety profile. The clinical development program included 20 clinical trials with over 1900 individuals exposed to lumateperone. The program demonstrated the efficacy for lumateperone in two positive well controlled trials in patients with schizophrenia. The unique pharmacology of lumateperone supports the observed benefits across a wide range of symptoms, including social function and depression, and supports its favorable safety profile. Here, we review the discovery of lumateperone's unique biological effects and its clinical actions in the treatment of schizophrenia.

Abbreviations

AMPA α-amino-3-hydroxy-5-methyl-4-isoxazolepropionic acid
AMPH amphetamine
cAMP cyclic AMP
DOI 2,5-dimethoxy-4-iodoamphetamine
DOPAC 3,4-dihydroxyhphenylacetic acid
EPS extrapyramidal motor symptoms
HVA homovanillic acid
LS Mean least squares mean
NMDA *N*-methyl-D-aspartate
PANSS positive and negative syndrome scale
PET positron emission tomography
PFC prefrontal cortex
PSP personal and social performance scale
SERT serotonin transporter
SSRI selective serotonin uptake inhibitor
TH tyrosine hydroxylase

1. Introduction

Paul Greengard, although principally known as a distinguished academic scientist actually started his scientific career in cyclic nucleotide research as a pharmaceutical scientist at Geigy Research Laboratories in the 1950s. Paul believed strongly in the need to translate academic research into therapies to address disease. But he was also never going to fit into the compartmentalized nature of pharmaceutical research taking direction from an executive more concerned about market share than the latest kinase to be discovered. After stints at Albert Einstein and Vanderbilt University Paul took a post as a Professor in the Department of Pharmacology at Yale and subsequently went to Rockefeller University in 1983 where he remained at the helm of the Laboratory of Molecular and Cellular Neuroscience until his death.

2. Paul Greengard and the founding of Intra-Cellular Therapies Inc (ITCI)

Throughout Paul's career he served on the advisory boards of several pharmaceutical companies such as Synaptic Pharmaceuticals, and he chaired the Scientific Advisory Board of Sugen, being instrumental in the development of the tyrosine kinase inhibitor which became known at Sutent. For a number of years he was a consultant to the neuroscience division of Aventis. However during all this time he had never founded a biotech company and more importantly he wanted the chance to guide its scientific direction. With his former post-doc, Allen Fienberg, the two started Intra-Cellular Therapies in April 2001. Paul began meeting with venture capitalists and a chance meeting with Dr. Sharon Mates led to her appointment as CEO and the third founder of Intra-Cellular Therapies. Veteran venture capitalist Moshe Alafi joined the group as the fourth founder. With a little help in finding lab space at Columbia's Audubon biotech incubator from co Nobel Laureate (2000), Dr. Eric Kandel, Intra-Cellular Therapies opened its doors in June 2002 with a handful of young scientists and a technician. They began working on Paul and Allen's initial idea dubbed *CNSProfile*™ a name used to describe all of the phosphorylation changes that a particular CNS drug might make in numerous brain signaling pathways. The idea was to map all of the changes produced by known antipsychotics and antidepressants. Those changes in phosphorylation that were common to various drugs were thought to illuminate a pathway integral to antipsychotic or antidepressant action for example. The work was a novel way to provide a rational basis to drug discovery in psychiatry as opposed to the chance way in which drugs such as chlorpromazine had been developed in the 1950s. The information gained through *CNSProfile*™ was used to identify ITI-007, later named lumateperone and branded CAPLYTA. From the beginning of Intra-Cellular Therapies in 2002 to his passing in 2019 Paul maintained an interest in all aspects of the company's growth. Today the company maintains a focus on cutting-edge science and novel therapies keeping Paul's vision clearly in mind.

3. Introduction to lumateperone for the treatment of schizophrenia

Schizophrenia is associated with a tremendous individual and societal burden, with acute schizophrenia having the highest burden, as defined as disability-adjusted life years, among 235 unique physical and mental health disorders (Salomon et al., 2015). The treatment of schizophrenia often requires lifelong pharmacotherapy. Because the causes of schizophrenia remain unclear, antipsychotic treatments focus on symptom reduction. Blockade of dopamine receptors is the cornerstone of antipsychotic control of psychosis, hallucinations, delusions, and related positive symptoms in patients with schizophrenia (Howes et al., 2009). However, excessive blockade of dopamine receptors can lead to debilitating adverse effects, including extrapyramidal symptoms (EPS), such as parkinsonism and akathisia, and hyperprolactinemia (Howes et al., 2009). Moreover, antipsychotic medications can also be associated with increased risk for metabolic and cardiovascular side effects (De Hert, Detraux, van Winkel, Yu, & Correll, 2011).

Lumateperone is a novel antipsychotic that simultaneously modulates serotonin, dopamine and glutamate neurotransmission, three key neurotransmitters implicated in schizophrenia. It achieves efficacy with a favorable safety profile. The clinical development program included 20 clinical trials with over 1900 individuals exposed to lumateperone. The program demonstrated the efficacy for lumateperone in two positive well controlled trials in patients with schizophrenia. The unique pharmacology of lumateperone supports the observed benefits across a wide range of symptoms, including social function and depression, and supports its favorable safety profile.

Dopamine neurotransmission is thought to be dysregulated in schizophrenia (Grace, 2016; Howes, McCutcheon, & Stone, 2015). All effective antipsychotics have affinity for dopamine D_2 receptors and reduce dopamine neurotransmission, either by post-synaptic receptor blockade or by presynaptic activation to reduce dopamine release. Antipsychotics that are dopamine D_2 receptor antagonists both pre- and post-synaptically (e.g., haloperidol, risperidone, olanzapine) effectively reduce dopamine neurotransmission by blocking post-synaptic receptors, but simultaneously increase dopamine release by blocking pre-synaptic receptors providing feedback to the cell to release more dopamine into the synaptic cleft. (Nakai et al., 2003) In contrast, antipsychotics that are partial agonists both pre- and post-synaptically (e.g., aripiprazole, cariprazine, brexpiprazole), effectively shut off dopamine release by activating the presynaptic receptors yet also partially stimulate the postsynaptic receptors (Burris et al., 2002). Either approach, on its own, requires relatively high levels of dopamine receptor occupancy, which can also result in extrapyramidal symptoms, such as parkinsonism and akathisia, as well as increased prolactin. Lumateperone uniquely acts as a presynaptic partial agonist and a postsynaptic antagonist at dopamine D_2 receptors (Snyder et al., 2015). By simultaneously blocking dopamine while reducing its release, lumateperone demonstrates antipsychotic efficacy at lower levels of D_2 receptor occupancy than that needed by other antipsychotics (Vanover et al., 2019). Lower D_2 occupancy is associated with lower risk for extrapyramidal symptoms and hyperprolactinemia (Howes et al., 2009).

The hallmark of second-generation antipsychotics is 5-HT_{2A} receptor antagonism combined with dopamine D_2 receptor blockade as it became more fully recognized that 5-HT_{2A} antagonism may enhance the antipsychotic efficacy mediated by D_2 receptor antagonism while reducing side effects (Li, Snyder, & Vanover, 2016). Lumateperone exhibits potent 5-HT_{2A} receptor antagonism with a higher ratio of 5-HT_{2A} to dopamine D_2 receptor occupancy than other antipsychotics (Snyder et al., 2015). Full occupancy of 5-HT_{2A} receptors with relatively low striatal D_2 occupancy by lumateperone at its therapeutic dose is associated with reduced D_2 mediated adverse effects relative to other antipsychotic drugs (Davis et al., 2015; Vanover et al., 2019). Unlike other antipsychotics, lumateperone also inhibits the serotonin transporter, a feature that it shares with the selective serotonin reuptake inhibitor, or SSRI, antidepressants.

Dysregulation of glutamate neurotransmission has also been associated with schizophrenia, yet no currently available antipsychotics address glutamate hypofunction (Howes et al., 2015). Lumateperone indirectly enhances glutamate neurotransmission downstream of dopamine D_1 receptor activation, which leads to increases of both NMDA and AMPA activity (Svensson et al., 2017). Lumateperone is the only antipsychotic drug shown to activate both NMDA and AMPA neurotransmission, perhaps owing to its ability to both modulate D_1 receptor mediated and block serotonin transporter (SERT) activity. These effects may further contribute to beneficial effects in patients with schizophrenia.

Current therapies for schizophrenia also have a number of off-target effects at serotonin$_{2C}$, histamine H_1, muscarinic cholinergic, and alpha-adrenergic receptors. These off-target actions likely contribute to weight gain, metabolic changes, orthostatic hypotension, tachycardia, and other adverse effects (Michl et al., 2014; Siafis, Tzachanis, Samara, & Papazisis, 2018). Lumateperone has minimal interactions with these off-target receptors and has minimal effects on body weight, glucose, lipids, and cardiac function.

4. Pharmacology of lumateperone

4.1 The biochemical pharmacology of lumateperone—A unique combination of receptor binding affinities

Lumateperone, or ITI-007, is 1-(4-Fluoro-phenyl)-4-((6bR, 10aS)-3-methyl-2,3,6b,9,10,10a-hexahydro-1*H*,7*H*-pyrido[3′,4′:4,5] pyrrolo[1,2,3-*de*] quinoxalin-8-yl)-butan-1-one, a tosylate salt (Fig. 1, Li et al., 2014; Snyder et al., 2015). It possesses high affinity binding to several receptors/transporters implicated in the therapeutic actions of antipsychotic medications, including serotonin 5-HT_{2A} receptors, dopamine D_2 and D_1 receptors, and SERT, as shown in Table 1. The binding affinities of several major atypical antipsychotic medications and the antidepressant medication, fluoxetine, derived from the NIMH Psychoactive Drug Screening Program Database or PDSP (http://pdsp.med.unc.edu/), are presented for comparison in Table 1. Interestingly, lumateperone shows few significant off-target binding interactions when tested against a selectivity panel comprised of 70 neurotransmitter receptors, enzymes, transporters, and channels (Snyder et al., 2015)

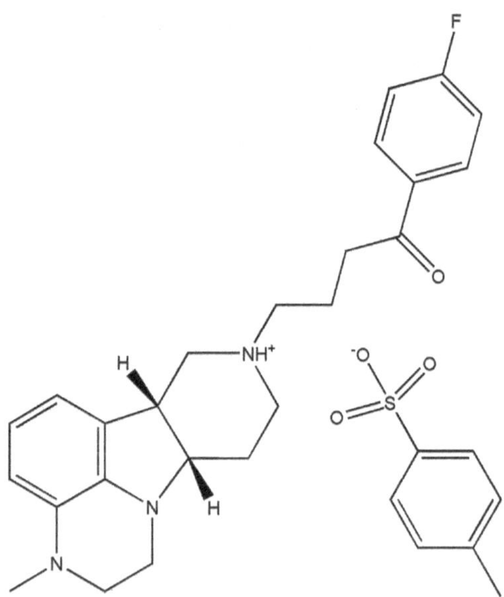

Fig. 1 The structure of lumateperone (also called ITI-007). Lumateperone is 1-(4-Fluoro-phenyl)-4-((6bR, 10aS)-3-methyl-2,3,6b,9,10,10a-hexahydro-1H,7H-pyrido[3′,4′:4,5] pyrrolo[1,2,3-*de*]quinoxalin-8-yl)-butan-1-one, the tosylate salt of IC200056. *Reproduced from Snyder, G.L., Vanover, K.E., Zhu, H., Miller, D.B., O-Callaghan, J.P., Tomesch, J., et al (2015). Functional profile of a novel modulator of serotonin, dopamine, and glutamate neurotransmission.* Psychopharmacology, 232, *605–621.*

Table 1 Receptor binding affinity of lumateperone (ITI-007) as measured by radioligand displacement assays: comparison with marketed antipsychotic and antidepressant medications.

Receptor	ITI-007[a]	Risperidone[b]	Olanzapine[b]	Aripiprazole[b]	Fluoxetine[b]
5-$HT2_A$	0.5	0.5	2.5	9	141
D_2	32	5.9	31	1.6	>10,000
D_1	52	564	128	1170	>10,000
SERT	33–72	>1000	>1000	240–405	0.9–20
Ratios					
D_2/5-$HT2_A$	**60**	**12**	**12.4**	**0.18**	**>70**
Receptor					
H_1 histamine	>1000	14	2	28	1240
5-$HT2_C$	173	63	7.1	130	69
α_1-adrenergic	73	2.3	60	26	2260
Ratios					
H_1/5-$HT2_A$	>2000	28	1	3	8.8
5-$HT2_C$/ 5-$HT2_A$	320	126	3	14	0.5
α_1/5-$HT2_A$	135	5	24	2.9	16

[a]Binding affinities were determined as described in Methods.
[b]Binding affinities for other compounds were derived from the NIMH Psychoactive Drug Screening Program (PDSP) Database (http://pdsp.med.unc.edu).
Reproduced from Snyder, G.L., Vanover, K.E., Zhu, H., Miller, D.B., O-Callaghan, J.P., Tomesch, J., et al (2015). Functional profile of a novel modulator of serotonin, dopamine, and glutamate neurotransmission. *Psychopharmacology, 232*, 605–621.

supporting the conclusion that the compound has high selectivity for key neurotransmitter receptors (serotonin and glutamate) and SERT.

Notably, as pertains to the safety profile of the compound, lumateperone possesses low affinity for several receptor targets that have been thought to be associated with liabilities for certain of the metabolic and cardiovascular complications of chronic antipsychotic treatment with current treatments. For example, lumateperone displays low binding affinity to the 5-HT_{2C} subtype of serotonin receptor, $\alpha 1$-adrenergic receptor, H_1 histaminergic receptor and muscarinic receptors (Li et al., 2014; Snyder et al., 2015) (Table 1). Drug interactions with both 5-HT_{2C} and H_1 receptor interactions have been shown to result in a disrupted metabolic profile leading to obesity and type II diabetes (Kroeze et al., 2003; Matsui-Sakata, Ohtani, &

Sawada, 2005; Nasrallah, 2008). Second generation antipsychotic drugs, in particular, like olanzapine, have potent effects at these receptors and result in profound weight gain (i.e., >50 pounds/year) in concert with elevated plasma cholesterol, glucose, and free fatty acids. Cardiovascular effects of major antipsychotic agents are also a concern; H_1 histaminergic and α-adrenergic receptor effects of these drugs are associated with cardiac liabilities, cognitive impairment, sedation, orthostatic hypotension, blurred vision, constipation, dizziness, and loss of bladder control (Lieberman et al., 2005). Lumateperone displays uniformly low affinity for these off-target receptors compared to most second-generation antipsychotic drugs (Table 1).

One of the most striking biochemical features of both first- and second-generation antipsychotic agents, as exemplified by the data in Table 1, is their high binding affinity to dopamine D_2 receptors in the brain. Functional cell-based assays employing recombinant human serotonin 5-HT_{2A} or dopamine D_2 receptors confirmed that lumateperone is a potent (nM) antagonist at both of these major targets. Notably, the affinity of lumateperone for SERT, an important target for antidepressant activity, is higher than other antipsychotic agents profiled (Table 1) including newer agents, such as brexpiprazole. As stated above, lumateperone separates from other widely-used antipsychotic medications as lacking high affinity binding to certain receptors implicated in major side effect liabilities, namely the histamine H_1 receptor and the serotonin 5-HT_{2C} receptor. Histamine H_1 receptor binding has been linked to profound sedation by antipsychotic medications (Reynolds & Kirk, 2010). Both histamine H_1 receptors and 5-HT_{2C}-type receptors also have been linked to abnormal lipid metabolism and excessive weight gain in medicated psychotic patients (Patel et al., 2009; Reynolds & Kirk, 2010). The low comparative affinity of lumateperone for these receptors is shown in Table 1; lumateperone possesses a high selectivity (i.e., >2000-fold) for 5-HT_{2A} receptors relative to histamine H_1 receptors and for 5-HT_{2C} receptors (~320-fold 5-HT_{2A} /5-HT_{2C} binding ratio).

A final, and potentially key feature of lumateperone's biochemical signature is the high (~60-fold) ratio of binding for D_2/5-HT_{2A} receptors. The potency of the compound toward 5-HT_{2A} receptors relative to D_2 receptors is greater than that of several antipsychotic medications surveyed, including risperidone (~10-fold ratio), olanzapine (~12-fold ratio), and aripiprazole (~0.18-fold ratio). These data suggest that, preclinically and clinically, escalating the dose of lumateperone will fully engage serotonin 5-HT_{2A} receptors before significant dopamine D_2 receptor blockade (and possible motor side effects) is achieved.

4.2 Discovery of novel phosphorylation patterns using the CNSProfile™ platform

High affinity binding interactions of antipsychotic agents with dopamine D_2 receptors are therapeutically important for the management of psychotic features and mania. However, potent antagonism of dopamine D_2 receptors in the striatum (caudate-putamen in humans) profoundly disrupts the normal homeostasis of dopamine neurotransmission in the these basal ganglia structures, and results in persistent and severe movement disorders, known as extrapyramidal movement disorders, or EPS, which limit the long-term utility and compliance for many antipsychotic drugs. Importantly, all first-generation (typical) and most second generation (atypical) antipsychotic agents exhibit liability for disturbances of dopamine neurotransmission and resulting EPS symptoms, including akathisia.

We evaluated lumateperone for its involvement in striatal dopamine neurotransmission using a biochemical method based on the measurement of dopamine-mediated protein phosphorylation sites on key effector proteins in rodent striatum. This platform, known as *CNSProfile*™, used, time- and dose-dependent changes in protein phosphorylation state to gauge activation state of the dopamine system on substrates reporting from primarily pre-synaptic or primarily post-synaptic striatal locations. As an example, tyrosine hydroxylase (TH), the rate-limiting enzyme in dopamine biosynthesis, is located predominantly within the striatum in the terminals of nigrostriatal dopamine projections from midbrain cell bodies. TH activity is controlled by phosphorylation at a S40 residue under the regulation of dopamine D_2 receptors (autoreceptors) expressed on the dopamine terminals (Harada, Wu, Haycock, & Goldstein, 1996); blockade of these receptors by antipsychotic drugs (D_2 receptor antagonists) provides feed-forward signals indicating an absence of presynaptic dopamine availability and strongly increases S40 phosphorylation and dopamine synthesis while D_2 receptor agonists provide a negative feedback signal indicating an abundance of dopamine availability and strongly decrease S40 phosphorylation and dopamine synthesis. Thus, since S40 phosphorylation state of TH is excessively elevated by antipsychotic drugs (e.g., haloperidol) that result in adverse effects occurring as consequence of high occupancies of D_2receptors in the brain (i.e., EPS including akathisia), we reasoned that this site may be used to interrogate the potential of lumateperone for induction of these adverse motor side effects.

A panel of marketed drugs with antipsychotic activity, including lumateperone, were profiled for effects of S40 TH phosphorylation in mouse striatum. All drugs were tested in mice at dose levels corresponding to efficacy in behavioral paradigms used to detect antipsychotic activity (i.e., condition avoidance responding). As anticipated, drugs with potent D_2 receptor antagonist activity, like haloperidol and risperidone, increased S40 TH by several fold, consistent with their ability to block presynaptic D_2 autoreceptors. Other agents, known to possess partial agonist activity at D_2 receptors, like aripiprazole, in contrast, showed little discernible change in S40 TH levels at active dose levels Interestingly, lumateperone, given at a range of doses with in vivo antipsychotic-like activity in mice, had no significant effect on TH phosphorylation (Fig. 2). These data on TH phosphorylation suggested that lumateperone would have minimal effect on the normal balance of dopamine neurotransmission in striatum and minimal effect on extrapyramidal motor performance. We confirmed the hypotheses derived from TH phosphorylation studies using neurochemical measures of striatal dopamine turnover. Similar to its effects on TH phosphorylation, lumateperone had no significant effects on dopamine metabolism, as reported by the ratio of DOPAC metabolite to dopamine (Table 2) whereas, as expected, both haloperidol and risperidone increased striatal DOPAC to dopamine ratio several fold. Importantly, additional confirmatory results were obtained in mouse catalepsy assays; lumateperone produced no observable reduction in stepdown latency (i.e., catalepsy) at behaviorally-relevant doses (Fig. 3), in contrast to haloperidol and risperidone, which are well known to elicit catalepsy at antipsychotic-relevant dose levels. In summary, the biochemical actions of lumateperone at dopamine D_2-type receptors suggest a compound with the functional activity of a partial agonist at presynaptic D_2 autoreceptors. Importantly, the lack of effects of lumateperone on striatal dopamine metabolism and motor performance (catalepsy) conform to those of antipsychotics with demonstrated pre- and postsynaptic partial agonism at D_2 receptors, like aripiprazole (Burris et al., 2002; Nakai et al., 2003) and, more recently, cariprazine (Kiss et al., 2010).

4.3 Behavioral pharmacology of lumateperone

Lumateperone demonstrates efficacy in various animal paradigms associated with antipsychotic activity (Table 3). Lumateperone blocks stereotyped head twitch behavior elicited by the $5HT_2$ agonist, 2,5-dimethoxy-4-iodoamphetamine,

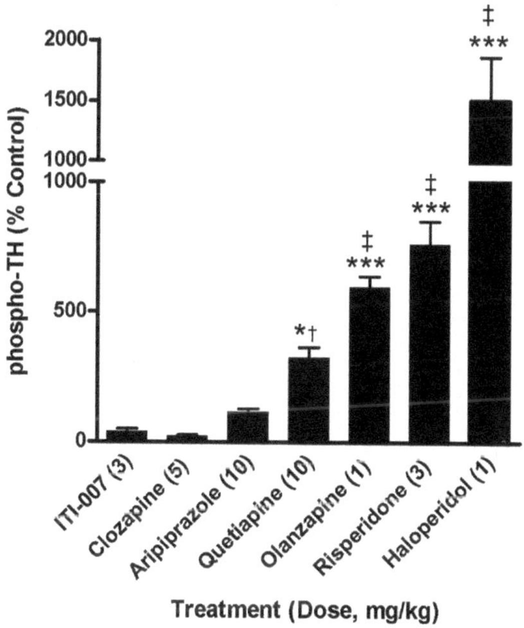

Fig. 2 Comparison of the effects of antipsychotic medications, including lumateperone (ITI-007), on the phosphorylation state of striatal TH in vivo. Mice ($N = 6$/treatment group) were treated acutely with behaviorally-efficacious doses of one of several antipsychotic medications, including ITI-007 (3 mg/kg, p.o.), clozapine (5 mg/kg, i.p.), aripiprazole (10 mg/kg, p.o.), quetiapine (10 mg/kg, i.p.), olanzapine (1 mg/kg i.p.), risperidone (3 mg/kg p.o.), or haloperidol (1 mg/kg i.p.) then killed 15, 30 or 60 min later. The change in phosphorylation state at serine (S) 40 of tyrosine hydroxylase (TH) was determined in striatal homogenates prepared from these mice using Western blotting with a phosphorylation-state specific S40 antibody. Phosphoprotein levels were normalized for the total level of TH in the sample as detected by a pan-TH antibody. Integrated changes in phosphorylation state were calculated, relative to control samples, over the 60 min period after drug treatment for each compound. $^{*}P < 0.01$; $^{***}P < 0.001$ compared with control, $^{‡}P < 0.001$ compared with ITI-007, clozapine, and aripiprazole; $^{†}P < 0.05$ compared with aripiprazole, ANOVA with Newman-Keuls post-hoc test. *Reproduced from Snyder, G.L., Vanover, K.E., Zhu, H., Miller, D.B., O-Callaghan, J.P., Tomesch, J., et al (2015). Functional profile of a novel modulator of serotonin, dopamine, and glutamate neurotransmission.* Psychopharmacology, 232, *605–621*.

(DOI), ($ID_{50} = 0.09$ mg/kg p.o.) consistent with its potency as a functional antagonist at $5HT_{2A}$ receptors. The compound blocks amphetamine (AMPH)-induced hyperlocomotion, consistent with its activity as a post-synaptic dopamine D_2 antagonist with an $ID_{50} = 1.5$ mg/kg (p.o.); lumateperone is similarly active in inhibiting the conditioned avoidance response in rats with an ID_{50} of 1.8 mg/kg (p.o.).

Table 2 Effect of acute (2h) or chronic (21d) daily treatment with haloperidol, risperidone, aripiprazole, or lumateperone (ITI-007) on HVA/DA and DOPAC/DA ratios in rat striatal tissue.

	Acute (2h) dosing				**Chronic (21d) dosing**			
Compound	**HVA/DA**		**DOPAC/DA**		**HVA/DA**		**DOPAC/DA**	
(dose in mg/kg)	**Mean**	**SD**	**Mean**	**SD**	**Mean**	**SD**	**Mean**	**SD**
Vehicle (0)	6.59	0.62	4.58	0.51	7.04	0.41	3.61	0.81
Haloperidol (3)	28.14[a,b,c]	2.08	22.68[a,b,c]	2.80	24.15[a,b,c]	4.89	17.00[a,b,c]	3.94
Haloperidol (1)	31.04[a,b,c]	1.84	19.69[a,b,c]	1.45	29.23[a,b,c]	4.85	18.26[a,b,c]	2.21
Risperidone (10)	23.06[a,b,c]	3.80	30.98[a,b,c]	2.68	36.39[a,b,c]	0.54	25.12[a,b,c]	1.91
Risperidone (1)	30.71[a,b,c]	1.86	14.35[a,b,c]	2.46	29.37[a,b,c]	2.26	16.35[a,b,c]	1.25
Aripiprazole (30)	11.20	0.90	11.89	0.96	12.32[a]	1.30	7.25[a,b]	0.80
Aripiprazole (3)	12.63	1.39	8.57	0.96	12.14[a]	1.71	8.27[a,b]	2.08
ITI-007 (10)	8.40	0.63	6.02	0.59	10.47	2.89	5.80	2.45
ITI-007 (3)	7.47	0.98	4.57	0.48	7.99	1.24	4.54	0.73
ITI-007 (1)	8.06	1.37	4.98	0.80	9.44	4.34	4.69	0.61

[a]$P < 0.05$ compared with vehicle alone.
[b]$P < 0.05$ compared with ITI-007(3).
[c]$P < 0.05$ compared with ITI-007 (10).
Reproduced from Snyder, G.L., Vanover, K.E., Zhu, H., Miller, D.B., O-Callaghan, J.P., Tomesch, J., et al (2015). Functional profile of a novel modulator of serotonin, dopamine, and glutamate neurotransmission. *Psychopharmacology, 232*, 605–621.

Other activities of lumateperone, which likely contribute to therapeutic efficacy, have been explored in animal paradigms. For instance, lumateperone has potent binding activity (70 nM, Table 1) at SERT suggesting antidepressant-like activity. Consistent with this hypothesis, lumateperone significantly reversed the effects of chronic social defeat exposure on avoidance behavior in mice (Fig. 4), an effect that is similar to that seen after chronic administration of antidepressant drugs such as imipramine and fluoxetine (Berton et al., 2006; Krishnan & Nestler, 2011; Snyder et al., 2015). Further, the potential of lumateperone for rapid acting antidepressant activity has been explored. Combination of antipsychotic drugs (like olanzapine) with antidepressant

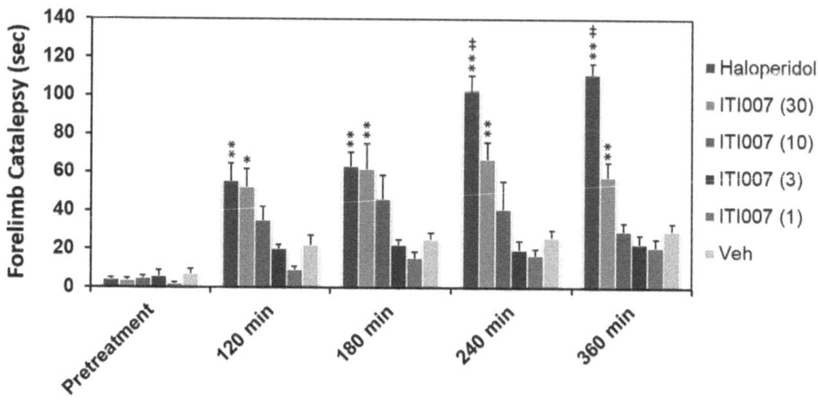

Fig. 3 Comparison of the effects of haloperidol and lumateperone (ITI-007) on motor performance as measured by forelimb catalepsy. Forelimb catalepsy was measured in mice using the bar grip test after animals received a single oral dose of vehicle (Veh) (0.5% methylcellulose in water, 6.7 ml/kg volume) or haloperidol (3 mg/kg) or lumateperone (ITI-007) (1–30 mg/kg) in vehicle solution. Catalepsy was reported in mice ($N = 4$/dose/drug) as the latency (in *sec*) to step both front paws down to the floor of the cage up to a maximum time of 120 s. Catalepsy scores were recorded for each mouse at 120, 180, 240, and 360 min after drug administration. Mean forelimb catalepsy time (in sec) was calculated across each group and time point. Data were analyzed using ANOVA with Newman-Keuls post-hoc test. Data are presented as mean ± SEM. $^{*}P < 0.05$; $^{**}P < 0.01$ compared with vehicle treatment. ‡ indicates statistically significant difference between haloperidol and ITI-007 treatments at $P < 0.01$ level. *Reproduced from Snyder, G.L., Vanover, K.E., Zhu, H., Miller, D.B., O-Callaghan, J.P., Tomesch, J., et al (2015). Functional profile of a novel modulator of serotonin, dopamine, and glutamate neurotransmission.* Psychopharmacology, 232, *605–621.*

Table 3 Functional activities of lumateperone in vivo in rodents.

Behavioral assay—rodent	ED50 (mg/kg, p.o.)
DOI-induced head twitches—inhibition	0.08
5-HT2A receptor occupancy in vivo	0.18
Conditioned Avoidance Responding (CAR)—Inhibition	1.8
AMPH-induced hyperlocomotion—inhibition	0.95
DA release in mPFC	Seen at 3, 10
DA release in striatum	Not seen 3 or 10
Catalepsy (step-down latency)	Not seen at <30

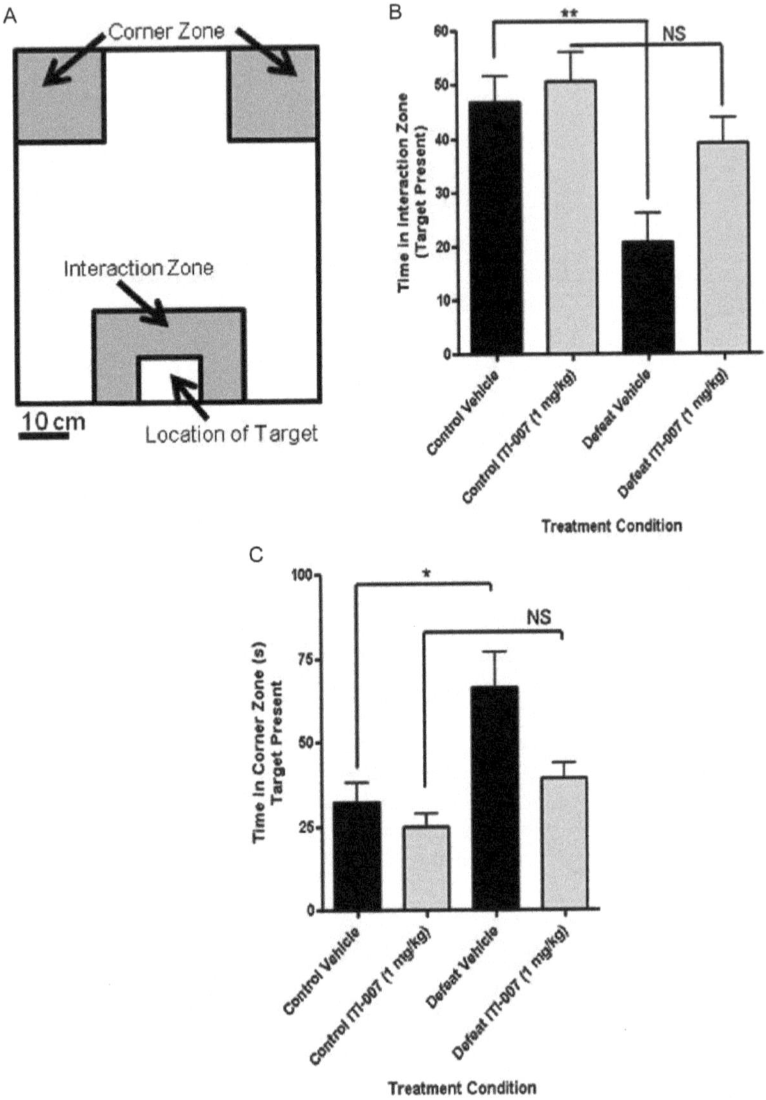

Fig. 4 Effect of chronic administration of lumateperone (ITI-007) on social behavior following repeated social defeat. Mice ($N = 8–12$/treatment group) were exposed to an aggressive resident mouse in the social defeat/resident intruder paradigm (as described in Krishnan & Nestler, 2011). They were then dosed once daily for 28 days, with either vehicle (5% DMSO/5% Tween-20/15% PEG400/75% water, 6.7 ml/kg volume) or lumateperone (ITI-007) (1 mg/kg, i.p.) in vehicle solution. On the day after the last drug or vehicle treatment mice were placed in the open field in the presence of a resident mouse (enclosed in a smaller cage) and the animal's behavior videotaped for 150 s. The time spent by each mouse in specified open-field quadrants, defined schematically in

agents (like fluoxetine) confer rapid acting antidepressant efficacy in animals and in depressed individuals. At the level of pyramidal neurons of the prefrontal cortex (PFC), this drug combination elicits enhanced glutamate neurotransmission in PFC slices mediated by activation of both NMDA-type and AMPA-type glutamate receptors (Björkholm, Jardemark, Schilström, & Svensson, 2015) an effect also seen with application of the rapid-acting antidepressant drug, ketamine (Björkholm et al., 2015). Lumateperone mimicked the actions of both ketamine and the combination of olanzapine + fluoxetine in rat PFC slices, significantly enhancing the conductance of NMDA and AMPA receptors (Svensson et al., 2017). This effect involves activation of a dopamine D_1 receptor, as the effect on glutamate neurotransmission is blocked by the D_1 receptor antagonist, SCH23390. Taken together, the animal data for lumateperone suggested preclinical activity as an antipsychotic agent with strong antidepressant activity and potential for rapid antidepressant benefit.

4.4 PET in healthy volunteers

In a clinical study using positron emission tomography (PET) in healthy volunteers, lumateperone, at a dose as low as 7 mg, exhibited high occupancy of 5-HT_{2A} receptors corresponding to essentially full saturation of cortical 5-HT_{2A} receptors at doses ≥ 7 mg, including the therapeutic dose of 42 mg (Davis et al., 2015). Lumateperone showed dose-related increases in D_2 receptor occupancy through 28 mg, the highest dose tested in healthy volunteers. Brain D_2 receptor occupancy levels were highly correlated with lumateperone plasma levels with extrapolated levels of approximately 40–50% striatal D_2 receptor occupancy at the efficacious dose of 42 mg. Moreover, lumateperone rapidly entered brain, exhibiting peak receptor occupancy within 30 min after a single oral dose. Serotonin transporter occupancy was similar to D_2 receptor occupancy. The goal was to achieve

panel (A) of the figure was determined by video-tracking. The total time (sec) spent by each drug treatment group in the Interaction Zone (panel B) in proximity to the resident mouse or, in the Corner Zones, at a distance from the resident mouse (panel C) was expressed as a mean (+SEM). *$P < 0.05$; **$P < 0.01$ compared with control Vehicle; NS, not significantly different from drug-treated control. *Reproduced from Snyder, G.L., Vanover, K.E., Zhu, H., Miller, D.B., O-Callaghan, J.P., Tomesch, J., et al (2015). Functional profile of a novel modulator of serotonin, dopamine, and glutamate neurotransmission.* Psychopharmacology, *232, 605–621.*

antipsychotic efficacy at the lowest level of D_2 receptor occupancy possible to minimize risk of EPS and hyperprolactinemia, while maintaining full $5\text{-}HT_{2A}$ receptor occupancy with serotonin reuptake inhibition. The data from the PET study in healthy volunteers provided proof-of-mechanism, confirmed the pharmacological action of lumateperone in human brain and were used to select doses for clinical studies. Lumateperone also binds to dopamine D_1 receptors in vitro, but these were not evaluated using PET in the healthy volunteer study due to a lack of a suitable ligand that could discriminate D_1 from D_2 receptor occupancies.

4.5 PET in patients with schizophrenia

To further the pharmacological characterization of lumateperone, D_2 receptor occupancy was evaluated using PET in patients with schizophrenia at plasma steady state (Vanover et al., 2019). At its therapeutic dose of 42 mg, lumateperone was associated with approximately 40% striatal D_2 receptor occupancy, lower than that of most other antipsychotic drugs which typically require >60% D2 receptor occupancy to achieve efficacy (Table 4). The relatively low striatal D_2 receptor occupancy at its therapeutic dose likely contributes to the favorable motor safety profile of lumateperone, with EPS and akathisia rates similar to placebo, and no hyperprolactinemia.

Table 4 Striatal dopamine D_2 receptor occupancy as measured by displacement of [^{11}C]-raclopride by lumateperone or other antipsychotics at efficacious doses in patients with schizophrenia.

Drug	Dose range	Mean D_2RO in Caudate and Putamen
Lumateperone	42 mg/day	~40%
Clozapine	75–900 mg/day	48–61%
Quetiapine	150–750 mg/day	30–62%
Ziprasidone	40–160 mg/day	56 to >59%
Risperidone	4 mg/day	72–81%
Olanzapine	5–60 mg/day	61–80%
Lurasidone	40–80 mg	>65%
Cariprazine	1.5–3 mg/day	69% to >90%
Aripiprazole	10–30 mg	88–90%

5. Efficacy of lumateperone for the treatment of schizophrenia

The antipsychotic efficacy of lumateperone was demonstrated in two positive, well-controlled clinical trials demonstrating statistically significant efficacy as measured by a decrease in the Positive and Negative Syndrome Scale (PANSS) total score by lumateperone 42 mg compared to placebo (Correll et al., 2020; Lieberman et al., 2016). The patient population evaluated in these studies was defined by a diagnosis of schizophrenia confirmed by a Structured Clinical Interview. Patients were also required to meet key inclusion criteria demonstrating a recent onset of acute exacerbation of symptoms at least moderate in severity.

The studies were conducted using a high level of rigor. To ensure appropriate diagnosis of schizophrenia and severity of illness for participants in the trials, both studies included an independent adjudication for eligibility; this entailed expert review of diagnosis and symptomatology by independent clinicians. Efficacy was measured using the PANSS (Kay, Fiszbein, & Opler, 1987), a well-validated, regulatory accepted, clinician-administered measure of schizophrenia symptoms, with a sufficiently large sample size to provide adequate statistical power. The mean baseline PANSS scores in these studies represented a moderately to markedly ill population, consistent with the target treatment population (Table 5). Additionally, patients were experiencing a recent acute exacerbation in positive symptoms. In an effort to reduce

Table 5 Clinical efficacy following treatment with lumateperone 42 mg (Studies 005 and 301) or risperidone 4 mg (Study 005) compared to placebo in patients with schizophrenia.

	Study 005[a]			Study 301[b]	
	Placebo	**Lumateperone**	**Risperidone**	**Placebo**	**Lumateperone**
Sample Size	***N*** **= 85**	***N*** **= 84**	***N*** **= 82**	***N*** **= 149**	***N*** **= 150**
Baseline PANSS Score	91.9	95.1	92.7	90.1	90.1
LS Mean Change from Baseline on Day 28	−7.4	−13.2	13.4	−10.3	−14.5
Effect Size	–	0.4	0.4	–	0.3

[a]Lieberman et al., 2016.
[b]Correll et al., 2020.

expectation bias and control the placebo-response, remote, central raters administered a structured clinical interview and rated the PANSS over a secure video conferencing system. Central raters were blinded not only to type of treatment, but also to duration of treatment at any given assessment.

5.1 Study 005 (Lieberman et al., 2016)

Study 005 was a randomized, double-blind, placebo- and active-controlled, inpatient clinical trial that randomized 335 patients with an acute exacerbation of schizophrenia. Patients were screened for up to a 7-day antipsychotic free period. Eligible patients were randomized equally across the four treatment groups. Intervention was dosed as oral monotherapy once daily in the morning for 4 weeks. Risperidone 4 mg was included as an active control, the most commonly prescribed antipsychotic for the treatment of schizophrenia in the United States at its most commonly used dose. For better tolerability of the active control risperidone and the high dose of lumateperone, a one-day dose titration was used to increase from 2 to 4 mg risperidone and from 42 to 84 mg lumateperone. No dose titration was needed for the 42 mg dose, which was well tolerated from Day 1. Following the last study assessment on the last treatment day, patients were stabilized on standard of care.

Treatment completion rates were high in this study relative to other controlled antipsychotic trials (Lieberman et al., 2005), with fewer discontinuations due to lack of efficacy for lumateperone than for placebo and fewer discontinuations due to adverse events with lumateperone than for risperidone. Importantly, the high treatment completion rates provide additional confidence in the efficacy results due to lesser impact of statistical corrections for missing data.

Lumateperone 42 mg met the primary objective in Study 005 and demonstrated antipsychotic efficacy as measured by a statistically significant greater reduction in PANSS total score compared to placebo at Day 28. Risperidone 4 mg also separated from placebo on the primary endpoint, performing as expected. The effect sizes of lumateperone 42 mg and risperidone 4 mg were similar in this study (0.4; Table 5), and similar to other recently approved antipsychotic drugs, with a similar trajectory of improvement over time.

A prespecified responder analysis was conducted with the proportion of patients meeting response criteria indicated by the clinically meaningful threshold for improvement of at least a 30% reduction in the PANSS total score. Subjects who discontinued were considered non-responders. Lumateperone 42 mg showed nominally significantly greater rates of response relative to placebo.

A secondary endpoint, the PANSS Positive Symptom Subscale, also demonstrated a benefit. Both lumateperone 42 mg and risperidone showed good control over acute positive symptoms with statistically significant mean reductions in the PANSS Positive Symptom Subscale scores at Day 28 compared with placebo.

In a small subgroup of patients with comorbid depression, defined as having Calgary Depression Scale for Schizophrenia (Addington, Addington, & Schissel, 1990) scores greater than 6 at baseline, lumateperone significantly reduced depression with a very large effect size (>1) compared to placebo, unlike risperidone. In this study risperidone failed to significantly reduce depression.

In a post-hoc analysis in Study 005, lumateperone 42 mg showed a statistically significant improvement compared to placebo on a cluster of PANSS symptoms that are associated with social function (Purnine, Carey, Maisto, & Carey, 2000). Risperidone also improved these symptoms, but to a lesser extent than lumateperone 42 mg.

5.2 Study 301 (Correll et al., 2020)

Study 301 was a randomized, double-blind, placebo-controlled, inpatient clinical trial that randomized 450 patients with an acute exacerbation of schizophrenia equally across three treatment arms. Intervention was dosed as oral monotherapy once daily in the morning for 4 weeks. No dose titration was needed for either lumateperone dose. Following the last study assessment on the last treatment day, patients were stabilized on standard of care.

As with Study 005, there were high treatment completion rates for Study 301, with fewer discontinuations due to lack of efficacy for lumateperone than for placebo and few discontinuations due to adverse events. Again, the high treatment completion rates provide confidence in the efficacy results due to lesser impact of statistical corrections for missing data.

Lumateperone 42 mg met the primary objective in Study 301 and demonstrated antipsychotic efficacy as measured by a statistically significant greater reduction in PANSS total score compared to placebo at Day 28. With a similar improvement in symptoms from baseline but a higher placebo response compared to Study 005, the antipsychotic treatment effect size for lumateperone in Study 301 was 0.3 (Table 5). Separation from placebo occurred as early as day 8 and was maintained through the end of the study. The lower dose, lumateperone 28 mg, showed numerical improvements from baseline, but did not separate statistically from placebo on the primary endpoint.

A responder analysis for Study 301 again showed greater rates of response for lumateperone 42 mg relative to placebo, for the prespecified response criteria. Additionally, lumateperone 42 mg met the key secondary objective, demonstrating statistically significant superiority compared to placebo in Clinical Global Impression scale for severity of illness (CGI-S; 1976) scores. These data indicate that the improvements seen by the clinicians represented clinically meaningful changes. Lumateperone also improved positive symptoms with separation from placebo on the PANSS positive subscale. The 42-mg dose demonstrated a significant effect as early as the first week of treatment that was maintained through the end of the study.

Based on the observations made in Study 005, social function was measured prospectively in Study 301 in two ways, a prespecified analysis for the PANSS-derived prosocial factor (Purnine et al., 2000) and the Personal and Social Performance scale (PSP; Patrick et al., 2009). Both doses showed improvements in social function and lumateperone 42 mg, specifically, demonstrated statistically significant separation from placebo in its reduction of the PANSS Derived Prosocial Factor at study endpoint.

Improvement in social function relative to placebo was also demonstrated on the PSP scale. While improvements in the PANSS-derived prosocial factor were centrally rated, the improvement in the PSP was based on expert clinician assessment at the site. The finding of improved social function as recognized by two independent clinicians is noteworthy, especially in as little as 4 weeks of treatment in an inpatient setting. This finding supports the potential of lumateperone to improve a broad range of symptoms associated with schizophrenia.

6. Efficacy summary

Lumateperone demonstrated efficacy for the treatment of schizophrenia in two positive well-controlled trials. The antipsychotic treatment effect size (0.3–0.4) in these studies for lumateperone is comparable to other recently approved antipsychotics, particularly after accounting for publication bias with a standardized mean effect of 0.38 (Leucht et al., 2017). In large meta-analyses, whereas some differences have been noted for efficacy among antipsychotics, treatment response can be largely differentiated based on safety profiles (Huhn et al., 2019).

7. Safety profile of lumateperone

Lumateperone was generally well tolerated in all clinical trials. It can be administered orally, once daily at its effective dose of 42 mg with no dose titration. Many other antipsychotics require dose titration due to limits in tolerability. Tolerability issues have also been associated with nonadherence of antipsychotics (Kane, Kishimoto, & Correll, 2013). The high treatment completion rates and low discontinuation rates attributable to adverse events with lumateperone in the efficacy trials suggest low rates of nonadherence due to lack of tolerability in real world use. In the placebo-controlled trials, treatment with lumateperone demonstrated a safety profile similar to placebo (Correll et al., 2020; Lieberman et al., 2016). The most frequent adverse events associated with lumateperone administered in the morning during clinical trials were somnolence and sedation, which were predominantly mild. In clinical practice, lumateperone may be administered in the evening to offset the risk of daytime sleepiness and be of potential benefit during the night.

In contrast to many other antipsychotics, lumateperone did not induce motor dysfunction, with rates of EPS, including akathisia, similar to placebo. Related to a lack of EPS, there is no need for cotreatment with benztropine to control motor sides effects, a concomitant treatment with its own side effects that is often administered with other antipsychotic drugs. Lumateperone also was not associated with hyperprolactinemia or other endocrine dysfunction. Body weight gain with lumateperone in short-term treatment trials were similar to placebo, as were changes in metabolic laboratory values. In contrast, many of the atypical antipsychotics cause weight gain, dyslipidemia, and changes in metabolic function that lead to Type II diabetes.

Thus, safety data from short- termed controlled and long-term open-label administration of lumateperone were consistent with a favorable safety profile.

8. Conclusion

Lumateperone (ITI-007, CAPLYTA™) is an antipsychotic agent, discovered and developed by Intra-Cellular Therapies, Inc. (ITCI) and approved for treatment of schizophrenia in adults in December 2019.

Substantial evidence of efficacy has been demonstrated with lumateperone 42 mg in two positive, large, randomized controlled trials. Lumateperone exhibits a favorable safety profile with body weight, metabolic profile, endocrine profile, and motor side effects similar to placebo. Somnolence and sedation associated with lumateperone use may be offset by evening administration. Characterized using intracellular assays inspired by the work of Paul Greengard, lumateperone exhibits a novel pharmacological profile and represents a new treatment option for schizophrenia.

Conflict of interest statement

The authors are current or former full-time employees of Intra-Cellular Therapies Inc. a clinical-stage pharmaceutical company engaged in the development of therapies for CNS diseases.

References

Addington, D., Addington, J., & Schissel, B. (1990). A depression rating scale for schizophrenics. *Schizophrenia Research*, *3*(4), 247–251. https://doi.org/10.1016/0920-9964(90)90005-R.

Berton, O., McClung, C. A., Dileone, R. J., Krishnan, V., Renthal, W., Russo, S. J., et al. (2006). Essential role of BDNF in the mesolimbic dopamine pathway in social defeat stress. *Science*, *311*, 864–868.

Björkholm, C., Jardemark, K., Schilström, B., & Svensson, T. H. (2015). Ketamine-like effects of a combination of olanzapine and fluoxetine on AMPA and NMDA receptor-mediated transmission in the medial prefrontal cortex of the rat. *European Neuropsychopharmacology*, *25*, 1842–1847.

Burris, K. D., Molski, T. F., Xu, C., Ryan, E., Tottori, K., Kikuchi, T., et al. (2002). Aripiprazole, a novel antipsychotic, is a high-affinity partial agonist at human dopamine D_2 receptors. *The Journal of Pharmacology and Experimental Therapeutics*, *302*, 381–389.

Correll, C. U., Davis, R. E., Weingart, M., Saillard, J., O'Gorman, C., Kane, J. M., et al. (2020). Efficacy and Safety of Lumateperone for Treatment of Schizophrenia: A Randomized Clinical Trial [published online ahead of print, 2020 Jan 8] [published correction appears in JAMA Psychiatry. 2020 Feb 19;:]. *JAMA Psychiatry*, 77(4), 349–358. https://doi.org/10.1001/jamapsychiatry.2019.4379.

Davis, R. E., Vanover, K. E., Zhou, Y., Brasic, J. R., Guevara, M., Bisuna, B., et al. (2015). ITI-007 demonstrates brain occupancy at serotonin $5\text{-}HT_{2A}$ and dopamine D_2 receptors and serotonin transporters using positron emission tomography in healthy volunteers. *Psychopharmacology*, *232*(15), 2863–2872. https://doi.org/10.1007/s00213-015-3922-1.

De Hert, M., Detraux, J., van Winkel, R., Yu, W., & Correll, C. U. (2011). Metabolic and cardiovascular adverse effects associated with antipsychotic drugs. *Nature Reviews. Endocrinology*, *8*(2), 114–126. https://doi.org/10.1038/nrendo.2011.156.

Grace, A. A. (2016). Dysregulation of the dopamine system in the pathophysiology of schizophrenia and depression. *Nature Reviews. Neuroscience*, *17*(8), 524–532. https://doi.org/10.1038/nrn.2016.57.

Harada, K., Wu, J., Haycock, J. W., & Goldstein, M. (1996). Regulation of L-DOPA biosynthesis by site-specific phosphorylation of tyrosine hydroxylase in at-20 cells expressing wild-type and serine 40-substituted enzyme. *Journal of Neurochemistry*, *64*, 629–635.

Howes, O. D., Egerton, A., Allan, V., McGuire, P., Stokes, P., & Kapur, S. (2009). Mechanisms underlying psychosis and antipsychotic treatment response in schizophrenia: Insights from PET and SPECT imaging. *Current Pharmaceutical Design*, *15*(22), 2550–2559.

Howes, O., McCutcheon, R., & Stone, J. (2015). Glutamate and dopamine in schizophrenia: An update for the 21st century. *Journal of Psychopharmacology*, *29*(2), 97–115. https://doi.org/10.1177/0269881114563634.

Huhn, M., Nikolakopoulou, A., Schneider-Thoma, J., Krause, M., Samara, M., Peter, N., et al. (2019). Comparative efficacy and tolerability of 32 oral antipsychotics for the acute treatment of adults with multi-episode schizophrenia: A systematic review and network meta-analysis [published correction appears in lancet. 2019 Sep 14;394(10202):918]. *Lancet*, *394*(10202), 939–951. https://doi.org/10.1016/S0140-6736(19)31135-3.

Kane, J. M., Kishimoto, T., & Correll, C. U. (2013). Non-adherence to medication in patients with psychotic disorders: Epidemiology, contributing factors and management strategies. *World Psychiatry*, *12*(3), 216–226. https://doi.org/10.1002/wps.20060.

Kay, S. R., Fiszbein, A., & Opler, L. A. (1987). The positive and negative syndrome scale (PANSS) for schizophrenia. *Schizophrenia Bulletin*, *13*(2), 261–276. https://doi.org/10.1093/schbul/13.2.261.

Kiss, B., Horvath, A., Nemethy, Z., Schmidt, E., Laszlovszky, I., Bugovics, G., et al. (2010). Cariprazine (RGH-188), a dopamine D3 receptor-preferring, D3/D2 dopamine receptor antagonist–partial agonist antipsychotic candidate: In vitro and neurochemical profile. *Journal of Pharmacology and Experimental Therapeutics*, *333*, 326–340.

Krishnan, V., & Nestler, E. J. (2011). Animal models of depression: Molecular perspectives. *Current Topics in Behavioral Neurosciences*, 7, 121–147.

Kroeze, W. K., Hufelsen, S. J., Popadak, B. A., Renock, S. M., Steinberg, S., Ernsberger, P., et al. (2003). H1 histamine receptor affinity predicts short-term weight gain for typical and atypical antipsychotic drugs. *Neuropsychopharmacology*, *28*, 519–526.

Leucht, S., Leucht, C., Huhn, M., Chaimani, A., Mavridis, D., Helfer, B., et al. (2017). Sixty years of placebo-controlled antipsychotic drug trials in acute schizophrenia: Systematic review, Bayesian meta-analysis, and meta-regression of efficacy predictors. *The American Journal of Psychiatry*, *174*(10), 927–942. https://doi.org/10.1176/appi.ajp.2017.16121358.

Li, P., Snyder, G. L., & Vanover, K. E. (2016). Dopamine targeting drugs for the treatment of schizophrenia: Past, present and future. *Current Topics in Medicinal Chemistry*, *16*(29), 3385–3403. https://doi.org/10.2174/1568026616666160608084834.

Li, P., Zhang, Q., Robichaud, A. J., Lee, T., Tomesch, J., Yao, W., et al. (2014). Discovery of a tetracyclic quinoxaline derivative as a potent and orally active multifunctional drug candidate for the treatment of neuropsychiatric and neurological disorders. *Journal of Medicinal Chemistry*, *57*, 2670–2682.

Lieberman, J. A., Davis, R. E., Correll, C. U., Goff, D. C., Kane, J. M., Tamminga, C. A., et al. (2016). ITI-007 for the treatment of schizophrenia: A 4-week randomized, double-blind, controlled trial. *Biological Psychiatry*, *79*(12), 952–961. https://doi.org/10.1016/j.biopsych.2015.08.026.

Lieberman, J. A., Stroup, T. S., McEvoy, J. P., Swartz, M. S., Rosenheck, R. A., Perkins, D. O., et al. (2005). Clinical antipsychotic trials of intervention effectiveness (CATIE) investigators: Effectiveness of antipsychotic drugs in patients with chronic schizophrenia. *The New England Journal of Medicine*, *353*, 1209–1223.

Matsui-Sakata, A., Ohtani, H., & Sawada, Y. (2005). Receptor occupancy-based analysis of the contributions of various receptors to antipsychotics induced weight gain and diabetes mellitus. *Drug Metabolism and Pharmacokinetics*, *20*, 368–378.

Michl, J., Scharinger, C., Zauner, M., Kasper, S., Freissmuth, M., Sitte, H. H., et al. (2014). A multivariate approach linking reported side effects of clinical antidepressant and antipsychotic trials to in vitro binding affinities. *European Neuropsychopharmacology*, *24*(9), 1463–1474. https://doi.org/10.1016/j.euroneuro.2014.06.013.

Nakai, S., Hirose, T., Uwahodo, Y., Imaoka, T., Okazaki, H., Miwa, T., et al. (2003). Diminished catalepsy and dopamine metabolism distinguish aripiprazole from haloperidol or risperidone. *European Journal of Pharmacology*, *472*, 89–97.

Nasrallah, H. A. (2008). Atypical antipsychotic-induced metabolic side effects: Insights from receptor-binding profiles. *Molecular Psychiatry*, *13*, 27–35.

Patel, J. K., Buckley, P. F., Woolson, S., Hamer, R. M., McEvoy, J. P., Perkins, D. O., et al. (2009). Metabolic profiles of second-generation antipsychotics in early psychosis: Findings from the CAFÉ study. *Schizophrenia Research*, *111*, 9–16.

Patrick, D. L., Burns, T., Morosini, P., Rothman, M., Gagnon, D. D., Wild, D., et al. (2009). Reliability, validity and ability to detect change of the clinician-rated personal and social performance scale in patients with acute symptoms of schizophrenia. *Current Medical Research and Opinion*, *25*(2), 325–338. https://doi.org/10.1185/03007990802611919.

Purnine, D. M., Carey, K. B., Maisto, S. A., & Carey, M. P. (2000). Assessing positive and negative symptoms in outpatients with schizophrenia and mood disorders. *The Journal of Nervous and Mental Disease*, *188*(10), 653–661. https://doi.org/10.1097/00005053-200010000-00003.

Reynolds, G. P., & Kirk, S. L. (2010). Metabolic side effects of antipsychotic drug treatment pharmacological mechanisms. *Pharmacology & Therapeutics*, *125*, 169–179.

Salomon, J. A., Haagsma, J. A., Davis, A., de Noordhout, C. M., Polinder, S., Havelaar, A. H., et al. (2015). Disability weights for the global burden of disease 2013 study. *The Lancet Global Health*, *3*(11), e712–e723.

Siafis, S., Tzachanis, D., Samara, M., & Papazisis, G. (2018). Antipsychotic drugs: From receptor-binding profiles to metabolic side effects. *Current Neuropharmacology*, *16*(8), 1210–1223. https://doi.org/10.2174/1570159X15666170630163616.

Snyder, G. L., Vanover, K. E., Zhu, H., Miller, D. B., O-Callaghan, J. P., Tomesch, J., et al. (2015). Functional profile of a novel modulator of serotonin, dopamine, and glutamate neurotransmission. *Psychopharmacology*, *232*, 605–621.

Svensson, T., Dutheil, S., Hendrick, J., Zhang, L., Wennogle, L. P., O'Gorman, C., et al. (2017). Lumateperone uniquely enhances glutamatergic neurotransmission athrough activation of both NMDA and AMPA channels via a dopmaine D1 receptor-dependent mechanism: Implications for treatment of mood disorders. In *American College of Neuropsychopharmacology annual meeting* (Poster #M76).

US Department of Health Education, and Welfare; ECDEU Assessment Manual for Psychopharmacology. (1976). *MD: US Dept of health education, and welfare*.

Vanover, K. E., Davis, R. E., Zhou, Y., Ye, W., Brasic, J. R., Gapasin, L., et al. (2019). Dopamine D2 receptor occupancy of lumateperone (ITI-007): A positron emission tomography study in patients with schizophrenia. *Neuropharmacology*, *44*, 598–605.

CHAPTER TWELVE

Uniting homeostatic plasticity and exosome biology: A revision of the conceptual framework for drug discovery in neurodegenerative diseases?

James K.T. Wang*
Dermalytica Inc., Wilmington, DE, United States
*Corresponding author: e-mail address: jktwang2@gmail.com

Contents

Advances in Pharmacology, Volume 90
ISSN 1054-3589
https://doi.org/10.1016/bs.apha.2020.10.002

Abstract

Neurodegenerative diseases (NDDs) are in need of new drug discovery approaches. Our previous systematic analyses of Huntington's Disease (HD) literature for protein-protein interactors (PPIs) and modifiers of mutant *Huntingtin*-driven phenotypes revealed enrichment for PPIs of genes required for homeostatic synaptic plasticity (HSP) and exosome (EV) function and exosomal proteins, which in turn highly overlapped each other and with PPIs of genes associated with other NDDs. We proposed that HSP and EVs are linked to each other and are also involved in NDD pathophysiology. Recent studies showed that HSP is indeed altered in HD and AD, and that presynaptic homeostatic plasticity in motoneurons compensates for ALS pathology. Eliminating it causes earlier degeneration and death. If this holds true in other NDDs, drug discovery in animal models should then include elucidation of homeostatic compensation that either masks phenotypes of physiologically expressed mutant genes or are overridden by their overexpression. In this new conceptual framework, enhancing such underlying homeostatic compensation forms the basis for novel therapeutic strategies to slow progression of NDDs. Moreover, if EVs are linked to HSP, then their ability to penetrate the brain, target cell types, deliver miRNA and other molecules can be leveraged to develop attractive drug modalities. Testing this new framework is posed as four questions on model development and mechanistic studies progressing from higher throughput platforms to mouse models. Similar approaches may apply to other CNS disorders including schizophrenia, autism, Rett and Fragile X syndromes due to potential links of their susceptibility genes to HSP and EVs.

Abbreviations

AD	Alzheimer's disease
ALS	amyotrophic lateral sclerosis
APP	amyloid precursor protein
Aβ	amyloid-beta
BDNF	brain derived neurotrophic factor
EV	extracellular vesicle
FDR	false discovery rate

FTD	frontotemporal dementia
HD	Huntington's disease
HSP	homeostatic synaptic plasticity
HTT	Huntingtin
mHTT	mutant HTT
LTD	long term depression
LTP	long term potentiation
NDD	neurodegenerative disease
NMJ	neuromuscular junction
PD	Parkinson's disease
PHP	presynaptic homeostatic plasticity
PPI	protein-protein interactor
SMA	spinal muscular atrophy
TTX	tetrodotoxin
YAC	yeast artificial chromosome

1. Introduction

Neurodegenerative diseases (NDDs), most prominently Alzheimer's (AD), Parkinson's (PD), but also Huntington's (HD) and a set of polyglutamine expansion disorders, amyotrophic lateral sclerosis (ALS), and spinal muscular atrophy (SMA), cause escalating human suffering and effective treatments largely absent. NDDs are progressive and manifest over years with a distinct spectrum of symptoms in the cognitive, motoric, and psychiatric realms, with a degree of overlap between the disorders (Van Bulck, Sierra-Magro, Alarcon-Gil, Perez-Castillo, & Morales-Garcia, 2019). With exceptions such as HD, SMA and a small number of familial NDDs associated with gene variants, the vast majority are sporadic with undefined etiology. The inheritable gene variants causing earlier onset or exacerbated disease progression have been intensively studied to reveal a fuller, albeit still muddled, picture of the pathophysiology underlying NDDs (Van Bulck et al., 2019). Therapeutic success has been scant, with disease modifying strategies succeeding only recently in the marketed antisense oligonucleotide drug for monogenic SMA (Neil & Bisaccia, 2019), with HD following in late stage clinical trials (Tabrizi et al., 2019). Drug discovery for NDDs is notoriously difficult, hampered at every stage by the lack of clarity on pathogenic mechanisms and of clinically validated targets. Indeed, promising lead candidates demonstrating efficacy in animal models built on NDD gene mutations (Harvey, Richie, Hoffer, & Airavaara, 2011) have thus far invariably failed in human clinical trials. This has led to reassessments of animal models and their usage, and to calls for standardization of best practices and new approaches (Götz, Bodea, & Goedert, 2018; Howland & Munoz-Sanjuan, 2014; Lutz, 2018; Morrice, Gregory-Evans, & Shaw, 2018; Mullane & Williams, 2019; Perrin, 2014; Puzzo, Gulisano, Palmeri, & Arancio, 2015). In this tribute to Paul Greengard's dedication to basic research with the ultimate goal to develop therapeutics for brain disorders, particularly AD and schizophrenia later in his distinguished career, I will discuss how a database-assisted, human insight- rather than algorithm-driven analysis of comprehensively curated HD literature showed that two as yet unconnected fields of biology, homeostatic plasticity and exosome biology, may be linked to each other and to HD and other NDDs (Wang, Langfelder, Horvath, & Palazzolo, 2017). Recent studies support and extend this hypothesis and suggest that the conceptual framework needs to be revised to address some of the long-standing scientific challenges in NDD drug discovery.

2. Challenges in NDD platforms and animal models for drug discovery

The challenges in drug discovery for NDDs begin with the target for drug screening and on to which animal model to test for *in vivo* efficacy prior to late preclinical development. With the dismal record of clinical failures, some have advocated revamping the process, from moving back to phenotypic from single target screening (Prior et al., 2014; Zhang, Luo, Zhou, Wang, & Zhong, 2014), to developing better animal models that address issues such as age-dependency of NDDs (Sun et al., 2020). Experimental models, particularly in animals, are subject to three forms of validation in drug discovery (Morrice et al., 2018). First is face validity, whether the "disease phenotypes" in the model are related to those in human patients; second is construct validity, whether the genetic or other alterations to produce the models are functionally relevant to those in human diseases; and third is predictive validity, whether candidates that ameliorate these putative disease phenotypes can succeed in human clinical trials. While failures of NDD animal models in predictive validity are partly due to a variety of procedural problems, such as the lack of standardized protocols, reproducibility and appropriate outcome measures, these are addressable as exemplified by the recommendations for HD and ALS (HD mouse models Field Guide at chdifoundation.org; Perrin, 2014), and will not be discussed here. I will instead focus on the closely linked construct and face validity, as no NDD platform fully satisfies either and it remains an actively debated topic.

On one end of the construct validity spectrum are uncommon monogenic diseases such as HD, an autosomal dominant disease caused by dynamic expansions of CAG (coding for glutamine) in the N-terminus of huntingtin (*HTT*) where repeat lengths 40 and higher are fully penetrant and inversely correlated with age of onset (Pandey & Rajamma, 2018). One might expect then that a "knock-in" mouse model of CAG repeats in the endogenous *Htt* gene could recapitulate the human phenotypes, yet such models even with CAG lengths expanded into hundreds show very mild phenotypes that are not practically usable for drug discovery. It is only with overexpression of human transgenes in Bacterial or Yeast Artificial Chromosome (YAC) platforms or of toxic fragments of mutant HTT (mHTT) that measurable phenotypes are obtained (Chang, Liu, Li, & Li, 2015). These phenotypes have similarities to some of the human disease symptoms but by no means fully recapitulate them. Most other NDDs cluster towards the other end of the spectrum where a limited number of genes implicated in rare familial form of the disorders are used to develop transgenic models. True for all NDDs is that the underlying pathogenesis and how it translates into disease symptoms and progression aren't clear, and therapeutic approaches have largely focused on single drug targets and specific hypotheses deduced from limited datasets. Arrival of the "omics" era has generated resources in genomic, transcriptomic, proteomic, metabolomic arena and encouraged a call for a unified approach to utilize them to tackle NDDs as part of a spectrum with overlapping pathogenic processes (Lam et al., 2020), albeit tempered by cautious counterpoint on their ultimate utility (Diaz-Ortiz & Chen-Plotkin, 2020). I will discuss in Section 3 how an effort by the CHDI Foundation, dedicated to developing HD therapies, to uncover unexplored areas of biology and thus potential new approaches for HD drug discovery yielded two such areas: homeostatic plasticity and exosome (or extracellular vesicle (EV)) biology.

3. Systematic analyses of PubMed data reveal links between homeostatic plasticity, EVs and NDDs

The cloning of the HD gene *HTT* in 1993 was pivotal in enabling the discovery of myriad of biological processes in which this ubiquitously expressed scaffolding protein is implicated (Saudou & Humbert, 2016). It also led to the identification in diverse experimental platforms from yeast to flies to rodents a large number of genes (*mHTT*-modifiers) that impact m*HTT*-dependent outcome measures such as cell death, protein aggregation and behavioral deficits. Yet, how expansion of CAG repeats in *HTT* leads to disease is still not clear. In an effort to discover unexplored areas of biology in HD, we developed a hypothesis-agnostic methodology to comprehensively curate the HD literature to first build a database of all *mHTT*-modifiers and protein-protein interactors (PPIs) of HTT, then iteratively analyze these datasets for their links to PubMed MeSH terms and biological functions to uncover previously unknown links to HD (Wang et al., 2017). This effort yielded a database of 1218 of m*HTT*-modifiers and 1619 HTT PPIs, with a significant overlap between the two of ~30% of each (false discovery rate (FDR) of 10^{-131} in enrichment analysis). We then analyzed these two HD datasets and the subset found in both for links to PubMed MeSH terms, published pathways and mechanistic gene sets such as KeGG and Gene Ontology, and confirmed multiple biological areas already known be involved in HD such as oxidative stress, protein processing and inflammation. Statistically much higher scoring (minimum FDR of 10^{-10} was our cutoff for detailed analyses of the hundreds of pathways and gene sets in enrichment analyses), however, are gene sets for biological functions not previously linked to HD, as follows (details in Wang et al., 2017):

3.1 The *mHTT*-modifiers and HTT PPIs are enriched for PPIs of genes required for HSP

The HD datasets contained genes required for multiple forms of homeostatic plasticity studied in both *Drosophila* neuromuscular junction (NMJ) and mammalian neuronal or mixed cultures, and of the 143 genes found in PubMed as of 2015 as required for distinct forms of HSP (presynaptic, postsynaptic, retrograde signaling, glial-neuronal, etc.) in these two platforms, half are also *mHTT*-modifiers and/or HTT PPIs. Moreover, PPIs for 65 of these HSP genes that segregate into eight distinct HSP signaling pathways (e.g. transcriptional regulation in presynaptic HSP; postsynaptic down-scaling; see table S6 in Wang et al., 2017) highly overlap each other, and the sum total of 3782 PPIs for these 65 HSP genes are in turn highly enriched with ~50% of *mHTT*-modifiers and of HTT PPIs (FDR of 10^{-151} and 10^{-243} respectively), clearly supporting a potential biological relationship between HTT and homeostatic plasticity. The first direct experimental support for this relationship is discussed in Section 4.4.

3.2 The *mHTT*-modifiers and HTT PPIs are enriched for PPIs of genes critical for EV functions, and for proteins carried in EVs

EVs are released and taken up at the *Drosophila* NMJ to mediate a specific form of synaptic plasticity (Budnik, Ruiz-Cañada, & Wendler, 2016; Maggio et al., 2019), and all 13 genes required for the release and uptake of exosomes in this specific EV function and 14 other genes required for EV life cycle in mammalian cells are also *mHTT*-modifiers and/or HTT PPIs (see table 1, Wang et al., 2017), and the 892 PPIs for the 13 EV synaptic function genes are again significantly enriched for the *mHTT*-modifiers and HTT PPIs (FDR of 10^{-62} and 10^{-112} respectively). Moreover, ~50% of the *mHTT*-modifiers and of the HTT PPIs are present in a database of 4019 proteins found in EVs (FDR of 10^{-92} and of 10^{-228} respectively) derived from various sources, almost all non neuronal, raising the intriguing possibility that many HTT-linked proteins and HTT itself, may well be carried in EVs, although mHTT in EVs has not been reported. As discussed in Section 6, many pathogenic NDD proteins are found in EVs, possibly for disposal but perhaps also as a route of "transmission" of toxicity. Finally, miRNA carried in EVs are also enriched for those that are differentially expressed in HD brain (table 3, Wang et al., 2017), again suggestive of a link between HTT and EV biology.

3.3 The HSP and EV PPIs highly overlap each other, and the common subset is even more enriched for *mHTT*-modifiers and HTT PPIs

Half of the 143 HSP genes are found in common with the EV synaptic function PPIs and the EV proteins, and 42% of the HSP PPIs (1600/3782) are also found in the two EV datasets (4469 total), and in these 1600 the enrichment of the HD datasets is even more pronounced (see fig S8, Wang et al., 2017). This suggests that EVs play as yet unknown roles in HSP, where retrograde signaling and transcellular coordination are prominent features (see Section 4.1), and that HSP and EV biology, particularly where they intersect, may be involved in HTT biology and pathophysiology.

3.4 The *mHTT*-modifiers and HTT PPIs highly overlap PPIs of other NDD-associated genes, and the NDD PPIs are highly enriched for the HSP and EV PPIs and EV proteins

We then expanded the analysis into other NDDs, including PD, AD, other polyglutamine NDDs, ALS and SMA, with the same strategy of curating

PPIs of disease-associated genes to perform enrichment analyses as with HTT. These NDD PPIs not only highly intersect the HTT PPI (see table 6.7, fig. 5, Wang et al., 2017), with FDR ranges from 10^{-21} for SMA to 10^{-224} for PD, but also each other (see table S11, Wang et al., 2017), with particularly striking enrichment of the PD PPIs (alpha-synuclein; PARK2) and of Tau in the HD datasets (44–57% of each), revealing a surprising degree of overlapping protein interactions between the NDD genes, centered on the scaffolding protein that is HTT (the 118 PPIs of Tau also highly overlap most other NND PPIs). Not surprisingly, then, all the NDD PPIs are also highly enriched for the HSP and EV PPIs, with even more striking overlap for the subsets found in common for HSP, EV, and HD (see table 8, fig. 6, Wang et al., 2017). An example of the degree of overlap between these datasets for the ALS PPIs is shown as a modified Venn Diagram in Fig. 1, note that the largest part of the 328 ALS PPIs is the 110 found in common between all three datasets from HD, HSP and EV (see Section 4.5 for details).

Thus, the large ~350 kDa HTT, well known as a scaffold protein with many interactors (Saudou & Humbert, 2016), forms an interactome enriched for PPIs of genes associated with familial forms of other NDDs. Moreover, these overlapping NDD interactomes also contain many PPIs of genes involved in HSP and in aspects of EV biology, and the high overlap of the latter two in each other suggests possible links between HSP and EVs

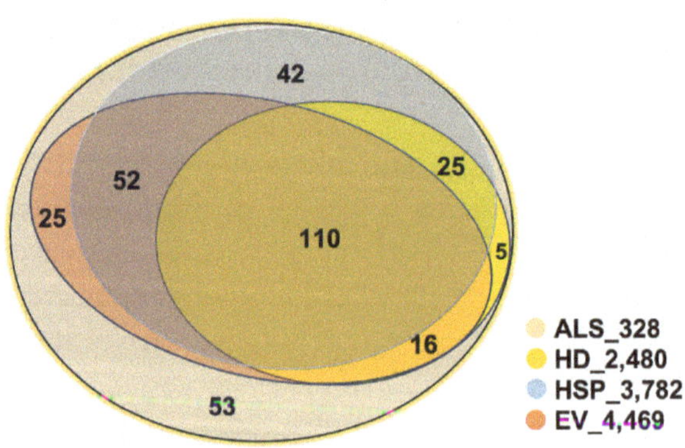

Fig. 1 Intersections of PPIs of ALS genes with the HD, HSP and EV datasets. A modified Venn diagram showing overlap of the ALS (PPIs of *SOD1*, *TARDBP* and *FUS*, 328 total) with the HD (mHTT-modifiers and HTT PPIs, 2480 total), the HSP (PPIs of 65 HSP signaling pathway genes, 3782 total); and the EV (EV synaptic signaling PPIs and EV proteins, 4469 total) datasets. Only genes found in common with the ALS set are shown: 156 from HD, 204 from HSP, and 187 from EV. The area of each set is approximately proportional to the set size, with the number of genes indicated. For example, 110 of the 328 ALS PPIs are found in common with all three other datasets, while 53 are not found in any.

that need to be experimentally verified. In the following sections, I will briefly discuss how homeostatic plasticity and EV biology may be relevant in NDDs, and how newly emerging evidence supporting a role for HSP in AD, HD and ALS suggests a revised conceptual framework for NDD drug discovery.

4. Importance of HSP in NDD: Background and emerging evidence

4.1 Homeostatic plasticity is a key feedback mechanism enabling proper brain functions

Synaptic plasticity is a critical physiological mechanism underlying complex brain functions, and the well-characterized Hebbian plasticity of long term potentiation (LTP) and long term depression (LTD) thought to mediate learning and memory is now joined by the non-Hebbian HSP as a critical enabling feedback mechanism to constrain LTP and LTD from runaway conditions and to enhance network stability (Turrigiano, 2012). Homeostasis as a concept is fundamental to biological systems, where a defined optimal operational range is maintained by multiple feedback mechanisms. Thus, it is assumed that complex neural circuits are regulated and constrained by robust homeostatic mechanisms in order to maintain proper functions even as perturbations escalate (Li, Park, Zhong, & Chen, 2019; Turrigiano, 2012). Detailed studies of homeostatic plasticity as multiple synaptic and cellular phenomenon such as synaptic up- and down-scaling, regulation of synapse number and intrinsic excitability, and the higher order, time domain-dependent metaplasticity that links Hebbian and non-Hebbian forms with a sliding threshold (Keck, Hübener, & Bonhoeffer, 2017; Li et al., 2019), only occurred in the last decade, with a large number of genes shown to be required for HSP on the synaptic and cellular levels (Frank, 2014; Turrigiano, 2012). Two platforms have been particularly productive: *Drosophila* NMJ where a powerful genetic tool kit enabled elucidation of presynaptic homeostatic plasticity (PHP) *in vivo* (Davis & Müller, 2015; Frank, James, & Müller, 2020), and mammalian neuronal cell cultures and more recently in brain slices utilizing genetic tools such as antisense reagents and KO animals (Diering & Huganir, 2018; Turrigiano, 2012; Zhai, Shen, Graves, & Surmeier, 2019). Several general conclusions can be drawn thus far: first, multiple forms of homeostatic plasticity such as PHP and synaptic scaling likely play important roles *in vivo,* even if it is still unclear how they are integrated for normal functions, partly due to the technical difficulties of teasing out the myriad processes in the complex whole organism; second, many of the genes critical for these forms of HSP are also well-known for their roles in Hebbian plasticity, suggesting a level of overlap and complexity in regulation, particularly for the metaplasticity that links Hebbian and homeostatic forms over the temporal domain, that have yet to be fully elucidated (Keck et al., 2017; Li et al., 2019); third, some of the HSP genes are mutated or are variants in neurological diseases, suggesting that disruption of homeostatic plasticity may play a role in neural pathophysiology (see Section 4.2); fourth, it follows that clearly delineated linkages of homeostatic processes to phenotypic outcomes in NDDs, such as behavioral outcomes that might be detectable earlier, will be critical determinants for drug discovery (Hulme, Jones, & Abraham, 2013) and that much more research is required.

As discussed in Section 4.5, a promising linkage between HSP and NDD phenotype has recently been made in ALS, where the primary degeneration is localized in the experimentally accessible and well-characterized NMJ with its PHP. Such linkages are lacking for NNDs rooted in the CNS due to the challenges of specific perturbation of HSP in complex circuits that can be directly linked to phenotypes, but an interesting possibility to consider is the homeostatic nature of sleep. Disruption of sleep and circadian rhythm has been documented for all NDDs (Herzog-Krzywoszanska & Krzywoszanski, 2019; Leng, Musiek, Hu, Cappuccio, & Yaffe, 2019; Zhang et al., 2020). In flies, sleep can be measured by time-dependent motoric assays (Dissel, 2020), and the fly platform has provided the foundational data for the synaptic homeostasis hypothesis (Donlea, 2019; Tononi & Cirelli, 2014), which states that the function of sleep is to downscale or reset the previous wake period's synaptic plasticity so that memory is consolidated and the circuits are reset for the next wake period. Recently, a pivotal study directly linked fly NMJ PHP to sleep, showing that the circadian regulators *Cul3* (a ubiquitin ligase) and *insomniac* are critical for retrograde signaling in PHP (Kikuma et al., 2019). This finding directly connects circadian regulators to PHP in the specialized NMJ for a role that occurs in the postsynaptic muscle. It also potentially expands the relevance of other elucidated PHP genes into CNS circuits that underlie complex behavioral phenotypes to which sleep belongs. The significance of this finding is further enhanced by the ability of mammalian orthologs of *insomniac*, KCTD2 and KCTD5, to directly substitute for its function in regulating fly sleep (Li et al., 2017), illustrating the strong evolutionary conservation of critical functions and signaling pathways from fly to mouse. The use of fly sleep as a surrogate

CNS homeostatic circadian-regulated outcome in the whole organism context is especially attractive given the genetic tools available in the fly platform, and this is further discussed in Section 8—3e.

4.2 Human genetic evidence implicating homeostatic plasticity in neurological disorders

A comprehensive curation of the literature completed by 2015 produced a list of 143 genes involved in various forms of HSP (Wang et al., 2017), which has already grown by the dozens since then. Some of these genes (Frank, 2014) are implicated in different NDDs when mutated or as genomic variants (see OMIM citation of each gene for primary references). Prominent examples include the voltage-gated calcium channel subunit Cav2.1 (CACNA1A; OMIM *601011), the human ortholog of the *Drosophila* gene cacophony that is required for PHP (Davis & Müller, 2015; Frank et al., 2020); polyglutamine expansion in this gene results in the autosomal dominant spinocerebellar ataxia type 6 (SCA6, OMIM 183086), one of nine polyglutamine disorders that include HD, and other mutations are associated with Episodic ataxia, type 2 (OMIM 108500) and Migraine, familial hemiplegic, 1 (OMIM 141500). Recent studies showed that the SAGA complex in glia which includes GCN5 provides epigenetic control over PHP in the NMJ (Wang, Morency, Harris, & Davis, 2020), and in the human ortholog STAGA, polyglutamine expansion in an integral member ataxin 7 results in SCA7 (OMIM *602301). Retrograde signaling in PHP engages transcription factors (Frank, 2014) that include *SMAD* and *PAX* members, and *SMN1* (OMIM 600354), mutation of which causes SMA, another monogenic NDD. These transcriptional regulators at least partly modulate expression of potassium channels of the Kv1 and Kv4 families that together with calcium channels regulate the readily releasable pool of transmitters (Lazarevic, Pothula, Andres-Alonso, & Fejtova, 2013); mutations in *KCNA1* (Kv1.1) cause Episodic Ataxia, Type 1 (OMIM 160120), and those in *KCND3* (Kv4.3) cause the very rare SCA19 (OMIM 607346). On the postsynaptic side, neurons with presenilin 1 KO or AD-linked mutation showed a defective synaptic upscaling in astrocyte cocultures (Pratt, Zimmerman, Cook, & Sullivan, 2011), suggesting a link between HSP and AD, as discussed further in Section 4.2. Recent data on the role of Sigma-1 receptor (S1R) in HSP (see Section 4.4) is another example as its mutation is associated with juvenile form of ALS (ALS16) and SMA2 (OMIM *601978). Thus, although many of these genes serve pleotropic biological functions, their involvement all along the signaling pathway for homeostatic plasticity and the association of their mutations with multiple NDDs suggest that disruption of HSP may be involved in pathophysiology of NDDs.

It should be pointed out that other nervous system disorders have also beenassociated with mutations in HSP genes. PHP signaling also includes the BLOC-1 and SNARE complexes at the active zone; and a member of the BLOC-1 complex has been implicated in schizophrenia (Dysbindin, *DTNBP1*, OMIM 607145). Two genes required for postsynaptic HSP are implicated in CNS disorders related to autism, *MECP2* (OMIM 300005) in Rett Syndrome and *FMRI* (OMIM 309550; Chen, Lau, & Sarti, 2014) in the Fragile X Syndrome and Fragile X-associated tremor/ataxia. FMR1 mutation has also been shown to block the retinoic-acid signaling pathway of HSP (Zhang et al., 2018). Interestingly, among the multitude of MECP2 actions, its deficiency alters HTT and HAP1-dependent axonal transport of brain-derived neurotrophic factor (BDNF) and of Amyloid Precursor Protein (APP), suggesting one more link among the NDDs and HSP (Roux et al., 2012). Recently, a strong link between PHP and a number of autism susceptibility genes have also been reported in the fly NMJ (Genç et al., 2020). In summary, the indirect evidence implicating homeostatic plasticity in multiple nervous system functions and pathologies is increasing and should spur further direct experimental verification and mechanistic elucidation.

4.3 Experimental evidence for a role of homeostatic plasticity in AD and PD

While the focus of much of AD therapeutic development has until recently been on the toxicity of Amyloid-beta (Aβ), much has also been learned about the effects of Aβ on a variety of synaptic functions, including Hebbian and non-Hebbian plasticity. The possibility of homeostatic compensation for degradation in circuitry function in AD has also long been debated (Frere & Slutsky, 2018; Jang & Chung, 2016; Peineau, Rabiant, Pierrefiche, & Potier, 2018; Small, 2004, 2008; Styr & Slutsky, 2018). Experimental evidence for involvement of specific forms of HSP in AD includes AMPAR downscaling in an AD animal model (Chang et al., 2006), Aβ exerting over-scaling (Gilbert et al., 2016), and the role of presenilin in synaptic upscaling (Pratt et al., 2011). There are also supportive data in more complex metaplasticity context, including defective age-dependent metaplasticity of LTP/LTD balance in an AD animal model (Megill et al., 2015); TNF-α mediated homeostatic inhibition of LTP (Singh, Jones, Mockett, Ohline, & Abraham, 2019); ryanodine receptor-mediated rescue of synaptic plasticity deficits (Li et al., 2017); and the altered LTP/LTD balance by the APP intracellular domain (Trillaud-Doppia & Boehm, 2018). Other indirect evidence on the molecular and cellular level include Aβ impacting signaling molecules PLK2 (Lee et al., 2017), SPAR and SNK (Sui, Zhan, Niu, Liang, & Li, 2017), EphAb/c-Abl (Vargas, Cerpa, Muñoz, Zanlungo, & Alvarez, 2018), CAMKII-mediated synaptic plasticity defects and dendritic loss (Opazo et al., 2018), and APP regulating Arc synthesis (Livingstone et al., 2019), all of which are involved in both Hebbian and homeostatic plasticity. Thus, APP and Aβ broadly impact multiple types of synaptic plasticity and functions, and further studies on how distinct forms of homeostatic plasticity may be involved in AD pathophysiology are needed.

Evidence for homeostatic plasticity is less robust in PD, with a few studies on a cellular level and others on the circuity level that infer homeostatic responses in striatal dopaminergic circuits, for example the impact on striatal neuron's intrinsic excitability after dopamine depletion (Azdad et al., 2009); MEF2 and activity-dependent spine loss (Tian, Kai, Hockberger, Wokosin, & Surmeier, 2010) and remodeling (Villalba & Smith, 2018). The homeostatic responses of spinal projection neurons to dopamine depletion in brain slices have been studied and reviewed in (Zhai et al., 2019).

4.4 Experimental evidence for the role of homeostatic plasticity in HD

Direct experimental evidence that HSP is altered in HD was only recently published (Smith-Dijak et al., 2019), where differences in synaptic upscaling were detected in cortical neuronal cultures from WT *vs* YAC128 mice expressing human 128Q-mHTT at 21 days *in vitro* and after 48 h of TTX exposure. At this stage, synaptic upscaling switches from predominantly postsynaptic insertions of additional AMPA receptors to a mix of enhanced presynaptic release and postsynaptic responses (Wierenga, Walsh, & Turrigiano, 2006). In WT neurons, there was a postsynaptic increase of mEPSP amplitude that did not reach statistical significance, together with a robust increase in mEPSP frequency due to formation of new synapses with mixed spine morphologies reminiscent of homeostatic scaling of dendritic morphology and volume to regulate Hebbian plasticity (Hobbiss, Ramiro-Cortés, & Israely, 2018). This latter response is blocked by BDNF, itself a key player in synaptic and homeostatic plasticity and in NDDs (Miranda, Morici, Zanoni, & Bekinschtein, 2019; Watt & Desai, 2010), suggesting that TTX inhibited activity-driven BDNF release. These homeostatic responses were absent in the YAC128 neurons, which are morphologically and electrically similar to

TTX-treated WT neurons, suggesting that upscaling is already induced by mHTT and/or it is occluded from responding to inactivity. Interestingly, pridopidine and 3PP, agonists of Sigma-1 receptor (S1R) which upregulates the BDNF pathway and stabilizes ER calcium levels, restored homeostatic responses in YAC128 neurons, indicating that the mHTT effects can be reversed and that S1R may be involved in calcium-dependent aspects of synaptic scaling. This is the first report at the cellular level of the impact of *HTT* expansion on HSP, and supports the likely impact of mHTT on homeostatic plasticity in the direct and indirect spiny projection neuronal pathways at the network level (Plotkin & Surmeier, 2015). These promising studies need to be extended to include other forms of HSP at the cell culture level, including the use of other HD animal models and co-culturing with glia to study its known effects on neuronal HSP, and at the fly NMJ presynaptic level *in vivo*. As discussed in Section 5, such studies will be the first to validate the role of HSP in a new NDD drug discovery framework. Finally, *S1R* mutations are implicated in juvenile form of ALS (ALS16) and SMA2 (OMIM *601978), and its removal from the *SOD1* mutant ALS model worsened the neurodegeneration and survival (Mavlyutov, Guo, Epstein, & Ruoho, 2015), further supporting an underlying link to HSP dysfunctions in multiple forms of NDDs.

4.5 Experimental evidence for the role of homeostatic plasticity in ALS

HSP has also been experimentally implicated in ALS. At the time of our 2014 analysis, only 3 genes (*SOD1*, *TARDBP*, and *FUS*) are most commonly associated with familial forms of ALS and possess significant number of PPIs, generating a total of 328 PPIs which significantly intersected with the HD, HSP and EV datasets (Fig. 1 Venn Diagram; FDR of 10^{-55}, 10^{-100}, and 10^{-61} respectively, with 110 of 328 PPIs found in all 3 and only 53 not found in any), and with other NDD PPIs (Wang et al., 2017). Since then, dozens more ALS-associated genes have been found (Mejzini et al., 2019), most prominently *C9ORF72* which we could not include at the time due to lack of known PPIs, is now shown to possess the most prevalent mutations in familial and genetic forms of ALS and importantly also in autosomal dominant frontotemporal dementia (FTD), which together with several other genes indicate certain commonality in the pathophysiology of these two distinct NDDs (one of these, SQSTM1, is indeed also a *mHTT*-modifier, a PPI of HTT and other NDDs, HSP and EV) (Ranganathan et al., 2020). An expanded hexanucleotide repeat (GGGGCC) in the first intron of *C9ORF72* results in repetitive RNAs that interfere with RNA processing and related functions, and in toxic dipeptide repeat proteins. As an NND with primary symptoms arising from motoneuron degeneration and progressive loss of motor control, ALS is perhaps the best-suited NND with which to test for involvement of PHP at the NMJ. Two important papers were published recently showing the critical roles of PHP in ALS. First, Perry et al. (Perry, Han, Das, & Dickman, 2017) examined seven *SOD1* and *C9ORF72 Drosophila* models of ALS, and three lines overexpressing the *C9ORF72* repetitive RNA complexes and/or dipeptide repeats met the selection criteria of specific and robust NMJ degeneration and loss of synaptic transmission. Yet these degenerating NMJs retained PHP functionality and most importantly, induction of PHP by genetic perturbation restored the NMJ synaptic strength and larval motor behavior back to WT levels. By contrast, activation of the Wallenda injury response pathway had no beneficial effect. Thus, pending confirmation in mammalian models, enhancing PHP may be a novel approach to consider as a disease modifying strategy for ALS.

The confirmation and additional important insights came from Orr et al. (Orr et al., 2020), who showed that in *Drosophila* NMJ basal PHP effectively compensates for ankyrin2-induced degeneration if the synaptic loss is less than 40%, so that synaptic transmission is near normal. This suggests that a similar compensation might have existed in fly models not chosen due to a lack of robust aberrant phenotype. As in the *C9ORF72* models PHP can be further induced in these NMJs. Most importantly, Orr et al. were able to translate these findings into a mouse model of ALS (*TDP-43* mutant) and of NMJ degeneration (*Zfp106* knockout), where significant neurodegeneration in the phrenic nerve NMJ is compensated for by PHP to maintain synaptic transmission, and further PHP can be experimentally induced. Moreover, deleting an essential mediator of PHP-the ENaC channel subunit *Scnn1a*- from motoneurons in the *Zfp106* model blocked PHP and dramatically accelerated degenerative phenotypes and shortened lifespan. This indicates that the apparently slow progressive course of the degeneration over the course of 100 days in these animals is partly due to the compensatory capability of PHP to counter and delay the onset, which the authors refer to as "homeostatic neuroprotection." However, it is still unknown in this mouse model whether further enhancement of an already active homeostatic compensation can delay degeneration and prolong survival beyond 100 days, and whether this also occurs in recognized ALS models. It is also an interesting question why PHP was only partially engaged in both the fly and mouse models as the degeneration worsened, as there appears to be a reservoir that can be further induced. If this is because there are physiological constraints in the whole organism context that occlude further induction, then it will be an issue that must be addressed before even considering homeostatic compensation induction as a therapeutic strategy. With that caveat aside, these data suggest that enhancing homeostatic plasticity may be a novel strategy for disease modifying therapies for NDDs. The remarkable conservation of not only the homeostatic mechanism but also of one of the key genes required for PHP from flies to mouse over 600 million years of evolutionary distance, despite large differences in biochemical and physiological features of the NMJ between the two species, is a testament to the importance of this and likely other forms of homeostatic plasticity.

5. Revised conceptual framework for drug discovery research in NDDs: Part 1

The first direct experimental evidence that PHP is compensating for pathogenic processes in ALS and that synaptic scaling is altered in HD, and likely also in AD, together with >170 genes shown to be required for distinct forms of homeostatic plasticity, suggest that the traditional conceptual framework for NDD drug discovery based on targeting modifiers of gene mutation-driven phenotypes in animal models needs to be reconsidered. The premise is that in progressive NDDs there are compensatory resistance by distinct forms of homeostatic plasticity to maintain normal functions until the limits of the system are breached. The gene mutations linked to familial forms of NDDs, even if rare, are instructive in that expression of most of the genes are wide in tissue distribution and early in age, yet the pathological manifestations of the NDD may be cell-type selective and delayed in time. These attributes of NDDs are certainly partly due to genetic background and the particular physiology of specific cell types that make them vulnerable over time, but another component may be homeostatic compensation capable of delaying the onset. Thus, even as more direct evidence on the role of HSP in NDDs is needed, it is time to consider anew the types of disease models deployed in basic research and in drug discovery given their poor track record in translating into clinical success. The common practice of driving ever higher expression of pathogenic genes until robust and thus measurable phenotypes are obtained or targeting the mutant gene only to putatively vulnerable neuronal types may in many cases drive the overly perturbed system outside the bounds of disease-relevant pathophysiology, likely contributing to the lack of translation into clinical success. The "homeostatic neuroprotection" idea suggests an alternative approach: that disease models should focus on the compensatory processes whether or not the mutant gene expression, especially when physiological, causes sufficiently robust phenotypes for drug discovery efforts. The key is to determine whether and which homeostatic process is compensatory in each NDD model, and if these appear relevant to the human disease context, they may form the basis for unifying face and construct validity in animal models. Ideally, such phenotypes can function as the experimental surrogates of what might be taking place in the human disease context over the span of decades and enable more successful drug discovery efforts. Before this approach can be even considered, however, extensive work will be needed to first test whether distinct forms of homeostatic plasticity are affected in each NDD, then to elucidate their compensatory ability and whether they are already occluded upon onset of pathology. Even then, by the nature of homeostasis whereby every action is countered by a reaction to maintain the status quo, the homeostatic process may itself be altered and set at a different level by the mutant gene and thus difficult to modulate. Moreover, long-term HSP appears to engage networks of long-lasting transcriptional changes, and it may well be a challenge to develop effective means of altering HSP as therapeutic strategies. One interesting possibility is EVs as discussed in Section 7 after the following introduction.

6. Do EVs and miRNAs play a role in homeostatic plasticity and NDDs?

Exosomes are 30–100 nm EVs formed through the endosomal pathway and carry a rich milieu of proteins, lipids, RNAs, and other molecules (Budnik et al., 2016). They are released from cells both as a means of waste management and also taken up by target cells as a means of intercellular cross-talk and coordination, adding yet another level of complexity to nervous system communication. We have previously speculated that EV biology plays a role in both HSP and in NDDs due to the extensive overlap of their interactomes. Interest in EVs in the nervous system has since gone up dramatically, certainly in NDDs due to their role in protein aggregation and proteostasis and as a means of transmission of toxic proteins (Guix, 2020; Li et al., 2020), their ability to cross the blood brain barrier (Saint-Pol, Gosselet, Duban-Deweer, Pottiez, & Karamanos, 2020), and thus possible use as a delivery method for therapeutic molecules and as discretely packaged diagnostic biomarkers (Wang & Zhang, 2020; Xia et al., 2019). Aspects of EV biology are also disrupted in genetic models of NDDs (Riva, Battaglia, & Venturin, 2019), including impaired biogenesis in an AD *APOE e4* model, and coupled with reduced release in a PD model (*PARK9/ATP13A2*); decreased number, intracellular trafficking and secretion in ALS/FTD (*C9orf72, MAPT, GRN*); and decreased secretion in HD (140Q-*HTT*). EVs also play important roles in neuronal-glial communication (Frühbeis, Fröhlich, Kuo, & Krämer-Albers, 2013). Finally, their ability to package and deliver miRNA is of particular interest because miRNAs can regulate expression of a multitude of target genes in a coordinated manner and are involved in NDD pathophysiology (Chen, Zhao, Zhao, & Li, 2017; Juźwik et al., 2019; Wu & Kuo, 2020). This is pertinent as many neuronal functions such as HSP require long-term, cell-type specific and coordinated transcriptional changes. Indeed, of the 52 miRNAs implicated in AD due to their effects on Aβ deposition, synaptic and autophagy deficits, aging, tau hyper-phosphorylation and neuroinflammation (Kou, Chen, & Chen, 2020), 41 are found in EVs (out of a total of 755 miRNA in EV cataloged as of 2015; Wang et al., 2017). 10 miRNAs that are dysregulated across multiple NDDs (Juźwik et al., 2019) are also all found in EVs. While the functional role of these miRNAs in EVs, if any, isn't known, their presence in EVs does add to the evidence that EVs may play multiple roles in NDDs and deserves further study. What is surprising, however, is that there is still no report directly implicating EVs in homeostatic plasticity, despite the involvement of retrograde signaling and of glial cells in HSP that EVs would be perfectly suited to mediate.

6.1 Indirect evidence that EVs and miRNA are involved in homeostatic plasticity

The possibility of EVs mediating transcellular signaling in HSP is particularly pertinent in the fly NMJ, where PHP involves a retrograde signal from muscle to motoneuron and epigenetic signaling from glia, and where Wnt and other morphogens are transported in EVs to mediate neurodevelopment and a specific form of plasticity akin to homeostatic responses but distinct from PHP (Budnik et al., 2016; Maggio et al., 2019), and where the fly ortholog of Arc forms retroviral capsid-like structures to bind mRNAs and are transported in EVs from neuron to muscle to regulate synaptic plasticity (Ashley et al., 2018). Arc is also well-known as a regulator of postsynaptic HSP (Béïque, Na, Kuhl, Worley, & Huganir, 2011). Thus, the fly NMJ platform, with its extensive genetic tools, is well positioned to determine if EVs play any role in PHP. Another intriguing link is that of the 12 miRNAs whose targets are required for multiple forms of HSP (Dubes, Favereaux, Thoumine, & Letellier, 2019) and that are linked to one or more neurological disorders including AD, ALS and HD, every single one can be detected in EVs, and 8 of the 12 are also differentially expressed in HD (Wang et al., 2017). Given the lack of direct experimental evidence, it is an important question to ask whether the roles of these miRNAs in HSP involve their transport in EVs, as discussed in Section 8.

7. Revised conceptual framework for drug discovery research in NDDs: Part 2

As enumerated above, the distinct advantages of EVs and miRNAs as means of therapeutic intervention are widely discussed. While our understanding of their biology is incomplete and the technologies required for their therapeutic development are still immature, it is an opportune time to place them alongside the traditional modalities of small molecules and biologics as studies on the relationships between HSP, EVs and miRNAs in NDDs are being carried out. Should HSP be shown to be compensatory for a particular NDD, the involvement of EVs and of miRNAs should be closely examined. While purely speculative, the ultimate therapeutic envisioned at this point will be a set of molecules that can enhance homeostatic compensation in NDDs by acting on conventional drug targets and/or by miRNA-mediated transcriptional regulation. These molecules will be carried in engineered or naturally derived EVs to target the appropriate cell types to counter the disease progression.

8. Testing, validating, and building out the revised conceptual framework

Much work remains to extend the encouraging initial data in HD and ALS to test and build out the still speculative conceptual framework of relying on compensatory homeostatic processes underlying NDD phenotypes as therapeutic strategies, with special attention to EVs and miRNA as potential mediators and future treatment modalities. Studies across the spectrum of NDDs will cross-leverage any commonalities in homeostatic compensation and EV biology, and they can be framed as four questions to be answered in a funnel shape with high throughput platforms triaging and prioritizing candidate genes and mechanisms into low throughput mouse *in vivo* models for validation. Thus, a first-pass survey of potential links between different forms of homeostatic plasticity, EV biology, and NDDs will lead to testing specific hypotheses *in vivo* in suitable or newly conceived animal models and finally to evaluating their potential for novel therapeutic approaches. The two primary higher throughput platforms will be the mammalian neuronal-glial cocultures, in which over 170 genes have been implicated in multiple forms of HSP, and *Drosophila* which provides the *in vivo* context with a powerful genetic tool kit to study behavioral outcomes, and in which PHP has been elucidated on the molecular level. Further justification for the fly platform is presented, followed by the four questions in Sections 8.1–8.4.

While the debate on NDD animal models is a long-standing one, the skepticism in industry is especially strong on the use of fly models as basis for drug discovery given their great evolutionary distance from human, even though this organism has provided a wealth of knowledge on the basic biology of NDDs. Our systematic and platform-agnostic analysis of the voluminous data on all HD platforms from yeast to flies, worms, cell cultures and mouse showed that there are indeed areas of convergence, wherein lies the highly conserved pathways despite the very different organismic context. This is particularly true for the HD fly *in vivo* screens which produced 243 m*HTT*-modifiers that highly intersected the HSP, EV, and NDD PPIs, supportive of the conservation of ENac channel as a key PHP regulator in ALS (Orr et al., 2020) and of key signaling pathways for critical functions such as homeostatic plasticity. That said, the current lack of clinical success deriving from rodent models argues that deployment of fly and other platforms, if at all, can only be justified in more innovative and integrated fashion. Still, given the well-stocked genetic toolkit, the ease and speed of the whole organism survival and behavioral assays, and their foundational nature for elucidating PHP on the molecular level, the fly platform is an excellent complement to the mammalian cell culture and *in vivo* assays for studying homeostatic plasticity. Indeed, the fact that two circadian regulators are critical for retrograde signaling from postsynaptic muscle in PHP suggests that the fly platform might enable the study of sleep as a surrogate readout of homeostatic plasticity at the whole organism behavioral level with which to evaluate the numerous HSP genes discovered in mammalian neuronal cultures. Moreover, the fly sleep assay can be integrated with additional CNS-based climbing behavior and survival/lifespan, providing an additional layer of validation of the genes and mechanism of interest before testing in the more laborious mouse disease models (see Sections 8.3 and 8.4 for additional discussion). A flow chart of this sequence is presented in Fig. 2, with details on each of the questions in Sections 8.1–8.4.

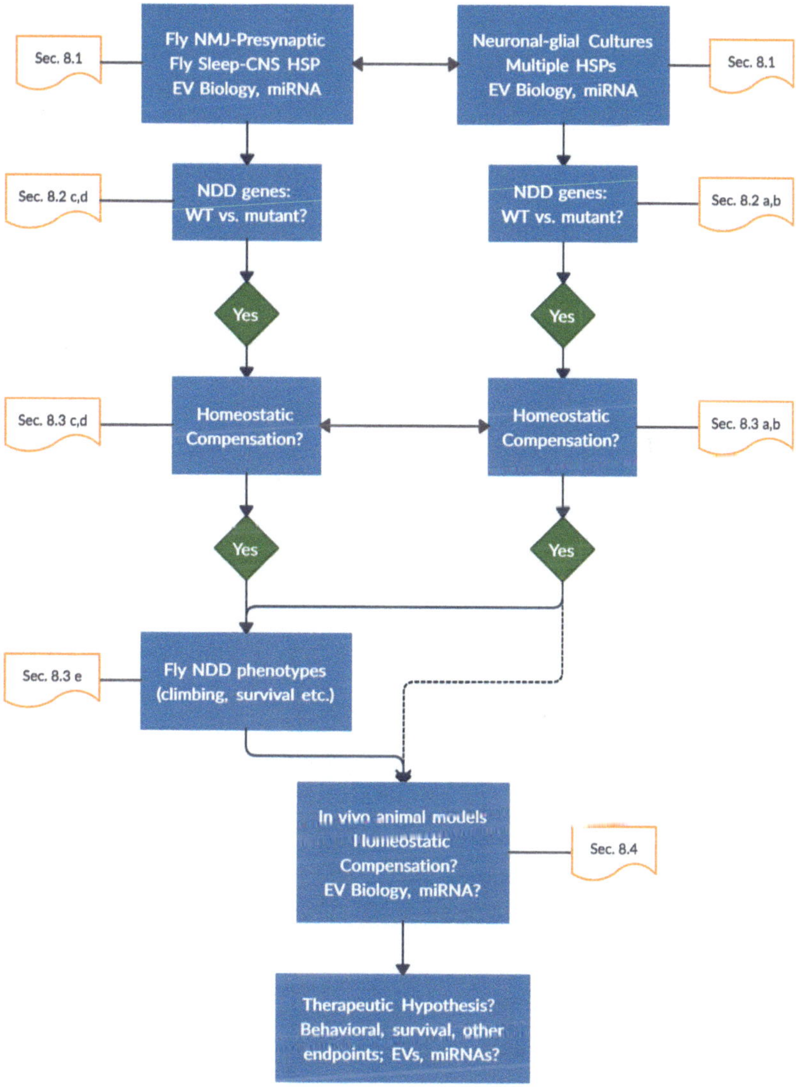

Fig. 2 A flow chart of the proposed studies to test, verify and build out a revised conceptual framework for NDD drug discovery. NO decisions are not shown, as the flow scheme is iterative in nature, and negatives can lead back to revisions of experimental plans. The outer boxes show the corresponding Sections in the text where each stage is discussed in detail.

8.1 Are EVs involved in different forms of homeostatic plasticity and how?

This is a straightforward question of whether EV is involved in different forms of homeostatic plasticity, independently of their roles in NDDs, and can be addressed in cocultures where EVs can be manipulated and their content analyzed, and in the fly NMJ where validated genetic tools to tease out EV biology and PHP are available. If EVs are indeed implicated, then elucidating their roles and specifically whether and which miRNAs are involved will inform and facilitate the studies posited for all the other questions.

8.2 How are any of the delineated homeostatic plasticity pathways, especially those in which EVs and miRNAs have been implicated, altered in each NDD genetic model?

2a. In the neuronal-glial cocultures expressing NDD genes, is there any difference in the multiple forms of HSP from WT controls in the basal state and when specific HSP signaling pathways are perturbed?

2b. What is the role of EVs and miRNA, particularly those found in Question 1, in cell culture HSP in the presence of NDD genes?

2c. In the fly larval NMJ, what is the impact of NDD genes on PHP?

2d. In the adult fly, what is the impact of NDD genes on the sleep phenotype?

Based on the direct link between two circadian regulators and retrograde signaling in the fly NMJ PHP (see Section 4.1), I propose to utilize sleep as a circadian form of homeostatic plasticity to probe its interactions with NDD gene mutations in the *in vivo* Drosophila behavioral context. Fly lines should express mutant NDD genes in both neurons and glia when appropriate to account for their crosstalk.

8.3 Does perturbing homeostatic plasticity compensation uncover or exacerbate phenotypes driven by mutant NDD gene expression?

A corollary to Question 2, here the question is whether perturbing homeostatic processes impacts outcomes driven by NDD gene expression or uncover those due to physiological NDD gene expression but otherwise obscured by homeostatic compensation. If unavailable, models of physiologically expressed NDD genes should be generated so that they can be compared to the existing ones that exhibit robust phenotypes.

3a–b. In cell cultures, a clear NDD gene-dependent biological effect may not be known, but EVs and miRNAs can nevertheless be examined as potential surrogate readouts.

3c–d. In flies, it is possible to control dosage of the NDD gene expression and then study the effects of perturbing HSP on the larval crawling behavior as a readout of NMJ function, and sleep as a surrogate readout of HSP in the CNS.

3e. To help prioritize for testing in the slower and lower throughput rodent animal models as posed in Section 8.4, genes of interest from both flies and cell cultures can be further interrogated in the classical adult fly climbing (negative geotaxis) and survival/lifespan assays as behavioral and degenerative readouts for NDD pathologies. While one cannot ascertain whether these assays reflect perturbation of homeostatic processes and/or unrelated mechanisms due to the challenges of teasing out homeostatic plasticity in complex circuits, positive data can still add to the confidence in moving to validation in mouse models. For drug discovery, testing candidate gene and mechanisms with only a plausible therapeutic hypothesis even in the absence of complete knowledge can still assist in a Go/No Go decision if positive and robust results from relevant animal models are obtained. Thus, as shown in Fig. 2, positive data from both mammalian cell cultures and fly sleep and other behavioral assays would support moving forward to mouse models, but that does not exclude a path bypassing the fly platform given sufficient rationale and supporting data.

8.4 Can *in vivo* phenotypes in animal models driven by mutant NDD gene expression and with underlying homeostatic compensation be identified and then reversed?

Answering Questions 2 and 3 should result in a large dataset in which convergence of the many NDD genes and platform results can be analyzed to prioritize the most promising homeostatic compensatory mechanisms and means of perturbation based on criteria that include mammalian conservation. These candidate mechanisms will be validated *in vivo* in animal models that express NDD genes in the context of perturbation of compensatory homeostatic plasticity, made even more feasible by the newer technologies for genetic manipulation such as CRISPR /Cas9. Therapeutic strategies to ameliorate the compensated disease phenotypes will likely be based on enhancing or activating specific compensatory mechanisms, possibly involving EVs and miRNA where appropriate. Success in answering this question will enable the formulation specific therapeutic hypotheses to guide the preclinical studies towards ultimate clinical validation of this revised drug discovery conceptual framework.

9. Conclusion

Drug discovery for NDDs thus far is a litany of expensive and time-consuming failures. Among the many challenges that are known and can be tackled, a revamped approach to the use of disease models from cells to animals is high on the to-do list. Systematic analyses of overlaps in protein interactomes of genes linked to NDDs, homeostatic plasticity and EVs suggest that there are biological relationships between them that if verified, could spur revision of the conceptual framework for NDD drug discovery. Thus, built on the premise that homeostatic plasticity processes are fundamental to proper functioning of the nervous system, and that when the system is perturbed by pathogenic genetic or environmental factors leading to slow progressive NDDs, "homeostatic neuroprotection" (Orr et al., 2020) helps to restrain and compensate to maintain normal functioning until a threshold is breached. In this framework, animal disease models will not rely solely on increasing genetic perturbation to obtain measurable pathological phenotypes with which to test candidates, as homeostatic compensation may have already been overcome and the results may fall outside the bounds of relevant pathophysiological context. Instead, the focus will be on the homeostatic compensations that either masked the impact of physiological expression of mutant genes or were overcome by their overexpression. If it can be shown that these homeostatic compensatory processes are still activatable and not occluded in the pathogenic context, then their enhancement may point to novel therapeutic strategies to slow the disease progression. The other part of the revised framework is the possibility of using exosomes or EVs as carriers to deliver candidate therapeutic molecules, in particular miRNAs that can mediate transcriptional modulation of the homeostatic processes of interest. Much more work is needed to test, verify and develop this still speculative framework, and a roadmap to obtain such data is framed as 4 questions, optimally to be answered in a systematic manner even if their scale and scope are obviously beyond the capability of any single laboratory. Indeed, it may require the organizational and resourcing capabilities of granting agencies and disease-focused foundations to coordinate and enable a community of investigators. Finally, it should be noted this framework may also apply to other nervous system disorders including schizophrenia, Rett Syndrome, Fragile X and autism due to their links to homeostatic plasticity and exosome biology. The ultimate validation of the utility of the framework of course will come in the form of success in clinical trials and approval of new disease modifying treatments much further down the road.

Conflict of interest

J.K.T.W is the President and a cofounder and stock holder in Dermalytica Inc. (Beverly, MA), a private biopharmaceutical company developing novel selective anti-microbial treatments for the skin.

References

Ashley, J., Cordy, B., Lucia, D., Fradkin, L. G., Budnik, V., & Thomson, T. (2018). Retrovirus-like Gag protein Arc1 binds RNA and traffics across synaptic boutons. *Cell, 172*(1), 262–274.e11. https://doi.org/10.1016/j.cell.2017.12.022.

Azdad, K., Chàvez, M., Bischop, P. D., Wetzelaer, P., Marescau, B., De Deyn, P. P., et al. (2009). Homeostatic plasticity of striatal neurons intrinsic excitability following dopamine depletion. *PLoS One, 4*(9). https://doi.org/10.1371/journal.pone.0006908.

Béïque, J.-C., Na, Y., Kuhl, D., Worley, P. F., & Huganir, R. L. (2011). Arc-dependent synapse-specific homeostatic plasticity. *Proceedings of the National Academy of Sciences of the United States of America, 108*(2), 816–821. https://doi.org/10.1073/pnas.1017914108.

Budnik, V., Ruiz-Cañada, C., & Wendler, F. (2016). Extracellular vesicles round off communication in the nervous system. *Nature Reviews Neuroscience, 17*(3), 160–172. https://doi.org/10.1038/nrn.2015.29.

Chang, R., Liu, X., Li, S., & Li, X.-J. (2015). Transgenic animal models for study of the pathogenesis of Huntington's disease and therapy. *Drug Design, Development and Therapy, 9*, 2179–2188. https://doi.org/10.2147/DDDT.S58470.

Chang, E. H., Savage, M. J., Flood, D. G., Thomas, J. M., Levy, R. B., Mahadomrongkul, V., et al. (2006). AMPA receptor downscaling at the onset of Alzheimer's disease pathology in double knockin mice. *Proceedings of the National Academy of Sciences of the United States of America, 103*(9), 3410–3415. https://doi.org/10.1073/pnas.0507313103.

Chen, L., Lau, A. G., & Sarti, F. (2014). Synaptic retinoic acid signaling and homeostatic synaptic plasticity. *Neuropharmacology, 78*, 3–12. https://doi.org/10.1016/j.neuropharm.2012.12.004.

Chen, J., Zhao, B., Zhao, J., & Li, S. (2017). Potential roles of exosomal MicroRNAs as diagnostic biomarkers and therapeutic application in Alzheimer's disease. *Neural Plasticity, 2017*. https://doi.org/10.1155/2017/7027380.

Davis, G. W., & Müller, M. (2015). Homeostatic control of presynaptic neurotransmitter release. *Annual Review of Physiology*, 77(1), 251–270. https://doi.org/10.1146/annurev-physiol-021014-071740.

Diaz-Ortiz, M. E., & Chen-Plotkin, A. S. (2020). Omics in neurodegenerative disease: Hope or hype? *Trends in Genetics, 36*(3), 152–159. https://doi.org/10.1016/j.tig.2019.12.002.

Diering, G. H., & Huganir, R. L. (2018). The AMPA receptor code of synaptic plasticity. *Neuron, 100*(2), 314–329. https://doi.org/10.1016/j.neuron.2018.10.018.

Dissel, S. (2020). Drosophila as a model to study the relationship between sleep, plasticity, and memory. *Frontiers in Physiology, 11*, 533. https://doi.org/10.3389/fphys.2020.00533.

Donlea, J. M. (2019). Roles for sleep in memory: Insights from the fly. *Current Opinion in Neurobiology, 54*, 120–126. https://doi.org/10.1016/j.conb.2018.10.006.

Dubes, S., Favereaux, A., Thoumine, O., & Letellier, M. (2019). MiRNA-dependent control of homeostatic plasticity in neurons. *Frontiers in Cellular Neuroscience, 13*, 536. https://doi.org/10.3389/fncel.2019.00536.

Frank, C. A. (2014). Homeostatic plasticity at the Drosophila neuromuscular junction. *Neuropharmacology, 78*, 63–74. https://doi.org/10.1016/j.neuropharm.2013.06.015.

Frank, C. A., James, T. D., & Müller, M. (2020). Homeostatic control of Drosophila neuromuscular junction function. *Synapse, 74*(1). https://doi.org/10.1002/syn.22133.

Frere, S., & Slutsky, I. (2018). Alzheimer's disease: From firing instability to homeostasis network collapse. *Neuron, 97*(1), 32–58. https://doi.org/10.1016/j.neuron.2017.11.028.

Frühbeis, C., Fröhlich, D., Kuo, W. P., & Krämer-Albers, E.-M. (2013). Extracellular vesicles as mediators of neuron-glia communication. *Frontiers in Cellular Neuroscience*, 7, 182. https://doi.org/10.3389/fncel.2013.00182.

Genç, Ö., An, J.-Y., Fetter, R. D., Kulik, Y., Zunino, G., Sanders, S. J., et al. (2020). Homeostatic plasticity fails at the intersection of autism-gene mutations and a novel class of common genetic modifiers. *eLife, 9*. https://doi.org/10.7554/eLife.55775.

Gilbert, J., Shu, S., Yang, X., Lu, Y., Zhu, L.-Q., & Man, H.-Y. (2016). β-Amyloid triggers aberrant over-scaling of homeostatic synaptic plasticity. *Acta Neuropathologica Communications*, *4*, 131. https://doi.org/10.1186/s40478-016-0398-0.

Götz, J., Bodea, L.-G., & Goedert, M. (2018). Rodent models for Alzheimer disease. *Nature Reviews Neuroscience*, *19*(10), 583–598. https://doi.org/10.1038/s41583-018-0054-8.

Guix, F. X. (2020). The interplay between aging-associated loss of protein homeostasis and extracellular vesicles in neurodegeneration. *Journal of Neuroscience Research*, *98*(2), 262–283. https://doi.org/10.1002/jnr.24526.

Harvey, B. K., Richie, C. T., Hoffer, B. J., & Airavaara, M. (2011). Transgenic animal models of neurodegeneration based on human genetic studies. *Journal of Neural Transmission (Vienna, Austria: 1996)*, *118*(1), 27–45. https://doi.org/10.1007/s00702-010-0476-6.

Herzog-Krzywoszanska, R., & Krzywoszanski, L. (2019). Sleep disorders in Huntington's disease. *Frontiers in Psychiatry*, *10*, 221. https://doi.org/10.3389/fpsyt.2019.00221.

Hobbiss, A. F., Ramiro-Cortés, Y., & Israely, I. (2018). Homeostatic plasticity scales dendritic spine volumes and changes the threshold and specificity of Hebbian plasticity. *iScience*, *8*, 161–174. https://doi.org/10.1016/j.isci.2018.09.015.

Howland, D. S., & Munoz-Sanjuan, I. (2014). Mind the gap: Models in multiple species needed for therapeutic development in Huntington's disease. *Movement Disorders*, *29*(11), 1397–1403. https://doi.org/10.1002/mds.26008.

Hulme, S. R., Jones, O. D., & Abraham, W. C. (2013). Emerging roles of metaplasticity in behaviour and disease. *Trends in Neurosciences*, *36*(6), 353–362. https://doi.org/10.1016/j.tins.2013.03.007.

Jang, S.-S., & Chung, H. J. (2016). Emerging link between Alzheimer's disease and homeostatic synaptic plasticity. *Neural Plasticity*, *2016*. https://doi.org/10.1155/2016/7969272.

Juźwik, C. A., Drake, S., Zhang, Y., Paradis-Isler, N., Sylvester, A., Amar-Zifkin, A., et al. (2019). microRNA dysregulation in neurodegenerative diseases: A systematic review. *Progress in Neurobiology*, *182*, 101664. https://doi.org/10.1016/j.pneurobio.2019.101664.

Keck, T., Hübener, M., & Bonhoeffer, T. (2017). Interactions between synaptic homeostatic mechanisms: An attempt to reconcile BCM theory, synaptic scaling, and changing excitation/inhibition balance. *Current Opinion in Neurobiology*, *43*, 87–93. https://doi.org/10.1016/j.conb.2017.02.003.

Kikuma, K., Li, X., Perry, S., Li, Q., Goel, P., Chen, C., et al. (2019). Cul3 and insomniac are required for rapid ubiquitination of postsynaptic targets and retrograde homeostatic signaling. *Nature Communications*, *10*, 2998. https://doi.org/10.1038/s41467-019-10992-6.

Kou, X., Chen, D., & Chen, N. (2020). The regulation of microRNAs in Alzheimer's disease. *Frontiers in Neurology*, *11*, 288. https://doi.org/10.3389/fneur.2020.00288.

Lam, S., Bayraktar, A., Zhang, C., Turkez, H., Nielsen, J., Boren, J., et al. (2020). A systems biology approach for studying neurodegenerative diseases. *Drug Discovery Today*, *25*, 1146–1159. https://doi.org/10.1016/j.drudis.2020.05.010.

Lazarevic, V., Pothula, S., Andres-Alonso, M., & Fejtova, A. (2013). Molecular mechanisms driving homeostatic plasticity of neurotransmitter release. *Frontiers in Cellular Neuroscience*, 7, 244. https://doi.org/10.3389/fncel.2013.00244.

Lee, Y., Lee, J. S., Lee, K. J., Turner, R. S., Hoe, H.-S., & Pak, D. T. S. (2017). Polo-like kinase 2 phosphorylation of amyloid precursor protein regulates activity-dependent amyloidogenic processing. *Neuropharmacology*, *117*, 387–400. https://doi.org/10.1016/j.neuropharm.2017.02.027.

Leng, Y., Musiek, E. S., Hu, K., Cappuccio, F. P., & Yaffe, K. (2019). Association between circadian rhythms and neurodegenerative diseases. *The Lancet. Neurology*, *18*(3), 307–318. https://doi.org/10.1016/S1474-4422(18)30461-7.

Li, Q., Kellner, D. A., Hatch, H. A. M., Yumita, T., Sanchez, S., Machold, R. P., et al. (2017). Conserved properties of Drosophila Insomniac link sleep regulation and synaptic function. *PLoS Genetics*, *13*(5). https://doi.org/10.1371/journal.pgen.1006815.

Li, Q., Navakkode, S., Rothkegel, M., Soong, T. W., Sajikumar, S., & Korte, M. (2017). Metaplasticity mechanisms restore plasticity and associativity in an animal model of Alzheimer's disease. *Proceedings of the National Academy of Sciences of the United States of America*, *114*(21), 5527–5532. https://doi.org/10.1073/pnas.1613700114.

Li, J., Park, E., Zhong, L., & Chen, L. (2019). Homeostatic synaptic plasticity as a metaplasticity mechanism—A molecular and cellular perspective. *Current Opinion in Neurobiology*, *54*, 44–53. https://doi.org/10.1016/j.conb.2018.08.010.

Li, X.-H., Zhang, J., Li, D.-F., Wu, W., Xie, Z.-W., & Liu, Q. (2020). Physiological and pathological insights into exosomes in the brain. *Zoological Research*, *41*(4), 365–372. https://doi.org/10.24272/j.issn.2095-8137.2020.043.

Livingstone, R. W., Elder, M. K., Barrett, M. C., Westlake, C. M., Peppercorn, K., Tate, W. P., et al. (2019). Secreted amyloid precursor protein-alpha promotes Arc protein synthesis in Hippocampal neurons. *Frontiers in Molecular Neuroscience*, *12*, 198. https://doi.org/10.3389/fnmol.2019.00198.

Lutz, C. (2018). Mouse models of ALS: Past, present and future. *Brain Research*, *1693*, 1–10. https://doi.org/10.1016/j.brainres.2018.03.024.

Maggio, S., Ceccaroli, P., Polidori, E., Cioccoloni, A., Stocchi, V., & Guescini, M. (2019). Signal exchange through extracellular vesicles in neuromuscular junction establishment and maintenance: From physiology to pathology. *International Journal of Molecular Sciences*, *20*(11), 2804. https://doi.org/10.3390/ijms20112804.

Mavlyutov, T. A., Guo, L.-W., Epstein, M. L., & Ruoho, A. E. (2015). Role of the Sigma-1 receptor in amyotrophic lateral sclerosis (ALS). *Journal of Pharmacological Sciences*, *127*(1), 10–16. https://doi.org/10.1016/j.jphs.2014.12.013.

Megill, A., Tran, T., Eldred, K., Lee, N. J., Wong, P. C., Hoe, H.-S., et al. (2015). Defective age-dependent metaplasticity in a mouse model of Alzheimer's disease. *The Journal of Neuroscience*, *35*(32), 11346–11357. https://doi.org/10.1523/JNEUROSCI.5289-14.2015.

Mejzini, R., Flynn, L. L., Pitout, I. L., Fletcher, S., Wilton, S. D., & Akkari, P. A. (2019). ALS genetics, mechanisms, and therapeutics: Where are we now? *Frontiers in Neuroscience*, *13*, 1310. https://doi.org/10.3389/fnins.2019.01310.

Miranda, M., Morici, J. F., Zanoni, M. B., & Bekinschtein, P. (2019). Brain-derived neurotrophic factor: A key molecule for memory in the healthy and the pathological brain. *Frontiers in Cellular Neuroscience*, *13*, 363. https://doi.org/10.3389/fncel.2019.00363.

Morrice, J. R., Gregory-Evans, C. Y., & Shaw, C. A. (2018). Animal models of amyotrophic lateral sclerosis: A comparison of model validity. *Neural Regeneration Research*, *13*(12), 2050–2054. https://doi.org/10.4103/1673-5374.241445.

Mullane, K., & Williams, M. (2019). Preclinical models of Alzheimer's disease: Relevance and translational validity. *Current Protocols in Pharmacology*, *84*(1), e57. https://doi.org/10.1002/cpph.57.

Neil, E. E., & Bisaccia, E. K. (2019). Nusinersen: A novel antisense oligonucleotide for the treatment of spinal muscular atrophy. *Journal of Pediatric Pharmacology and Therapeutics*, *24*(3), 194–203. https://doi.org/10.5863/1551-6776-24.3.194.

Opazo, P., Viana da Silva, S., Carta, M., Breillat, C., Coultrap, S. J., Grillo-Bosch, D., et al. (2018). CaMKII metaplasticity drives Aβ oligomer-mediated synaptotoxicity. *Cell Reports*, *23*(11), 3137–3145. https://doi.org/10.1016/j.celrep.2018.05.036.

Orr, B. O., Hauswirth, A. G., Celona, B., Fetter, R. D., Zunino, G., Kvon, E. Z., et al. (2020). Presynaptic homeostasis opposes disease progression in mouse models of ALS-like degeneration: Evidence for homeostatic neuroprotection. *Neuron*, *107*, 95–111.e6. S0896627320302786 https://doi.org/10.1016/j.neuron.2020.04.009.

Pandey, M., & Rajamma, U. (2018). Huntington's disease: The coming of age. *Journal of Genetics*, *97*(3), 649–664. https://doi.org/10.1007/s12041-018-0957-1.

Peineau, S., Rabiant, K., Pierrefiche, O., & Potier, B. (2018). Synaptic plasticity modulation by circulating peptides and metaplasticity: Involvement in Alzheimer's disease. *Pharmacological Research*, *130*, 385–401. https://doi.org/10.1016/j.phrs.2018.01.018.

Perrin, S. (2014). Preclinical research: Make mouse studies work. *Nature News*, *507*(7493), 423. https://doi.org/10.1038/507423a.

Perry, S., Han, Y., Das, A., & Dickman, D. (2017). Homeostatic plasticity can be induced and expressed to restore synaptic strength at neuromuscular junctions undergoing ALS-related degeneration. *Human Molecular Genetics*, *26*(21), 4153–4167. https://doi.org/10.1093/hmg/ddx304.

Plotkin, J. L., & Surmeier, D. J. (2015). Corticostriatal synaptic adaptations in Huntington's disease. *Current Opinion in Neurobiology*, *33*, 53–62. https://doi.org/10.1016/j.conb.2015.01.020.

Pratt, K. G., Zimmerman, E. C., Cook, D. G., & Sullivan, J. M. (2011). Presenilin 1 regulates homeostatic synaptic scaling through Akt signaling. *Nature Neuroscience*, *14*(9), 1112–1114. https://doi.org/10.1038/nn.2893.

Prior, M., Chiruta, C., Currais, A., Goldberg, J., Ramsey, J., Dargusch, R., et al. (2014). Back to the future with phenotypic screening. *ACS Chemical Neuroscience*, *5*(7), 503–513. https://doi.org/10.1021/cn500051h.

Puzzo, D., Gulisano, W., Palmeri, A., & Arancio, O. (2015). Rodent models for Alzheimer's disease drug discovery. *Expert Opinion on Drug Discovery*, *10*(7), 703–711. https://doi.org/10.1517/17460441.2015.1041913.

Ranganathan, R., Haque, S., Coley, K., Shepheard, S., Cooper-Knock, J., & Kirby, J. (2020). Multifaceted genes in amyotrophic lateral sclerosis-frontotemporal dementia. *Frontiers in Neuroscience*, *14*, 684. https://doi.org/10.3389/fnins.2020.00684.

Riva, P., Battaglia, C., & Venturin, M. (2019). Emerging role of genetic alterations affecting exosome biology in neurodegenerative diseases. *International Journal of Molecular Sciences*, *20*(17), 4113. https://doi.org/10.3390/ijms20174113.

Roux, J.-C., Zala, D., Panayotis, N., Borges-Correia, A., Saudou, F., & Villard, L. (2012). Modification of Mecp2 dosage alters axonal transport through the Huntingtin/Hap1 pathway. *Neurobiology of Disease*, *45*(2), 786–795. https://doi.org/10.1016/j.nbd.2011.11.002.

Saint-Pol, J., Gosselet, F., Duban-Deweer, S., Pottiez, G., & Karamanos, Y. (2020). Targeting and crossing the blood-brain barrier with extracellular vesicles. *Cells*, *9*(4), 851. https://doi.org/10.3390/cells9040851.

Saudou, F., & Humbert, S. (2016). The biology of huntingtin. *Neuron*, *89*(5), 910–926. https://doi.org/10.1016/j.neuron.2016.02.003.

Singh, A., Jones, O. D., Mockett, B. G., Ohline, S. M., & Abraham, W. C. (2019). Tumor necrosis factor-α-mediated metaplastic inhibition of LTP is constitutively engaged in an Alzheimer's disease model. *The Journal of Neuroscience*, *39*(46), 9083–9097. https://doi.org/10.1523/JNEUROSCI.1492-19.2019.

Small, D. H. (2004). Mechanisms of synaptic homeostasis in Alzheimers disease. *Current Alzheimer Research*, *1*, 27–32. https://doi.org/10.2174/1567205043480573.

Small, D. H. (2008). Network dysfunction in Alzheimer's disease: Does synaptic scaling drive disease progression? *Trends in Molecular Medicine*, *14*(3), 103–108. https://doi.org/10.1016/j.molmed.2007.12.006.

Smith-Dijak, A. I., Nassrallah, W. B., Zhang, L. Y. J., Geva, M., Hayden, M. R., & Raymond, L. A. (2019). Impairment and restoration of homeostatic plasticity in cultured cortical neurons from a mouse model of huntington disease. *Frontiers in Cellular Neuroscience*, *13*, 209. https://doi.org/10.3389/fncel.2019.00209.

Styr, B., & Slutsky, I. (2018). Imbalance between firing homeostasis and synaptic plasticity drives early-phase Alzheimer's disease. *Nature Neuroscience, 21*(4), 463–473. https://doi.org/10.1038/s41593-018-0080-x.

Sui, H., Zhan, L., Niu, X., Liang, L., & Li, X. (2017). The SNK and SPAR signaling pathway changes in hippocampal neurons treated with amyloid-beta peptide in vitro. *Neuropeptides, 63*, 43–48. https://doi.org/10.1016/j.npep.2017.03.001.

Sun, M., McDonald, S. J., Brady, R. D., Collins-Praino, L., Yamakawa, G. R., Monif, M., et al. (2020). The need to incorporate aged animals into the preclinical modeling of neurological conditions. *Neuroscience & Biobehavioral Reviews, 109*, 114–128. https://doi.org/10.1016/j.neubiorev.2019.12.027.

Tabrizi, S. J., Leavitt, B. R., Landwehrmeyer, G. B., Wild, E. J., Saft, C., Barker, R. A., et al. (2019). Targeting huntingtin expression in patients with Huntington's disease. *New England Journal of Medicine, 380*, 2307–2316. https://doi.org/10.1056/NEJMoa1900907.

Tian, X., Kai, L., Hockberger, P. E., Wokosin, D. L., & Surmeier, D. J. (2010). MEF-2 regulates activity-dependent spine loss in striatopallidal medium spiny neurons. *Molecular and Cellular Neurosciences, 44*(1), 94–108. https://doi.org/10.1016/j.mcn.2010.01.012.

Tononi, G., & Cirelli, C. (2014). Sleep and the price of plasticity: From synaptic and cellular homeostasis to memory consolidation and integration. *Neuron, 81*(1), 12–34. https://doi.org/10.1016/j.neuron.2013.12.025.

Trillaud-Doppia, E., & Boehm, J. (2018). The amyloid precursor protein intracellular domain is an effector molecule of metaplasticity. *Biological Psychiatry, 83*(5), 406–415. https://doi.org/10.1016/j.biopsych.2016.12.015.

Turrigiano, G. (2012). Homeostatic synaptic plasticity: Local and global mechanisms for stabilizing neuronal function. *Cold Spring Harbor Perspectives in Biology, 4*(1). https://doi.org/10.1101/cshperspect.a005736.

Van Bulck, M., Sierra-Magro, A., Alarcon-Gil, J., Perez-Castillo, A., & Morales-Garcia, J. A. (2019). Novel approaches for the treatment of Alzheimer's and Parkinson's disease. *International Journal of Molecular Sciences, 20*(3), 719. https://doi.org/10.3390/ijms20030719.

Vargas, L. M., Cerpa, W., Muñoz, F. J., Zanlungo, S., & Alvarez, A. R. (2018). Amyloid-β oligomers synaptotoxicity: The emerging role of EphA4/c-Abl signaling in Alzheimer's disease. *Biochimica et Biophysica Acta (BBA) Molecular Basis of Disease, 1864*(4, Part A), 1148 1159. https://doi.org/10.1016/j.bbadis.2018.01.023.

Villalba, R. M., & Smith, Y. (2018). Loss and remodeling of striatal dendritic spines in Parkinson's disease: From homeostasis to maladaptive plasticity? *Journal of Neural Transmission, 125*(3), 431–447. https://doi.org/10.1007/s00702-017-1735-6.

Wang, J. K. T., Langfelder, P., Horvath, S., & Palazzolo, M. J. (2017). Exosomes and homeostatic synaptic plasticity are linked to each other and to Huntington's, Parkinson's, and other neurodegenerative diseases by database-enabled analyses of comprehensively curated datasets. *Frontiers in Neuroscience, 11*, 149. https://doi.org/10.3389/fnins.2017.00149.

Wang, T., Morency, D. T., Harris, N., & Davis, G. W. (2020). Epigenetic signaling in glia controls presynaptic homeostatic plasticity. *Neuron, 105*(3), 491–505.e3. https://doi.org/10.1016/j.neuron.2019.10.041.

Wang, L., & Zhang, L. (2020). Circulating exosomal miRNA as diagnostic biomarkers of neurodegenerative diseases. *Frontiers in Molecular Neuroscience, 13*, 53. https://doi.org/10.3389/fnmol.2020.00053.

Watt, A. J., & Desai, N. S. (2010). Homeostatic plasticity and STDP: Keeping a neuron's cool in a fluctuating world. *Frontiers in Synaptic Neuroscience, 2*, 5. https://doi.org/10.3389/fnsyn.2010.00005.

Wierenga, C. J., Walsh, M. F., & Turrigiano, G. G. (2006). Temporal regulation of the expression locus of homeostatic plasticity. *Journal of Neurophysiology, 96*(4), 2127–2133. https://doi.org/10.1152/jn.00107.2006.

Wu, Y.-Y., & Kuo, H.-C. (2020). Functional roles and networks of non-coding RNAs in the pathogenesis of neurodegenerative diseases. *Journal of Biomedical Science*, *27*, 49. https://doi.org/10.1186/s12929-020-00636-z.

Xia, X., Wang, Y., Huang, Y., Zhang, H., Lu, H., & Zheng, J. C. (2019). Exosomal miRNAs in central nervous system diseases: Biomarkers, pathological mediators, protective factors and therapeutic agents. *Progress in Neurobiology*, *183*, 101694. https://doi.org/10.1016/j.pneurobio.2019.101694.

Zhai, S., Shen, W., Graves, S. M., & Surmeier, D. J. (2019). Dopaminergic modulation of striatal function and Parkinson's disease. *Journal of Neural Transmission*, *126*(4), 411–422. https://doi.org/10.1007/s00702-019-01997-y.

Zhang, M., Luo, G., Zhou, Y., Wang, S., & Zhong, Z. (2014). Phenotypic screens targeting neurodegenerative diseases. *Journal of Biomolecular Screening*, *19*(1), 1–16. https://doi.org/10.1177/1087057113499777.

Zhang, Z., Marro, S. G., Zhang, Y., Arendt, K. L., Patzke, C., Zhou, B., et al. (2018). The fragile X mutation impairs homeostatic plasticity in human neurons by blocking synaptic retinoic-acid signaling. *Science Translational Medicine*, *10*(452). https://doi.org/10.1126/scitranslmed.aar4338.

Zhang, F., Niu, L., Liu, X., Liu, Y., Li, S., Yu, H., et al. (2020). Rapid eye movement sleep behavior disorder and neurodegenerative diseases: An update. *Aging and Disease*, *11*(2), 315–326. https://doi.org/10.14336/AD.2019.0324.

Kolibri 360 GmbH
Ferdinand-Jühlke-Straße 7
99095 Erfurt, Deutschland
produktsicherheit@kolibri360.de